PARA-STATES AND MEDICAL SCIENCE

D1232189

Critical Global Health

Evidence, Efficacy, Ethnography

A SERIES EDITED BY VINCANNE ADAMS AND JOÃO BIEHL

Para-States and Medical Science

MAKING AFRICAN GLOBAL HEALTH

P. Wenzel Geissler, editor

DUKE UNIVERSITY PRESS *Durham and London* 2015

Library of Congress Cataloging-in-Publication Data
Para-states and medical science : making African global health / P. Wenzel Geissler, editor.
pages cm — (Critical global health)
Includes bibliographical references and index.
ISBN 978-0-8223-5735-3 (hardcover : alk. paper)
ISBN 978-0-8223-5749-0 (pbk. : alk. paper)
ISBN 978-0-8223-7627-9 (e-book)
1. Medical care — Research — Africa. 2. Medical policy — Africa. 3. AIDS (Disease —
Treatment — Africa. I. Geissler, Wenzel. II. Series: Critical global health.
RA440.87.A35P36 2015
362.1096 — dc23
2014024287

The index was prepared with the generous support of the Department of Social Anthropology, University of Oslo.

Cover art: Photo collage (*above*) Guillaume Lachenal, Institut d'Enseignement Médical, 2007, Kinshasa, Democratic Republic of the Congo; (*below*) John Manton, termite-eaten records, 2006, Uzuakoli, Nigeria.

CONTENTS

A Life Science in Its African Para-State

P. Wenzel Geissler

The twenty-first century is an age of *para* phenomena, not simply in the sense of a "millennial" age of mirage, specter, and occult imaginaries (e.g., see Comaroff and Comaroff 2000), but also in its reliance on absent presences. The prefix, denoting "beside, near, behind, and from" as well as "opposed and contrary to," captures a conflation between original and copy, object and imprint or shadow—or between model, mold, and cast object—that challenges contemporary social scholarship. *Para-* helps us to avoid alternative descriptors such as *post-* or *anti-* as in postdemocratic, postdevelopment, antipolitical—which draw attention to important features but miss the peculiar sense of things changing without losing their form. Democracy becomes para-democracy when its institutions and routines persist but democratic control evaporates, which is different from twentieth-century anti- or non-democracies, for example, in their various military guises, but yet not postdemocratic; the economy becomes a para-economy if informal or illegal transactions, and formal ones cease to be distinguishable, and when this conflation operates across economic scale, from African bicycle mechanics to British MPs; even contemporary "revolutions" have a whiff of para-about them—neither fundamental political-economic ruptures nor obvious counterrevolutions. The remnants of older social and political forms appear sometimes as "mere" performance, empty shells, and sometimes solid and durable; insidious changes rather than obvious ruptures can be observed anywhere: more of the same things, and yet something very different.

In this edited volume we are particularly interested in the *para-state* in Africa—the ways in which the state, albeit changed or in unexpected ways, continues to work as structure, people, imaginary, laws, standards, and so on. The term helps us to avoid older normative understandings of the state, as well as the resulting misleading notions of "weak" or even "disappearing" African statehood. The state, the authors in this collection agree, remains indubitably present and potent—if not always in control or fulfilling legitimate expectations of control. Specifically, we shall explore the para-state through one of its foundational fields of action and main manifestations in the lives of its citizens: medical science.

Biomedical Science in Africa

Medical and medical-related bioscientific knowledge has been generated from and applied to tropical Africa for over a century, transforming global medical knowledge and health in Africa. Medical science, government, and citizenship were intertwined in this process, evolving from early twentieth-century concerns with the health of imperial soldiers and settlers and the maintenance of the African workforce, through visions of health care as part of the Christian mission endeavor, to mid-twentieth-century projects of melioration and progress embodied by the British Colonial Welfare and Development Acts of 1940 and 1945 and subsequent postcolonial developmentalism and internationalism (Packard 1989; Comaroff and Comaroff 1991; Vaughan 1991; Ranger 1992; Iliffe 1998; Hunt 1999; Harrison 2004; Tilley 2011).

While medical science's structures resembled those of other life sciences—linking metropolitan institutions and collections to imperial stations and experimental sites—and shared their legitimizing narratives about enhancing the (ex-)colonies' value and uplifting their inhabitants' lives by triggering development, what marks biomedical science is its particular moral valence. Preoccupied with saving lives and reducing suffering, medical research is a science of human life itself, which intertwines technical, political, and moral action, as early missionaries were the first to appreciate. Further removed from economic calculus than, say, agriculture, livestock, or plant sciences, medicine's good is hard to contest. Medicine occupies the high ground, and other life sciences often bolster their moral justification with claims to medical, life-sustaining effects beyond economics (often through arguments of nutrition, from colonial cash cropping to current GMO debates).

The "developmental state" of the late colonial and early postcolonial era tightly intertwined health, medical science, government and population, and social good. In theory a textbook biopolitical regime (if in reality less extensive and coherent [Vaughan 1991]), it envisioned government-paid and regulated doctors and scientists, networked from metropolitan centers and capital cities to the margins of emerging national territories, conducting research on citizens to produce knowledge, which government then used to improve the health of the citizenry. Implicit to this was a particular notion of scientific knowledge as tool to improve human lives, of the state as an advocate of its people, and of citizens as default subjects of research and government.

Some historians of Africa observed that this developmental nation-state was only a brief moment in the African longue durée; an imposition lacking the European original's underlying experience, and presumably with less lasting effects (e.g., Vaughan 1991; Cooper 2002). While nation-building processes in Africa and Europe were obviously different, such historical relativization of the African state should not distract one from its promissory character. For generations of Africans, the state has shaped what the world looks like, where one places oneself in it, and where one wants it to move. Its institutions and processes have proven surprisingly durable, but it is collective hopes and individual aspirations attached to the state that had the most long-lasting imprint on African lives and institutions (which might be the case in original European nation-states as well). In particular state medicine and medical science continue to emanate not simply power and sometimes fear, as Masquelier (2001) had it, but civic purpose and hope for (better) life (Prince 2013).

In recent decades this quintessentially modern tie between government and medicine has been affected by changes: epidemics of HIV, cancer, and noncommunicable diseases emerged; care facilities decayed, services were privatized, and market-inspired funding mechanisms and private insurances expanded; nongovernmental, transnational interventions became vital sources of disease-specific health care; and scientific research was, together with other life science work, reconstituted alongside decaying public institutions (see, e.g., Langwick 2011; Livingston 2012; Marsland and Prince 2012; Prince 2013; Prince and Marsland 2013). Doctors move between government hospitals and private practices to gain livable incomes; patients with little hope of obtaining medicines from their government seek treatment from NGOs and research organizations; and medical scientists court global drug trials and seek international scholarships. As a consequence of this situation, visions of scientific government and government science have turned into nostalgic memories of past hopes in many postcolonial countries (e.g., Mbembe and Roitman 1995; De Boeck 1998; Werbner 1998a;

Ferguson 1999; Masquelier 2001; Geissler 2011; Tousignant 2013; Droney 2014), and long-standing African misgivings about bioscientific technologies and associated economic interests have expanded from popular rumors to public arguments about the political economy of science (e.g., Feldman-Savelsberg, Ndonko, and Schmidt-Ehry 2000; White 2004; Fairhead, Leach, and Small 2005; Yahya 2007; Nordling 2012; see also Kelly and Fassin in this volume).

Despite these societal changes, the state has not disappeared. As the cases in this collection show, it remains tangible in the many people enrolled in its workforce, its buildings and circulations, and its habitual procedures and paper trails; it also remains present in people's claims for care, in state providers' determination to define policies and standards, and even in foreign donors' insistence on working through state "partners." And the state also persists in people's memories of (better) functioning government services, which far from being "mere" nostalgia direct their longings for a better future. All this is not quite the same as the developmental state of old, but it is not yet something altogether different either—hence the *para-* tag as analytical parenthesis.

The loosening of the biopolitical compound between state, medicine, and science has also opened creative spaces. New formations of government (for example, NGOs, transnational sovereigns, global philanthropy, humanitarian interventionism, public-private partnerships, pharmaceutical multinationals, nationalist anti-science) and new modes of collectivization (sometimes labeled "biological," "therapeutic," "pharmaceutical," or even "clinical trial citizenship" [Rose 1996; Ecks 2005; Nguyen 2005; Rose and Novas 2005]) have filled some of the spaces vacated by the nation-state without providing a similarly totalizing collective whole. The aim of this edited volume is to explore the place of medical and related life science work in Africa within these changed frames, trying to avoid tropes of totalizing rupture, and keeping the state in view, attending to its partial, residual, or lingering, lateral, mimetic, or mediated, that is, *para*, effect in contemporary biopolitics. Medical experimentation and intervention have been critical in the making of twentieth-century, modern Africa; they remain central for our understanding of twenty-first-century Africa and its place in a world in which life as such has become a focus of government and knowledge production.

A Sense of Change

The millennial present feels different from the time of our childhoods during the last third of the twentieth century. This sense of discontinuity has been given different labels, depending on disciplinary origins, political orientation, and geographical location, focusing on different facets of a diffuse experience, or trying to capture convergences between disparate phenomena. Some broad terms have equally rapidly expanded their currency and lost purchase: *globalization*—for some producing homogeneity, for others diversification—provided an encompassing but somewhat vacuous analytical concept during 1980s and 1990s; *neoliberalization* was then helpful to foreground concrete political-economic processes—global and national wealth redistribution and evolving class conflicts—but tends toward economic determinism, capital-conspiracy narratives, or overstretching causalities, which obscures attendant political opportunities (see Ferguson 2010).

Different *post-* concepts such as *post–Cold War, postsocialist, post-nation-state, post-democracy*, or, from an African vantage point, *post-postcolonial* (Ombongi 2011) or *second postcolonial* (Comaroff and Comaroff 2000) focus on historical comparison, but by emphasizing rupture they lose specificity; they also raise the question of whether we really are *post-* in the sense of beyond, and what we are in rather than after. Other descriptions focus instead on exemplary contemporary phenomena, such as humanitarianism and emergency (Fassin and Pandolfi 2010; Bornstein and Redfield 2011), nongovernmental politics (Feher 2007), biosecurity and epidemic preparedness (Dry and Leach 2010), or bioeconomies (e.g., Rajan 2006; Cooper 2007). This array of interrelated "key traits" of the contemporary configuration then raises questions about the proportional weight of particular phenomena, causal connections, and points of convergence.

Irrespective of the labels, for those who gained consciousness in the 1960s and 1970s, it suffices to switch on the kitchen radio to realize that ours, indeed, is a different world: delimited military-cum-humanitarian interventions in global zones of abandonment and global scares about emergent infections and travelling, drug-resistant pathogens transform the face of public (now "global") health; persistent low-level conflicts at ever-shifting margins, suicide bombings, drones, and extrajudicial rendition and executions reference a new face of politics; and impoverished and diseased masses, dependent upon transnational food and treatment programs points toward an emerging global economy of survival.

In Africa this experience of rupture is accentuated by political and economic upheavals and violence (see, e.g., De Boeck 1994, 1998; Ferguson 1999). "Things fall apart" again, including the modernist edifice that Chinua Achebe once had accused of disrupting an older social fabric. Nostalgic (or ironic) comparison between the present and one's grandparents' 1960s and 1970s is common in everyday conversations, political discourse, popular literature and music, and reflections about professional practice (see, e.g., Simpson 1998; Werbner 1998b; McGregor 2005; Nyairo 2005; Prince 2006), and not least among academics and scientists whose conditions of life and work have radically changed (see Arnaut and Blommaert 2009). Such temporalities of contrast do not merely account for historical processes and experiences but also give—interwoven with the materiality of present life and traces of pasts—texture to the present and orientation to actions and aspirations (De Boeck 1998; Tousignant 2013).

This particular sense of time and of one's place in time—the temporality of things-having-changed—marks contemporary social experience. Looking back, the past before the change, whatever content and value one gives it, lies behind the rupture: the time of the long 1980s, between the postcolonial then and an as yet unclear now. The para-state idiom aims to grasp this layering of temporal experience. In its temporal sense, *para-* also refers to the blurred vision produced by the filter of change; neither post one thing and not yet quite something else, *para-* captures a sense of historical uncertainty, a temporality of doubt framed by the figure of historical contrast.

New Biopolitical Forms in Africa

One characteristic of the present is its focus on life. Many new social forms have physical well-being and optimization, scientific knowledge of life, the utilization of bodily materials, and mere human survival at their core. Concerns with epidemics and pharmaceutical treatments; humanitarian emergencies and interventions; and the prominent role of the life sciences in economic value creation, in imaginaries of progress (and threat), and in debates about ethical values share an interest in life as such.

The government of life has been a feature of modern biopolitics throughout the past centuries; what, according to Rose (2001, 5), is different in the present is that "the ideal of an omnipotent social state that would shape, coordinate, and manage the affairs of all sectors of society has fallen into disrepute. The idea of 'society' as a single, if heterogeneous, domain with the national culture, a national population, a national destiny, coextensive with a national territory and the powers of a national political government has entered a crisis. In this new configuration the political meaning and salience of health and disease have changed." As a result of this, bodies are no longer approached collectively, as in old-style public health, but as containers of "somatic individuality" (Rose 2001), bearers of traits and risks, and targets of individual management and maximization. Taking these insights to Africa implies a shift: while among Western middle classes the new vital politics may be primarily about optimization, for many others, including many Africans, life is increasingly about survival. Somatic individuality is here less about striving for physical perfection than about an individualized struggle to keep the body going (see Marsland and Prince 2012).

This difference notwithstanding, Africa is particularly suitable for exploring the new vital politics. Contemporary political-cum-economic-cum-epidemiological changes of science and care, academia and government are more visible here than in European post-welfare societies, where lasting infrastructures, bureaucratic institutions, and administrative habits maintain a façade of stability and where decaying structures are overwritten by new ones. The proliferation of "nongovernmental politics" (see Feher 2007) is more obvious where kleptocratic governments have turned their backs on their nations. Privatization and reduced government budgets hit hard among people without personal equity; class contradictions become more radical here, separating those participating in global opportunities from the majority without access to education and employment and those who rely upon decaying public provisions from those who benefit from new private insurances and care providers. People's survival depends here on innovative biopolitical forms—refugee camps or food drops, vaccination campaigns, treatment programs, or clinical trials.

Africa has for long been described as a "laboratory" (Tilley 2011), a site of knowledge production and "experimental governmentality" (Bonneuil 2000), where medical (and other life science) practices were tried out together with novel social orders. In fact, the trope of experimentation predates historical analysis and derives from the colonial lexicon itself (see Lachenal 2010). Recent decades witness an intensification and enlargement of experimentation, from small-scale experiments, which served as pilots for larger programs, to large-scale experimental interventions, producing and validating evidence as they go (see Nguyen 2009; Rottenburg 2009).[1] In the near-absence of government health care, experimental formations have become vital for people's survival and well-being; this includes experimentation sensu stricto, clinical trials, which provide health care and treatment. Medical experimentation has thus a particular place in contemporary Africa, referencing a wider spectrum of novel biopolitical forms between nation-state and medical science, which can be discerned more clearly and earlier in Africa than elsewhere.

The Nation-State Past

The origin and counterpoint for the designation of the present as para-state is the nation-state, in which territory and population, home and people fall in one and in which the influence of government extends from centers of power and knowledge toward the margins. Life as an object of knowledge and of regulation had a particular place in the modern nation-state, familiar from Foucault's studies of "biopower." Irrespective of its actual historical realization, this mid-twentieth-century vision of the government of life—represented, for example, by the British social theorist Richard Titmuss (1907–1973), whose work shaped the National Health Services in Britain and postcolonial Africa (Oakley 2004)—has been steadily eroded by the replacement of society (as in people, territory, and state) with market as organizational metaphor and the spread of the liberal dichotomy of the state versus the people (rather than the idea of the former as democratic embodiment of the latter).

Over the course of a few decades, the generation of scientific knowledge, previously a privilege of state institutes and universities, has been changed by new modalities of funding, management, and audit and new notions of intellectual ownership and value; simultaneously, the utilization of scientific knowledge has been progressively privatized and moved out of the taken for granted core domains of national government—health care and education. These changes affect the lives of citizens and their understanding of the nation as the principal space of rights, claims, and obligations: gradually the modern republic disappears from view. As noted, African institutions and idioms of nationhood of recent origin, dependent upon external funding and riddled by historical contradictions (see, e.g., Bayart, Ellis, and Hibou 1999), suffered particularly from these political-economic assaults.

This said, African nation-states are not simply "weakened" (see Roitman 2004) or reduced to an image or a specter (e.g., Masquelier 2001). The state remains in existence, embodied by millions of civil servants, the institutions they work in, and the regulations and standards they uphold; it is revealed in the control and force it exercises over its boundaries and its people, and it serves as projection of expectations and claims and memories of past hopes. In many if not most African countries the state "works" less well for the majority of its people than it should (and maybe did, at some point), if *working* implies availing the possibilities of education or health care to the population at large, but the state's place in biopolitical order has changed, not diminished.

A Para-State

To capture this transformation, our title uses the shorthand *para-state*. This term has historically shifting meanings; according to the *Oxford English Dictionary*, a *para-state* is "an organization which takes on some of the roles of civil government or political authority; an agency through which the state operates indirectly; [also] an industry which is partially state-run," while a *para-statal* is "an organization or industry, now esp. in some African countries, having political authority and serving the state indirectly" (OED, online). In Africa the term historically often refers to state-owned industries and state interventions into the market, such as commodity boards. This use of *para-state* denotes an ambiguous conflation between state and non-state spaces—the state meddling in non-state spaces to bolster its power—which is antithetical to 1980s liberal economic policies (e.g., Colclough and Manor 1993; Tangri 2000).

Our own use of the term shares connotations of ambiguity and transgression, but it references the opposite operation: modeled upon a more recent version of para-statal reorganization, it describes a chunk of the original nation-state that is parceled out and run differently, shaped by market operations. This para-state "takes on some of the roles" of the nation-state without being part of or coextensive with it, evolving next to, around, or in the interstices of the state, thriving in its cordoned-off segments, upon the traces and detritus of the state, and interpreting memories and visions of nation and state toward different ends.

The *para-* prefix references—as in other *para-* phenomena, such as para-science or para-politics—a creative relationship between new (bio)political forms and the state. The para-state emerges at times within the ruins or carcass of the older nation (for example, new regulatory, ethics, or patenting agencies implanted by global policies into older government structures);

it evokes images and memories of past forms or projects older visions and hopes onto the emergent structures of the future (as in resurrections of nationalist rhetoric in neoliberal economics); at times it revitalizes, zombie-like, partially and temporarily, older state structures or limbs of those structures (for example, HIV clinics within neglected hospitals, research outfits in decaying universities); at other times it utilizes, sometimes drains, what is left of state institutions (for example, recruiting drug trial participants from public clinics or hiring qualified professionals from government hospitals into disease control programs).

At the same time, the para-statal formation creates new organisms, unexpected life forms and associations, homunculi and phoenixes, such as the South African HIV Treatment Action Campaign, which challenges the nation-state on its own grounds, calling for scientific progress and demanding the equal distribution of its fruits (see Robbins 2008) or the momentary rebirth of an assertive nation-state, as in Fassin's example in this volume of the South African government's attacks against transnational science in defense of its territory and people (see Comaroff and Comaroff 2000). Even when these new formations reject or attack outright the biopolitical institutions of the nation-state (proposing an activist nongovernmental alternative), the nation-state remains the point of reference. This is why the term *para-state*, retaining the state in focus by directing one's gaze slightly beside its original locus, seems suitable as a cover under which to explore the novel biopolitical spaces on the African continent.

Para-Statal Organizations

Specifically, we take the term from the para-statal scientific institutes, which were founded across Africa in the late 1970s as a new institutional form of the life sciences after the decline of national universities and government research bodies and in response to new transnational funding opportunities and changed scientific interests, practices, and technologies. These para-statal bodies are nominally "national": linked to ministries and with politically appointed chairs, their names and rhetoric evoke the nation, and their legitimacy—scientific validity, ethic justification, and legal and economic accountability—is predicated upon this nation-state connection.[2] Yet, at the same time, they are not integrated into governmental processes and resource flows or the national educational project—they don't implement policy, spend tax revenue, or provide degrees.[3] Instead, they are commonly constituted as corporations, holding private property rights and assets and generate income and profits independent of the government budget. Apart from basic infrastructure, they are not government funded, and although nominally national, they depend upon transnational agencies and private partners' support. They are collaborators: entities that can only exist in conjunction with something else, enacted and stabilized through practices glossed as *collaboration*—the contemporary version of the social contract— as implied by the prefix *para-*, "analogous or parallel to, but separate from or going beyond, what is denoted by the root word" (*OED*, online).

As the chapters in this collection illustrate, much bioscientific work in Africa today is conducted in para-statal frames, relating to but not part of the state, labeled variously as *public-private partnership, collaboration, statutory institution, nongovernmental organization, local partner*: HIV positive populations (and care providers) depend upon treatment programs run by nations outside Africa, creating para-statal sovereignty and citizenship (see Nguyen and Poleykett in this volume); scientists in public African universities link, through citizens' viral materials, to private U.S. university researchers, founding new interstitial institutions and appropriating spaces left by receding national science (see Lachenal and Poleykett in this volume); para-statal research institutes in conjunction with a Euro-American national public health institution create scientific research stations and field sites (see Gerrets, Geissler, and Kelly in this volume); civil servants gain their living, expertise, and identity oscillating between state employment and transnational collaborations (see Whyte and Poleykett in this volume); patients move between attachments to transnational health care experiments and national referral institutions, making new associations in between (see Meinert and Poleykett in this volume); an African public institution conjoined with foreign private charities or corporations runs disease eradication programs (see Beisel in this volume); and all of a sudden, the allegedly dead nation-state raises its mighty head in nationalist (or Pan-Africanist) resilience to transnational scientific and economic intrusions (see Fassin, Kelly, and Geissler in this volume).

What can be designated as *para-state* is more or less prominent in different countries and with regard to different institutions—and more or less camouflaged by nationalist discourse, which has a different historical rooting and salience in different African nations; in some cases, institutional segments of the nation-state are used or revived; in others, state forms are copied, referenced, or translated; and in other cases again, state functions are picked up temporarily by non-state others. Moreover, the "slippery" (Gerrets in this volume) para-forms may look differently—and indeed operate to different effect—depending on one's vantage point: for some they appear as genuinely national institutions, for others as fraudulent mirages of statehood, for others again as spaces in which (some) Africans play the games of foreign donors or as territories of opportunity that can be utilized, albeit indirectly, by national scientists for collective social interests. The diverse phenomena grouped by the term *para-state* have in common that the state remains an absent presence; like the blind spot at the center of the eye, the state is always part of the picture.

Collaborative Sites

An exemplary materialization of para-state science are the large, well-equipped, and highly productive research sites, which are featured in many of the chapters in this book, that have grown in most countries of sub-Saharan Africa since the 1980s, constituted of nominally national African institutions and governmental, public, or charitable bodies and leading universities in Europe or the United States (see, e.g., Crane 2011). They mark the northern partners' spheres of interest in terms of study populations, clinical sites, and geographical-administrative areas, and they invest in infrastructure such as buildings, laboratories, transportation, and staff within the demarcated and securitized spaces they control.[4] While some of them have antecedents in the late colonial period (see, e.g., Kelly and Poleykett in this volume), most of them emerged during the past three decades.

As several chapters in this collection point out, rather than integrating research work into the existing geography of national health care provision, referral systems, public health programs, or national academic institutions, these sites often create separate spaces that provide perfect technical and managerial conditions for scientific work (International Organization for Standardization [ISO] accredited laboratories, high standards of health care and surveillance, controlled accounts, adherence to ethical regulations), set apart from the decaying governmental infrastructures around them. Due to their monopolization of technology, expertise, and participant access, they increasingly concentrate world-leading epidemiological laboratories and research. This constitutes a shift, not only with respect to the developmental nation-state of immediate postcoloniality but also from the situation thirty years ago, when medical research was conducted by a multitude of overseas and (African) national students and researchers using national infrastructure and attached to national ministries of health or universities.

Despite their impressive structures, these research sites are not permanent, depending for resources and expertise on time-limited externally funded projects. The looming threat—characteristic for transnational outsourcing, for example, of manufacturing industries—that the foreign partners move on to a different site and country means that national governments exercise only limited de facto control over these new entities.

The elusiveness of such science sites is part of their very constitution, which leaves many questions unanswered. *Collaborative partnership* emphasizes equality, symmetry, and mutual independence and glosses over divergent interests, inequalities, and dependencies, as well as ambiguities and contradictions (Okwaro and Geissler 2015; for participants' perspectives see also Molyneux et al. 2005). Who leads the collaboration? Who employs staff? Whom do staff, participants, and wider publics perceive as in control? Who is responsible for research outcomes and long-term effects and side effects? And who takes care of participants after a trial or in the case of adverse events? From these unanswered questions arises a configuration of power, which seems harder to contest (by actors or anthropologists) than older regimes of experimentation—for example, imperial scientific domination or contemporary for-profit clinical trials—where contradictions and conflicts of interest were more obvious.[5]

Given the independence of these entities from the nation-state, why is the state still necessary for para-statal science? The answer is that it provides legitimacy and rationale to the scientific undertaking: the national government retains legal responsibility and liability for research activities; it underwrites regulatory rules and provides ethics approval; it sets laboratory, pharmaceutical, and professional standards (although increasingly transnational standards such as ISO and Good Clinical Practice [GCP] are adhered to).[6] It allows legitimate access to citizens' bodies and avails public medical facilities for the recruitment of participants, for clinical trial procedures, and for the referral of participants after the end of research projects. And finally, it serves as the ultimate destination of findings, which ideally translate—after circulation through global scientific journals and health policy agencies—into national health policies.[7] Thus the state remains crucial to the activities, but it no longer functions as one center around and from which activities are assembled.[8]

The Archipelago of Science

Para-state science sites are unlike national centers—public universities, referral hospitals, or government ministries—of nation-state science. These radiated across territory and population, extending the purview of scientific knowledge, making the population known, and applying and distributing knowledge to it. Instead, the para-statal configuration consists of networks of enclaves—specialized laboratories, clinical research centers, donor-run patient support centers, research wards, experimental huts and villages, and demographic surveillance systems. These are dotted across the nation, linked to one another and transnational circulations of expertise, data, resources, and policy, which crisscross the globe without necessarily touching upon national structures of knowledge generation and use. Thus, epidemiological and demographic data produced in collaborative surveillance systems is analyzed by transnational scientists and institutions, before it is shared with local administration or national authorities; research wards cannot change care standards in surrounding hospitals or dispense care after the end of a trial; laboratories and data-processing units are established in air-conditioned high-quality buildings or pre-equipped containers adjacent to crumbling health facilities; transnational scientists working in these sites train their (African and overseas) graduate students in leading European and American universities, rather than national universities. While Thomas Moore's archetypically modern republic of Utopia was an island governed from its center reaching out to its shores, the para-state configuration is in this instantiation an archipelago of well-protected islands of modern science and government, enclosures in which the fruits of modernity—wealth, health, opportunity, innovation, freedom—are confined and contracted (Geissler 2013).

From a certain angle, this may not look so different from the past: isolated mission hospitals in the jungle (see Manton in this volume), and colonial nutrition experiments in the desert (see Kelly in this volume). As historians of colonial medicine have shown (e.g., Vaughan 1991), African public health and care provisions have always been patchy, and academic institutions have always remained somewhat separate from their surroundings (see, e.g., Nyamnjoh 2004); there has never been a totalizing African republic of knowledge and welfare. The radical difference between the present archipelago and previous configurations is then not just the geographical forms—that science sites are not at the center of any territory, that bound-

aries are fortified, and that circulatory flows are global—but the direction-
ality of relations between "islands" and remaining territory: early colonial
hospitals were envisaged as bridgeheads for the arrival of modernity; developmental state experimental sites were envisaged as "pilots" for the scientific government of national territory—both being mere starting points
for larger projects. Contemporary enclosures of evidence production operate more like localized "sensors" of a global system; like weather stations,
enclaved "surveillance systems" feed data into global knowledge streams,
and while one hopes that this knowledge will have a benefit, somewhere and
eventually, the connection between sensor and its surrounding is neither
that between starting point and trajectory nor between model and reality.

The image of the archipelago emphasizes the isolation and separation
of its constituent islands, and it is indeed one important trait of scientific
spaces, like the above mentioned research stations, that they are fortified
and accessible only to some. The way they are construed—administratively
as well as architectonically—does pose an obstacle to localized circulation.
At the same time, their boundaries are also always constituted by movement
across them: by staff members entering in the morning and leaving in the
evening; by research participants and biological specimens being brought
there, and formal and informal information being taken outside; by clinicians moving between their commitments to transnational science, the government health care system, and their own private practices; by pharmaceuticals, money, and other forms of value circulating beyond their limited
spaces. In other words, while these are enclosures, they are anything but
hermetic, and their boundaries are demarcated in processes of continuous
transgression. Rather than merely tracing new boundaries and discerning
novel regimes, ethnography is to attend to these processes and pay attention
to the less obvious relations between enclaves and the surrounding territory.

Science in Its Neoliberal Landscape

The archipelago of enclosures, superseding older versions of modernity
as expanding, colonizing, encompassing, and improving territories and
populations, is not limited to scientific production. Enclosures, enclaves,
spaces of exception have been described by anthropologists such as Ferguson (2006) and Ong (2006) as characteristic expressions of a twenty-first-
century political economy, reflected in phenomena as diverse as resource
extraction arrangements, export production zones, and urban condomini-

ums. The fact that publicly funded public health science and gold mines, sweatshops, and high-class urban enclaves share a similar geography today seems no coincidence; yet, as overarching causalities of the "neoliberalization" type have limited explanatory value, the task for the anthropologist remains to figure out relationships and interactions between similar patterns.

Widening economic differences, reflected in shrinking African government budgets (further decreased by decades of misuse of funds), play a role. As national academic, scientific, and medical institutions lose their ability to perform their tasks, integration with well-resourced external institutions becomes more challenging, and the greater the discrepancy between resource rich entities and their surroundings, the greater is the need to control flows. Such economic effects are sharpened by the imprint of external partners' policies and ideology: if the mandate of a foreign organization is, for example, to protect the health of its own population, then building a sustainable African national health system is not on the agenda; if the imaginary of a big charity is focused on quick technological fixes achieved with high, targeted capital input, this does not favor health system integration.

Global technological, medical, and scientific developments contribute to these separations: bioscientific research has come to depend upon high-end technology with a rapid turnover and innovation rate—automated laboratory tools, sequencing equipment, MRI scanners, the newest diagnostic tests and reagents, high-speed data networks—and global rather than national standards, which carry high costs and complex international supply, maintenance, and training arrangements. If good science needs high capital input and innovation, driven and funded by global centers of excellence (such as Euro-American academia), then a structure of globally interconnected scientific enclaves imposes itself.

Technological shifts are accompanied by changed management and the evaluation and audit of science: if valid outcomes—vital for sustained funding—are defined by publication in few world-leading journals and translation into global policy recommendations by transnational agencies, rather than in relation to local circulation, clinical practice, and public health intervention, then the gap between transnational science production and national public health contexts necessarily widens (see, e.g., Feiermann 2011).

Finally, enclosures and scientific experiments share a topography and temporality. In order to achieve validity, experiments are confined to a particular place, different from the world at large (see, e.g., Gieryn 1983; Shapin 1988): the scientific laboratory, or the experimental "field," with its demarcated territory and population. Spatial boundaries come with limitations in time: the experiment runs until it has achieved its predetermined outcome (open-ended experiments would imply different epistemology and political economy). The contemporary emphasis on valid experiments—epitomized in the proliferation of "randomized controlled trials" in public health research and beyond it into social and economic policy—rather than, for example, clinical, observational, or operational research, enforces the topography of enclosure. The convergence between the topography of science and other political-economic processes can thus partly be explained with the particularities of the experiment itself. Experiments constitute states of exception, which anthropologists like Aiwa Ong (2006) or Mariella Pandolfi (e.g., Fassin and Pandolfi 2010), among others, identified as critical to the contemporary political-economic order, exemplified by phenomena as diverse as humanitarian emergencies and export production zones. Emergency interventions and economic zoning—experiments in their own right—are based on a state of exception, limited to a particular "hot spot" and the time of a "crisis." As Nguyen and others show in their contributions to this collection, the global scientific response to the HIV crisis provides an exemplar for the convergence between experiment, emergency, and wider political economy and the processes of deterritorialization these entail.

New Collectives

In step with the deterritorialization of bioscientific work in para-statal science, the collective that is the target of bioscience—the source and destination of its knowledge—has changed. The national citizenry, which was central to the nation-state's efforts at generating and utilizing scientific knowledge, is turned into an assemblage of individual bearers of bodies and ailments, rights and claims, such as HIV "clients" in transnational treatment programs or clinical trial "volunteers." If these "somatic individuals" recollectivize in the process of their engagement with, for example, medical research, they do so not as one citizenry but as multiple and shifting new collectives: "peer groups," "patient advocacy groups," "community" representatives and advisory boards, and the like (see, e.g., Prince 2012a, 2012b). These multiple, overlapping, and ephemeral biosocial collectives are governed by similar biopolitical techniques like the ones employed by the older, disciplining nation-state: registration and identity cards, statistics and demography, laboratory values and bodily measurements, enhanced with contemporary biometrics, data networks, and satellite-based surveillance technology. And just like their common biopolitical ancestor, the national population, these collectives generate subjectivity, as exemplified by "HIV identities" (see Dilger 2009; Nguyen 2009) or by clinical trial participants' sense of belonging (see Fairhead, Leach, and Small 2005; Geissler, Kelly, Pool, and Imoukhuede 2008).

What is different is their topography and timeline: the new biopolitical technologies do not usually create, or aim for, one larger, lasting collective—as in the unitary civic public of the nation-state people, defined in terms of shared residence, biogenetic ties, language, or history—which can serve as a frame for political contestation and intentionality, as a target for education and science, and as a space to negotiate effects and distribution of scientific outcomes.[9] Instead, they continuously evoke overlapping entities, which come and go, shrink and enlarge, overlap and merge—akin to media publics, constituted by ongoing processes of address, reception, and (mis)translation. These multiple publics are still subject to governmentality, but they are not governed in one overarching direction—for example, population well-being or improvement—but in many different (usually short-term) directions, shaped by contested interests.

Some anthropologists have attempted to capture these novel collectives in the idiom of multiple (biological) citizenships (e.g., Biehl 2004); while this can be fruitful (e.g., Petryna 2002), this becomes problematic if an inflation of plural citizenships questions the privileged position of citizenship as social and political aim. Reserving the term *citizenship* for the latter encompassing project, by contrast, allows for the comparison of the implications and possibilities offered by diverse collectives and the assessment of their contribution to a larger emancipatory political project or not. Citizenship then remains a placeholder for an unfulfilled project, rather than a handy label. In a similar vein, the notion of the public—as in public health and public science—might best be reserved for particular formation of medical science and for a political direction in this regard.

Anthropologies of Public Science

The interest, across this edited volume, in the changing role of the state is linked to the fact that all contributions are about *public* health science: publicly funded and publicly accountable biomedical work. Indubitably, the texture of "the public" has changed and its umbilical tie with the nation-state has loosened (see, e.g., Prince and Marsland 2013). If the public evoked in Richard Titmuss's writings on public health in postwar Britain referenced one lasting project, contemporary publics are multiple and have less defined territories: they may cover fragments of the older national public, combine pieces from different locations across levels of scale, or escape topographical and scalar location altogether. They wax and wane, merge and split up, are evoked and disbanded. And the distinction between public and private appears today often less obvious than in older versions of public health.

Yet, there remains an important conceptual and political difference between public science—as in spending tax revenue and being accountable to democratic institutions, led by publicly employed scientists publishing in academic journals, and referencing the social justice project of "public health"—and scientific research or health services for profit, conducted by pharmaceutical and biotech corporations. The promiscuous paradigm of "public-private partnership" and collaboration, discussed above, and the intrusion of corporate funding and models of intellectual property into academic institutions should not distract from this analytical and political distinction. Precisely because public science is today threatened, its particular frames and its actors' intentions deserve attention—as reminders of past aspirations and to give orientation in ongoing struggles about the politics of science and health.

Recent anthropological literature on transnational medical research has focused on nonpublic medical charting of the "free market conversion of clinical research" (Elliott 2010) or even the emergence of "biocapitalism" (Rajan 2006), showing that global outsourced markets of human experimentation have grown in recent years, being driven by the pharmaceutical industry's search for surplus value, and that poorly regulated clinical trials have become part of the valorization of the human body in contemporary global bioeconomies (e.g., Cooper 2008; Fortun 2008; Fisher 2009; Petryna 2009; Abadie 2010). Even if this literature might exaggerate the significance of bioeconomies, biological innovation-cum-exploitation is indeed a salient feature of contemporary public imaginaries of global futures—hence the resonance of the recent novels of, for example, Margaret Atwood (2003, 2009) or Kazuo Ishiguro (2005).

However, it is no coincidence that most of these analyses focus not on Africa but on Eastern Europe and Southeast Asia, where (since the early 1990s) poor medical care provision is combined with an underpaid but well-trained medical workforce and reasonably well organized public medical institutions. Just as with other "free market conversions," the new bioeconomy does not seem to work in quite the same way in most of Africa. Contrary to dark tales of the *Constant Gardener* type (Le Carre 2000) (echoing the 1960s Tuskegee scandal [Reverby 2009]), in which Euro-American scientists, paid by inscrutable global corporations or, with equally sinister connotations, the U.S. government and army, experiment on black people to generate profits from vulnerable, disposable bodies, most medical research in Africa today is open to public scrutiny, publicly funded (albeit not necessarily by the national government of the population enrolled of the trial), and by and large free from immediate corporate profit interests.[10]

To say that this research is more "public" is not simply to say that it is morally superior, but it poses different analytical and political challenges. For example, the aimed-for outcomes of public health research are more varied than those of industry research and development. Although (public) drug and vaccine trials have become more common in Africa in recent years—partly in response to some large charities' preference for pharmaceutical rather than public health solutions (see, e.g., Biehl 2007)—much bioscience experimentation in Africa is not after valuable new drugs but aims for affordable prevention strategies (see, e.g., Gerrets in this volume) or commercially marginal "adapted" medical solutions (see Kelly, Beisel, and Fassin in this volume).

The specificity of the African case lies, moreover, in the fact that most medical research in Africa today is conducted in collaborations between government institutions and public academic institutions in Africa and Europe and North America.

These institutions are usually mandated to pursue "public health" aims of equitable improvements to health, and although even public universities of course also pursue other, more managerial agendas, these stated intentions shape public representations of research institutions, personal justifications of scientists and other science workers, and the practices that produce public research, for example, justifying funding proposals, gaining ethics approval, motivating participants, negotiating research practices, and disseminating findings.

Such transnational collaborations are certainly shaped by unequal power and resources but not directly by profit calculations. In some trials, pharmaceutical multinationals contribute drugs or partial funding and thereby gain influence on the trial protocol and management, but even this involvement is often less for direct value creation motives qua experiment than for reasons of corporate image and tax savings.[11] In these constellations, patterns of black and white, exploited and exploiter, are less clear-cut and thus more interesting for social anthropology: the world of public scientists and doctors trying to generate knowledge between disparate locations and across wide differences of wealth and power—aiming for better knowledge and a common good—is closer to our own than that of multinational pharmaceutical companies. Public health science constitutes, in principle, a critique of the conditions of inequality that cause much ill health and that commercial drug research and development, by contrast, uses for profit maximization. This difference is not trivial.

In order to critically scrutinize changing public health research, and to give political thrust to such scrutiny, the promise of public science, as in public good and public health, needs to remain a conceivable reality. Just as the nation-state cannot be discarded but is needed as a contrast to and ingredient in emergent forms of collectivization, sovereignty, and citizenship, the *public* of public health, singular, serves as a heuristic device and political orientation. Seeing public science in Africa not as a mere version of contemporary "biocapitalism," on a continuum with the use of humanity as source of primary accumulation, but as something different, pointing to different histories and social processes, guides analyses toward different political struggles. Public health science today is situated and implicated by the inherent, growing contradictions of the global political economy—on occasion threatened by being engulfed by it—but not coextensive with it.[12]

Parallels of Private and Public Science

Once we recognize these different structures and intentionalities, interpenetration and parallels between industry and public health science can be explored ethnographically. This may bring into view private scientists concerned with public interest or even resisting excessive profit maximization (e.g., Petryna 2009; see also Sleeboom-Faulkner and Patra 2011), private companies manipulating the idea of the public for profit (e.g., Hayden 2007), pharmaceutical companies gaining influence in public HIV research (Nguyen in this volume), which in turn may open potential (publicly funded) drug markets, and public universities competing in markets of research funding and policy influence (Crane 2011); and on a personal level, we see scientists make careers in public health research, attain degrees, make livelihoods, invest for old age, and educate their children.

There are also striking topographical parallels between public and private science: industry clinical trials have become dispersed; no longer centered in Euro-American medical school hospitals, trials are spread between specialized subcontractors in diverse locations, from cheap U.S. motels to postindustrial neighborhoods in South Asia; data (and profits) are concentrated in Switzerland or the United States, involving global transfers of resources, equipment, drugs, biological material, and data (Abadie 2010; Rajan 2006). A similar deterritorialization can be observed in public health research, though the motives are less unequivocal: for example, "multisite" clinical trials have become the new standard in HIV prevention and vaccine research, combining findings from multiple subpopulations spread across continents in order to accelerate findings and enhance their validity and applicability. Connected to this, much funding is invested into global networks of "demographic surveillance areas"—interlinked field research enclaves with highly controlled populations available for tightly regulated transnational trials. And while some biological materials still travel across the globe to specialized laboratories in leading universities, increasingly analyses are conducted on-site, in well-equipped collaborative research laboratories, from where data is pooled in northern public institutions, universities, or research consortia.

Connected to these shifting geographies composed of globally networked enclaves, the temporality of public health science changed: originally conceived within a long-term project of national melioration, and attending to entire human lifetimes, today timeframes are more limited. Experiments such as clinical trials have fixed endpoints, when data collection ends and research clinics cease to exist and patients—who have completed their role in the trial but not necessarily gained health—leave the trial clinic's care. Moreover, recruitment for multisite trials is a race against time, in which sites compete to attract upcoming trials—sources of funding and future output—or to contribute as many participants as possible to a global pool, before the globally determined sample size has been achieved—and thereby gain recognition and authorship. Such trials are not directly shaped by competitive pharmaceutical markets and their search for profit, and their participants or their specimens are not adequately described as commodities; yet there are obvious elements of market competition and managerial logic here, and the relationship with trial participants shows similar spatiotemporal traits as competition-driven pharmaceutical research and development.

Another parallel development pertains to the role of scientists in public and private health research: just as global drug development is operated by an anonymous bureaucracy to which individual clinicians are mere "phantom investigators" with little control or scientific creativity (Fisher 2009), scientists in large-scale public health trials are often far removed from actual clinical engagements, which are conducted as routine work by a local workforce, structured by detailed "standard operation procedures" (a concept adapted from the military lexicon), and global standards set by the ISO or the International Conference on Harmonisation (ICH) and overseen by site-PIs, so-called principal investigators who, contrary to their designation, are hired by the transnational trial management after the research protocol has been developed and approved and who thus bear little resemblance to the original principal investigator, as motor of intellectual innovation.[13] Again, while this process of "outsourcing" is not driven by profit maximization motives, similarities with dispersed and routinized practices of pharmaceutical research and development are striking.

Finally, commercial and public research operate within the same context of economic, political, and scientific-technical inequality and face similar ethical and political problems—standards of care, regulatory weakness, exposed populations. It does make a difference whether those conducting an experiment use poor participants, bad health care, and weak oversight to reduce costs and liability or whether they actively try to strengthen African regulatory authorities, improve standards of care within the limits of public budgets, and employ globally agreed upon ethics codes (however weak these may be) to protect vulnerable participants. Yet irrespective of the actors' different intentions, it remains a source of political contradiction that people suffering a high prevalence of disease and few medical provisions rely upon clinical trials for their survival or that health professionals on low salaries in under-resourced facilities are dependent upon medical research to make ends meet and find professional satisfaction. This contradiction is obvious when it is cynically manipulated as a source of private gain; it becomes more interesting when this constellation is engaged by actors (and institutions) despite their stated intentions: when mobile public scientists with egalitarian convictions engage these structures to produce public science—with the ultimate aim of reducing inequality and the suffering it creates; or when African scientists enact scientific partnerships, keenly aware of the fundamental inequalities that remain unaddressed by this idiom (Okwaro and Geissler 2015; see Redfield 2012; Wendland 2012). These contradictions, arising from trying to do the right thing in the wrong context—trying to do something—produce public health science in Africa today. The ethical and political choices faced by public scientists under these conditions might not always differ from those involved in for-profit pharmaceutical trials (see Petryna 2007; Patra and Sleeboom-Faulkner 2009); the difference is that whereas pharmaceutical research and development works in spite of personal dilemmas, public health research needs to address these contradictions; it cannot afford ignoring them if the *public* in public health is to make sense in the long term (Geissler 2013, 2014).

Ethnographies of Biopolitical Longing

Apart from the deliberate focus on public rather than private science, and connected to that on Africa, the chapters in this book—resulting from the authors' ongoing conversation about medical science in Africa over several years—share some premises. First, none of the chapters portrays science as a complexity-reducing tool of (postcolonial) domination or (developmental) discipline; the anthropological "critique of biomedicine" is by and large absent. Partly this move away from the anxieties of 1980s medical anthropology critique is because post-Foucauldian and post-Marxist analyses have become a foundation of our thinking, and partly because our interest has shifted back to the possibilities and responsibilities of science. It also may be shaped by the experience of fieldwork in an age of receding, crumbling medical services and growing medical needs, and among people who if anything long for rather than loath the discipline and control that public health was once said to emanate (e.g., Lupton 1995). Indeed, most of the authors in this collection share a commitment to bioscience and public medicine—engaging an ethics of (always ambivalent and contested) "promise" rather than of suspicion and containment (see Fortun 2005). Even Nguyen's "deconstructing" analysis of HIV interventions in this volume aims ultimately for "meaningful long-term investment in public health." Little can be heard here of the medical relativism of old, where people knew better than doctors and biomedicine was just one, tainted and "reductionist," knowledge among many; by contrast, the authors seem to accept the primacy and the desirability of medical science.

An associated shift applies—for many of the chapters—to perceptions of nation and state. The authors do not position "the state," with its biomedical technologies, in opposition to people or locality, as in the "state versus people" imaginary of liberal anthropology (e.g., Scott 1998). Instead, they share an interest in the mutual, open-ended constitution of health and larger collective forms and in the political possibilities of collectives engaged or evoked by scientific and medical action, including the collectives of state and nation. Beyond the celebration of ever-multiplying collectivities—publics, citizenships, sovereignties, "civil society"—they point toward the question of what it is that marks the singular national collective, and the nation-state, among this emergent multitude. This does not mean that all authors agree on a particular collective form—beyond political commitment to the pursuit of health as collective project—or unanimously long for the lost national collective of public health. But their analyses open up the way toward a new look of the nation as a particular frame for scientific work and public health.

The first two chapters, by Nguyen and Manton, set the stage with two contrasting arguments, one charting a radically transformed biopolitical landscape, the other one expressing doubts about its novelty. Reflecting on U.S.-funded HIV treatment programs, Nguyen discerns a new transnational regime in which African lives rely upon sovereignty beyond the control of "their" nation-state. Legitimate domination is here not only exercised through taking lives but also to maintaining them. The scope of AIDS relief, dwarfing national medical budgets, combined with its sense of emergency, amounts to a "government by exception": "experimentality" as global health's new mode of governmentality. One could discuss whether the present constellation is "unprecedented" or extends colonial biopolitics and whether it comprises "entire populations," since HIV sufferers remain a minority, and whether this description underrates the persistent purchase of the nation-state in citizens' lives (as well as other sources of government—for example, churches). Yet Nguyen's hypothesis of a new mode of African medical-shaped governmentality provides an inspiring lead into the subsequent chapters.

Manton, the only historian, expectedly objects to any "bland description" of the historical process in terms of grand transformations. He questions the contrast between the present constitution of science outside and beyond the state and an imaginary past of "successful integration of research and public health" around the monolithic figure of the nation-state. After a sensitive ethnographic description of a Nigerian leprosarium in the present—ant-eaten patient files registering the dysfunction of health care and science, and the suffering of patients, doctors, and scientists—Manton examines the interactions between university laboratory, pharmaceutical industry, and mission medicine in early postcolonial Nigerian leprosy research. He reveals a "collage of non-state actors" not dissimilar from the contemporary para-state and argues that the "reach of the state . . . always relied on the arms of missionaries, adventurers and capitalists." This is a caveat against too clear-cut descriptions of the present by contrast to the past (and of the historical process as radical shift). At the same time, Manton's cautious approach helps us to capture the prehistory of the present para-state in the "infancy of the elaboration of new global research relationships and capacities."

The chapters by Lachenal and Geissler both engage critically with narratives of historical rupture—"neoliberalization" as extended biopolitical regime—one pointing to the futility and ineffectiveness of the supposedly disciplinary regime, the other tracing historically sedimented contradictions within its territory. Lachenal's analysis of "extractive, privatized, and internationalized" Cameroonian virus research draws attention to a symptomatic, if not obvious, trait of contemporary science: "medical nihilism," reflected in "non-interventionist interventions," that is, outbreaks of intense but ineffective action, hyped-up "hotspots," public health as performance and spectacle set against a backdrop of nonexistent or extremely deficient "real" public health. While such nihilism can be found in the colonial past (see Lachenal 2010), Lachenal suggests that it has become a central feature of the present. His description of highly publicized, well-funded, and self-consciously urgent "virological extraction" by entrepreneurial scientists from U.S. and European universities resembles the economic nihilism of speculative finance, underlining parallels between scientific and political-economic changes (despite the fact that the "virus hunting" is funded by Euro-American and Cameroonian state agencies, interspersed with specific commercial interests). Patterns of non-intervention, hubris, and absurdity in projects such as "viral forecast" and "epidemic preparedness" pose a challenge to late twentieth-century understanding, inspired by Foucault, of African public health as a "disciplinary" project. What emerges instead is a new pattern of biogovernment, maybe even (pace Nguyen's hypothesis) an "anti-governmentality." Lachenal emphasizes that his observations are derived from particularly futile "non-interventions" and suggests that on-going HIV mass-treatment programs—instituted after this fieldwork—go beyond a mere "specter" of public health. Despite the obvious difference between life-sustaining treatment for millions and the imaginary of future viral threats, Lachenal's attentiveness to "nihilism" is helpful to provide a constructive critique of hubris and absurdity, even within seemingly more efficacious interventions, for example, the Presidential Emergency Program for AIDS Relief (PEPFAR), a "historic commitment . . . the largest by any nation to combat a single disease" (PEPFAR website).

The logic of "non-intervention" could also be examined around the transnational clinical trial site described by Geissler, where three decades of major scientific discoveries that shaped global health policy effected few lasting improvements of the local health system. Instead, Geissler conducts an archaeological search, on the grounds of this "collaborative" site, for traces of alternative practices and imaginaries of public health research, contrasting to or conflicting with those dominating the present. Within the landscape of a research site dominated by hierarchies of collaboration and, seemingly, by one dominant model of transnational science associated with the era of neoliberalization, he traces different pasts (and past futures) that reveal nationalist visions of public health, contradictions and recalcitrance, and lasting claims for scientific melioration. Following some of the narrative fault lines embedded in this place of science, he opens up for diverse readings of the present and of future possibilities.

The next two pairs of chapters attend to the workings of bioscientific intervention. Gerrets and Whyte question the alleged disappearance of the state—one by attending to the nation's persistent role as institution and vector of intentionality, the other by attending to the lasting appeal of government civil service. Whyte draws our attention to the many Ugandans who still are employed by government, derive vital sustenance from this, and dispense government services. This group continues to exercise societal influence, in spite of growing economic instability, and new, shifting, employment opportunities in the expanding nongovernmental sector and transnationally funded AIDS interventions. Exploring "working-class citizens'" (including health care workers') experience, Whyte shows how the comparison between different ways of making a living—between the relative stability but poor remuneration of state employment and the lack of security in other kinds of work—forms a part of contemporary Ugandans' lives and choices. The stability of government work not only pertains to government employees but also forms the backdrop to everybody else's thinking about work, employment, and public health under conditions of generalized insecurity—be it in the informal business sector or in the world of temporary NGO contracts. Throughout Whyte's account runs the notion of the "original Uganda," which references, in the parlance of older Ugandans, the pre–civil war nation, marked by stable government employment and collectively shared hopes in science-based futures. It is this "original" that across dysfunctional African nation-states lives on, both in the persistence of nation-state institutions and their employees and as memory and counter-foil to present developments. As several of the chapters show, people, funds, and expertise move between state and non-state spaces, and government employment and newer forms of work—for example, public health inter-ventions, medical research—often depend upon one another: pensionable employment in a university or ministry of health can serve as stable basis for temporary engagements with transnational interventions, and the legiti-macy bestowed by public sector employment and standards can be trans-ferred to nongovernmental opportunities and converted to higher yields.

These movements are obvious in Gerret's ethnography of collaborative malaria research by Tanzanian and U.S. public institutions—a somewhat atypical "public-private partnership," involving bilateral government inter-actions and little private enterprise. His case presents a step up in scale in the experimentalization of public health, maybe indicative of emerging systems of global health governance: rather than citizens' bodies, what is intervened upon here is the body of the nation (presumably unbeknown to patient-citizens)—its health policies, procurement, and clinical management. Ger-rets confronts the "hybrid" quality of para-state science head-on—but ar-rives at surprising outcomes: flexibility and openness, even "slipperiness," function here as foundations of transnational collaboration, but these quali-ties serve at the same time to promote a public, civic, and national agenda rather than particular interests external to the nation. In response to the moot trope of "inevitable globalization" (e.g., Kickbush 2003), Gerrets ar-gues that transnational "global health" is necessary to counter the nation-state's inability to deal with global (infectious) disease problems, and he reveals the lasting, crucial importance of nation-state government for al-legedly "global" interventions, documenting the lasting appeal of the nation to public health actors (see also Wendland 2012). Gerrets shows those who argue that "global health" governance furthers the neoliberal demise of the nation-state and undermines sovereignty how state institutions and actors negotiate opportunities arising from "slippery" global partnerships to fur-ther not only individual interests but also visions of social good, articulating civic commitments that can no longer be realized through emaciated nation-state structures alone: "the partnership's malleability and its planners' faith in flexibility and ambiguity opened up new opportunities for representatives of public sector institutions to assert their claims and pursue their interests, fostering a para-statal space that enabled the state to reassert authority corroded during the preceding era of neoliberal reforms." The "slippery space" of para-state health science, then, is not opposed to the nation-state—as a panacea against its dysfunction or as a nail in its coffin: "The para-state space was at times quite distant from the state but on other occasions barely distinguishable from it." In addition to this caveat against simple imaginaries of contrast and shift, Gerrets draws our attention to "the variable forms that para-state spaces take across different historical and political economic context": postsocialist Tanzania, different from, for example, neighboring Kenya or Uganda, maintains stable and visible government institutions, and Tanzanian doctors, scientists, and patients share decades of mass education and primary health care, which produced a particular vision of civic space, nation, and citizenship (see Langwick 2011).

The next two chapters, by Poleykett and Meinert, use ethnography of HIV research to attend to affective and relational dimensions, which further complicate narratives of rupture and transformation. Poleykett sets out to trace postcolonial "survivals" of sanitary regulation in contemporary transnational HIV research in Senegal. At first sight, her old state clinic, with a long-established cohort of prostitutes, providing archived data, insufficient care facilities, and regulatory means of enforcement to U.S.-based HIV research teams, lends itself to a simple narrative of biopolitical domination, combining postcolonial governmentality and twenty-first-century bioscience. However, looking closely at the "porous boundary between regulation and research," observing everyday work at the clinic and in trials, Poleykett finds herself unable to discern any "single project" of "research piggybacking" on postcolonial governmentality: "the two bureaucratic forms do not come together as part of a concerted effort and their interweaving is much more a product of care, obligation, reciprocity, curiosity, and creativity than cynical or opportunistic profiteering." Somewhat counterintuitively, Poleykett observes that disciplinary medical practices, and even their architectural framing by a distinctly colonial edifice, are appreciated *as* care, which is reminiscent of recent discussions about *care* in the social sciences (Mol 2008) that fosters "deep mutual respect and care" between prostitutes and staff and a sense of belonging and citizenship: "the pleasures of membership" within which even invasive clinical practices instill "feelings of security and pleasure." For the mostly female state employees, mediating regulation, research, and care provides new opportunities and responsibilities, resembling other anthropologist's observations about changing gender roles and social-professional mobility in transnational bioscience sites (see Meinert in this volume); in this case extra resources available from transnational collaboration do not simply represent additional income but also enable circulation and opportunities to meaningfully deploy professional capacity. For the research participants, on the other hand, membership in the trial clinic allows new forms of association, like the formation of a radical sex worker organization, which gradually gains independence from the trial, enabling lay expertification and political struggle.

Meinert's ethnography of one family's engagements with a HIV research project conducted by the world's largest public health agency in collaboration with a Ugandan para-statal research institute shows that experimental networks intersect, extend, and play off against existing associations, expand and break existing relations and groups, and establish new ones. The research project creates new, bounded spatial formations on various levels of scale: through intensified technologies of surveillance, a "study area" is demarcated within which study participants must reside in order to benefit from trial care and transport, a well-equipped "clinical research center" is carved out of the government hospital compound, and special rooms are set aside for research patients in the hospital ward. Yet while these constitute enclosures, Meinert observes that their boundaries are crossed and that they also serve as embodiments of the desires, hopes, and expectations that patients and doctors initially bring to the bioscientific project—thus they constitute manifest structures of ex- and inclusion and discipline, but they also point beyond the present condition. Meinert also remarks upon the peculiar experimental temporality discussed above—research procedures, employment contracts, laboratory and clinical facilities, and not least antiretroviral treatment (ART) are time-limited—and shows how patients and professionals think critically about these limitations, weighing short-term opportunities against long-term needs. The denizens of the experimental regime explore and use its opportunities rather than simply succumbing to experimental governmentality. Moreover, although the HIV experiment does constitute a rupture in governmental practices and people's lives, there are continuities too: the family Meinert stays with, which is drawn into multiple engagements with the antiretroviral (ARV) experiment (including the anthropologist's choice of residence), is a chief's family with a mission background; experimentality is mapped here upon older forms of governmentality; all protagonists continue to reckon with the nation-state, partly as memory, reference point for comparison with the past, partly as enduring contemporary structures, and partly, still, as a project, a hope for how things should become. Meinert's careful documentation of the persistence of the state and the national collective in people's lives contrasts sharply with the obliviousness to the state in the cited American researcher's claims that there isn't any national health system. Together with the preceding ethnographic chapters, Meinert's case complicates the patterns drawn by historical ruptures, spatial enclosures, and temporal limitations.

The collection ends with three chapters engaging the changing nation itself: a multinational corporation taking the role of the nation, the performance of nation-state territory in the operation of scientific models, and a case of two nation-states, South Africa and the United States, engaging in a contest on the territory of public health, science, and rationality. Beisel's example of a transnational gold-mining company that takes on national malaria control provides an extreme case of para-state science. Rather than a simple tale of corporate power usurping the nation-state, corporation and state fuse here, but the nation remains a source of legitimacy and authority, convincing citizens to submit to control practices by company employees and the Global Fund to avail US$158 million to a corporate responsibility program. There are some ruptures away from old-style nation-state public health: funding and expertise circulate in transnational networks, actions are governed by a company, interventions are time-limited projects, workers are company employees on temporary contracts. But there are also continuities, underlined by the aesthetic similarities between contemporary spray men and colonial public health spray teams. Public health interventions, notably in the developmental nation-state era, were marked by infinite, not rarely futile, iterations of action and experiment (for example, sleeping sickness control [Hoppe 2003; Malowany, Geissler, and Lwoba 2011]; public health administration [Lachenal 2010]; malaria and onchocerciasis eradication [Geissler 2011]; agriculture and nutrition [Bonneuil 2000]). The fusion between intervention and investigation in the contemporary campaign revives older features of national public health, maybe by contrast to the 1990s detached transnational science as mere provider of evidence, to be "translated" via policy back into action.[14] Similarly, the way in which Beisel's control program engages its population—"top-down," aiming for education and behavioral change—seems to refer back to older forms of government-led public health, prior to the era of "participation" and "community engagement." Beisel denounces the democratic deficit of such authoritative public health, especially in the hands of a mining company—legitimate claims to company responsibilities are conveniently ignored. Yet it remains to be debated whether Beisel's recommendation to conduct malaria control as "real-world experiment" instead, drawing civic negotiation into scientific decision making, would remedy this democratic deficit. One might argue that the novelty of the current situation lies less in a particular form of "public engagement" in specific experimental activities (or the lack of it) and more in the lack of democratic organization and institutionalization of science on a national level of scale—due to the roles played by the multinational mining corporation and the Global Fund. To remedy this democratic deficit, the inclusion of citizens into the nitty-gritty of a particular experiment may not be sufficient—potentially deflecting from the larger political task—to establish democratic governance.

Making explicit historical comparisons, Kelly explores how experimentation by British scientists in the miniature "laboratory nation" of the Gambia articulates nationhood, expertise, and public health around the Second World War and in the present—the beginning and end of British-Gambian science. Relations between science and territory, and model and reality, have changed: the first experiment constructs a microcosm envisioned to be subsequently expanded across territory, a "pilot" for national welfare and development. The second experiment disconnects expert knowledge and national concern: transcending scalar modeling, it aims for translation into global policy; it is an exemplar of contemporary deterritorialized experimentation, by contrast to past governmental science (but see Beisel in this volume for corporate-cum-national public health as another possible realignment in the present). Underlying this change are continuities: both trials are part of the same British institutional setup; both are technical-cum-social experiments, which emplace scientific innovation, taking into account local social and economic practices, incorporating populations and using local staff; and scientific work relies in both cases upon particularities of place (and the laboratory scale of the mini-nation itself). Moreover, both experiments rely upon institutional assemblages: although funding changed from public sources to transnational big charity "collaboration" with the nation-state, unstable alliances and unpredictable realignments are here found already before decolonization, which thereby becomes prehistory rather than historical contrast (see also Manton in this volume). This pattern of continuity-in-change is personified by the village health workers used in the recent experiment: created after the 1978 Alma Ata conference to build primary health with local volunteers as a national bottom-up project, they are revived in 2004 as transnational research staff on temporary contracts; continuously linking government, people, and the UK Medical Research Council (MRC), they embody a new regime in an old form (see also Kelly 2011). Eventually, both experiments fail to produce the anticipated extension in scale—one due to economic pressures, the other due to environmental conditions—and while one results in a shift (back) from adapted technology to a plantation economy, the other ends with a decision to close down the research site altogether. At the end of her chapter, Kelly directs our imagination beyond the contemporary biopolitical regime: the MRC station is closed because, as Kelly argues, "long-term commitment to the Gambia is anachronistic . . . as research has less and less to do with specific places than with experimental networks"—the archipelago turns into a mirage. Intertwined with this further deterritorialization of science, the nation returns with a vengeance—maybe as a backlash—in the Gambian president's militant (indeed violent) stance against multinational pharmacology and AIDS treatment (see Cassidy and Leach 2009). Like other antiscientific neo-nationalist public health outbursts elsewhere in Africa (see Fassin in this volume), this may serve as a reminder of the risks entailed by visions of return to the national collective of public health.

Fassin's "political biography of Nevirapine" charts the rise and fall of a wonder drug for the prevention of maternal transmission of HIV. The narrative of media-amplified scientific and political hype—transnational scientists and organizations build momentum around a health intervention and temporarily silence objections to full-scale "roll-out"—is familiar from the history of public health, from malaria eradication in 1955 to male circumcision in 2007. What is new in Fassin's story is the role played by the state: this young nation-state calls for caution against the progress of science, even stops experimentation; it aligns itself with marginal scientists rather than dominant scientific institutions; it poses national public health concerns—about drug resistance and the budget and the demographic effects of targeted HIV interventions—in opposition to a popular, rights-based demand for the extension of scientific discoveries. These public health arguments are intertwined with a nationalist discourse about protecting Africans from global exploitation, black bodies from white experiments; opposition to global science becomes part of the nationalist struggle against racially defined transnational exploitation. This peculiar disjuncture between dominant science and national government is played out jointly with a third force, that of postliberation popular activism, which, while originally politically aligned with the new government, finds itself now scientifically opposed.

While this narrative, the author claims, has no simple moral, it serves like the Gambian case as a caveat against the assumption that nation-state governments are either naturally aligned with science—sharing one modern rationality—or that the millennial nation-state has left the field of science to transnational experts and agencies. Here the state is a prominent science actor; by opposing the global rational consensus of scientists, the state reasserts its independence. This move appears on the surface as contrary to the widespread claims that the state's role is weakening, notably in the field of health and science; this state is gaining strength, and it uses the biomedical controversy to make nationalist and in the broader sense "Africanist" assertions. Instead of positioning itself on the side of seemingly self-evident rationality, in this political constellation rationality and evidence are open to scientific and political contestation. Fassin's observations underscore, again, the importance of history, implying both local specificity and global causality, to specific para-statal configurations. The fact that South Africa won independence recently and late, when the nation-state no longer provided the universally dominant model of political imagination, is the key to understanding the southern African biography of Nevirapine. Moreover, the constellation engaging nation-state government, transnational scientists, and African clinicians and activists has its own historicity and evolved and changed dramatically over a short period of time.

———————

The chapters below share attention to concrete practice, experience, and relations—within and beyond science—and respect for specific historical trajectories and places. Originating from different disciplines, they are committed to new ways of integrating history and anthropology: interrogating historical remains ethnographically—be it Manton's patient records or Geissler's remains of older research stations; situating the ethnographic record within larger historical movements; and attending to historical comparisons drawn by the studied people. The chapters below constitute a critical conversation about the proposition that the postmillennial present constitutes a radical shift away from the mid-twentieth-century past. While several chapters attend empirically to both past and present, all contributors draw attention to certain convergent peculiarities of the present, "para-state" configuration—notably territorial, temporal, and scalar changes—and describe reconfigurations of familiar biopolitical entities—experimentality, transnational sovereignty, and alternative citizenships.

While most observe discontinuities, the authors' attention shifts quickly back to continuities, recurrences, traces, and memories. Framed by the two opening chapters, Nguyen's euphoric incantation of radically "novel forms" of sovereignty and biopolitical domination and Manton's historical-archaeological caveat against such claims to novelty, the contributors leave the classic anthropological-historiographic pendulum of continuity versus discontinuity to swing elsewhere and trace, instead, lines and lineages between past and present, applying the narrative of para-statal transformation as a heuristic device.

In this process, they qualify the initial proposition. Almost all emphasize the continued relevance of the nation-state—as institutional framing, a source of legitimacy and authority, providing resources and study populations, as an association of people and source of livelihoods, as a rhetorical device and project. Rather than postulating the replacement of the state by other forms of organized power, attention shifts to how it is that the state still works for science. Taking classic Foucauldian biopolitical governmentality as a starting point, the authors are then less interested in demonstrating how the older biopolitical apparatus morphs into an even more menacing disciplining machine—although Nguyen's text alerts us to this somewhat threatening possibility. Instead, the idea of an extension of biopolitical discipline from past into present is problematized (together with the idea of totalizing governmentality), with reference to the contradictions, persistent weaknesses and failures, resistances, and surprising outcomes produced by "disciplinary" technologies. This opens an agenda for future research. What happens if science and government go different ways rather than colluding in a disciplinary project? How are seemingly absolute biometric forms of surveillance and control used and sabotaged? How do we deal with unpredictable processes of collectivization and consciousness, arising unintended from regulation and surveillance? Where does civic commitment reside, if it can emerge from industry health interventions or post-neoliberal public-private partnerships? And, if the present is unpredictable, what is to happen next? Is the para-state of science the last step before science is definitely disentangled from territory and population, as Kelly suggests? Are we moving toward "global health" nihilism, performance and specter, or toward a global, transnational military-therapeutic complex—or both? What then about the manifold reformulations of the strong nation, be it through mining company public health or through counterfactual rejection of global scientific consensus? Is there hope for alternative outcomes, scope for contradiction and struggle? True to the implications of the *para-*prefix, the para-state opens a space not only of menace and uncertainty but also of wonder and surprise.

Notes

This collection is the outcome of collaborative events supported by a Leverhulme Research Leadership Award (F/02 116/D). The index was prepared with the generous support of the Department of Social Anthropology, University of Oslo. Chapters 4 and 10 draw on materials generated as part of research funded by the Wellcome Trust (GR077430 and GR081507 respectively).

1 For Nguyen, contemporary experimentality represents "an inversion of the classical model whereby evidence of efficacy permits intervention"; in the contemporary case, "intervention drives the need for self-validating evidence" (2009). This proposition may overemphasize change—did not colonial agricultural and economic interventions also function as experiments, continuously generating new data (see Bonneuil 2000)?—and overrates the significance of HIV; yet a strikingly new feature of contemporary African experimentality is that it often is inserted directly into national government; Nguyen's example of PEPFAR programs is a case in point (for other HIV-related examples see the chapters by Fassin and Meinert), but also the malaria trial discussed by Gerrets, in this volume, manipulates—viral style—entire government structures into an experimental configuration.

2 As the historian of science Hutchinson shows in a forthcoming PhD thesis, the foundation of the new para-statals in the late 1970s was also in important ways a nationalist moment, irrespective of the early neoliberal context, and the overall outcomes of the scientific transformation that it engendered during subsequent decades (Hutchinson, forthcoming; see also Tousignant 2013; Droney 2014).

3 It is precisely because contemporary collaborative science is not integrated in structures of academic education that "capacity building" has become a central concern of these institutions and their funders (see, e.g., Marjanovic et al. 2012). Although it certainly is laudable that the training of African scientists has become an integral part of some funders' policies, capacity building—usually not providing lasting support for national academic institutions and involving small numbers, often gaining degrees from European and American universities—remains an unanswered challenge.

4 Financial investments in these sites are considerable. Although total funding amounts are difficult to assess because funding may be transferred along different channels—core infrastructure funding, specific project funding from diverse funders, expatriate salaries, training programs for individual scientists, and so on—but for the larger sites, annual transfers can amount to tens of millions of dollars. The annual core grant for one such station in Kenya, for example,

amounted to about $30 million in 2008, excluding expatriate salaries and separate project grants, dwarfing government budgets for medical research.

5 The hard-to-grasp quality of the para-statal situation is evidenced by the allegedly "local" organizations that have emerged over the last few years around the major research centers, combining HIV care provisions (alongside but separate from government health facilities) with scientific research. Nominally "local," underlined by African language names, these are managed and staffed by leading North American universities (acting as their subsidiaries) and subsidised by HIV aid moneys, notably from PEPFAR, which formally cannot be used for research but for "evaluation" of ongoing interventions.

6 Good clinical practice (GCP) is a regulatory protocol, issued by the International Conference on Harmonisation (ICH), which details practical procedures, including those pertaining to ethical matters (consent, incentives, etc.) around clinical trials. It has been endorsed by the World Health Organization (WHO) and by the U.S. Federal Drug Administration (FDA), which is responsible for licensing pharmaceuticals to the world's largest pharmaceutical market, and it is therefore of crucial importance to the conduct of clinical trials all over the world, shaping widespread ideas about what the ethics of medical research are about (see, e.g., EMEA 2002).

7 While the rationale for transnational public health research remains, obviously, to inform policy, this process is complicated—probably more so than when research was conducted by government institutions themselves. In the contemporary configuration, data usually have to travel several times around the globe, for processing and analysis, for peer-reviewed publication, and finally to get approval from organizations like the FDA or WHO, before they are turned into national policy, and even then material conditions and resource limitations can make implementation of findings difficult. In response to this hiatus, "research-to-policy" has emerged as an academic specialization, complete with its own dedicated journals, aiming to facilitate the process and thereby to maintain the legitimacy and purpose of transnational public health research (see, e.g., Gilson 2008).

8 Research in emergency situations (civil war, refugee camps, disease outbreaks) is an exception from this state reliance, as in these cases humanitarianism or international or corporate sovereignty may take the place of nation-state.

9 This might be particularly the case in Africa. For a contradicting Southeast Asian case of contemporary biomedical nationalism, see, e.g., Reubi (2010).

10 This does not mean that exploitative pharmaceutical experiments, which utilize weak regulatory and medical structures, high disease burdens, and treatment-naïve populations to conduct experiments with little oversight, do not occur in Africa. The 1996 Pfizer Trovan trial during a meningitis outbreak in Nigeria is the often cited example. See Sarah Boseley, "WikiLeaks Cable: Pfizer 'Dirty Tricks to Avoid Clinical Trial Payouts,'" *Guardian*, October 12, 2010, http://www.guardian.co.uk/business/2010/dec/09/wikileaks-cables-pfizer-nigeria;

see also the forthcoming anthropological work of Morenike Folayan and Kris Peterson on the subject.

11 While northern agencies invariably portray their work as economically disinterested, motivated by social good, some African para-statal research bodies have embraced a more entrepreneurial ethos of product development and profit generation in a bid to justify their existence in the changed climate of neoliberal restructuring (e.g., Langwick 2011).

12 Cory Hayden's (2003, 2007) work on bioprospecting benefit sharing and on pharmaceutical production in Mexico analyses anthropologically the repositionings and transformations of public-private divides, guided by an understanding of the public as political project.

13 The emergence of the African "site-PI" results from a paradoxical interaction between multisite trials designed and managed by a central northern agency and increasing political pressure toward greater "local" African participation. Thus, major American agencies insist today that PIs are recruited among African scientists in collaborating institutions, while at the same time centralizing the process of research design and analysis in locations and among scientific staff outside of Africa.

14 Hence, rather than epitomizing a radically new form, Beisel's case inserts itself in an ongoing chain of transformation, beginning with malaria spraying as part of national and municipal public health, moving through transnational malaria science and policy from the 1960s WHO "eradication" to the 1990s bed net trials sometimes directly involving chemical industry, to today's contemporary fusion of corporate-cum-national responsibility (which, in turn, reveals ties back to much older forms of corporate malaria control) (see Schumaker 2011).

References

Abadie, Roberto. 2010. *The Professional Guinea Pig: Big Pharma and the Risky World of Human Subjects*. Durham, NC: Duke University Press.

Agamben, Giorgio. 1998. *Homo Sacer: Sovereign Power and Bare Life*. Palo Alto, CA: Stanford University Press.

Arnaut, Karel, and J. A. N. Blommaert. 2009. "Chthonic Science: Georges Niangoran-Bouah and the Anthropology of Belonging in Côte d'Ivoire." *American Ethnologist* 36, no. 3: 574–90.

Atwood, Margaret. 2003. *Oryx and Crake*. London: Bloomsbury.

Atwood, Margaret. 2009. *The Year of the Flood*. London: Bloomsbury.

Bayart, Jean-François, Stephen Ellis, and Béatrice Hibou. 1999. *The Criminalization of the State in Africa*. Bloomington: Indiana University Press.

Biehl, João. 2004. "The Activist State: Global Pharmaceuticals, AIDS, and Citizenship in Brazil." *Social Text* 22, no. 3: 105–32.

Biehl, João Guilherme. 2007. "Pharmaceuticalization: AIDS Treatment and Global Health Politics." *Anthropological Quarterly* 80, no. 4: 1083–126.

Bonneuil, Christophe. 2000. "Development as Experiment: Science and State Building in Late Colonial and Postcolonial Africa, 1930–1970." *Osiris* 15: 258–81.

Bornstein, Erica, and Peter Redfield. 2011. "An Introduction to the Anthropology of Humanitarianism." In *Forces of Compassion: Humanitarianism between Ethics and Politics*, edited by E. Bornstein and P. Redfield, 3–30. Sante Fe, NM: SAR Press.

Cassidy, Rebecca, and Melissa Leach. 2009. "Science, Politics, and the Presidential AIDS 'Cure.'" *African Affairs* 108, no. 433: 559–80.

Colclough, Christopher, and James Manor. 1993. *States or Markets? Neo-liberalism and the Development Policy Debate*. IDS Development Studies. Oxford: Clarendon Press.

Comaroff, Jean, and John Comaroff. 1991. *Of Revelation and Revolution*, vol. 1, *Christianity, Colonialism, and Consciousness in South Africa*. Chicago: University of Chicago Press.

Comaroff, Jean, and John Comaroff. 2000. "Millenial Capitalism: First Thoughts on a Second Coming." *Public Culture* 12, no. 2: 291–343.

Cooper, Frederick. 2002. *Africa Since 1940: The Past of the Present*. Cambridge: Cambridge University Press.

Cooper, Melinda. 2008. *Life as Surplus: Biotechnology and Capitalism in the Neoliberal Era*. Seattle: Washington University Press.

Crane, Johanna. 2013. *Scrambling for Africa: AIDS, Expertise, and the Rise of American Global Health Science*. Ithaca, NY: Cornell University Press.

De Boek, Filip. 1994. "'When Hunger Goes around the Land': Hunger and Food among the Aluund of Zaire." *Man* 29, no. 2: 257–82.

De Boeck, Filip. 1998. "Beyond the Grave: History, Memory, and Death in Postcolonial Congo/Zaïre." In *Memory and the Postcolony: African Anthropology and the Critique of Power*, edited by R. Werbner, 21–57. Postcolonial Encounters. London: Zed Books.

Dilger, Hansjorg. 2009. "Doing Better? Religion, the Virtue-Ethics of Development and the Fragmentation of Health Politics in Tanzania." *Africa Today* 56, no. 1: 89–110.

Droney, Damien. 2014. "Ironies of Laboratory Work during Ghana's Second Age of Optimism." *Cultural Anthropology* 29, no. 2: 363–84.

Dry, Sarah, and Melissa Leach. 2010. *Epidemics: Science, Governance and Social Justice*. Oxford: Earthscan.

Ecks, Stefan. 2005. "Pharmaceutical Citizenship: Antidepressant Marketing and the Promise of Demarginalization in India." *Anthropology and Medicine* 12, no. 3: 239–54.

Elliott, Carl. 2010. "The Mild Torture Economy." *London Review of Books* 32, no. 18: 26–27.

EMEA (European Medicines Agency). 2002. *ICH Topic E 6 (R1) Guideline for Good Clinical Practice*. London: EMEA.

Fairhead, James, Melissa Leach, and Mary Small. 2005. "Public Engagement with

Science? Local Understandings of a Vaccine Trial in the Gambia." *Journal of Biosocial Science* 38, no. 1: 103–16.

Fassin, Didier, and Mariella Pandolfi. 2010. *Contemporary States of Emergency. The Politics of Military and Humanitarian Interventions*. New York: Zone Books.

Feher, Michel. 2007. *Nongovernmental Politics*. New York: Zone Books.

Feiermann, Steven. 2011. "When Physicians Meet: Local Medical Knowledge and Global Public Goods." In *Evidence, Ethos and Ethnography: The Anthropology and History of Medical Research in Africa*, edited by P. W. Geissler and C. Molyneux. Oxford: Berghahn.

Feldman-Savelsberg, Pamela, Flavien T. Ndonko, and Bergis Schmidt-Ehry. 2000. "Sterilizing Vaccines or the Politics of the Womb: Retrospective Study of a Rumor in Cameroon." *Medical Anthropology Quarterly* 14, no. 2: 159–79.

Ferguson, James. 1999. *Expectations of Modernity: Myths and Meanings of Urban Life on the Zambian Copperbelt*. Berkeley: University of California Press.

Ferguson, James. 2006. *Global Shadows: Africa in the Neoliberal World Order*. Durham, NC: Duke University Press.

Ferguson, James. 2010. "The Uses of Neoliberalism." *Antipode* 41: 166–84.

Fisher, Jill. 2009. *Medical Research for Hire: The Political Economy of Pharmaceutical Clinical Trials*. New Brunswick, NJ: Rutgers University Press.

Fortun, Mike. 2005. "For an Ethics of Promising, or: A Few Kind Words about James Watson." *New Genetics and Society* 24, no. 2: 157–74.

Fortun, Mike. 2008. *Promising Genomics: Iceland and deCODE Genetics in a World of Speculation*. Berkeley: University of California Press.

Geissler, Paul Wenzel. 2011. "Parasite Lost: Remembering Modern Times with Kenyan Government Medical Scientists." In *Evidence, Ethos and Ethnography: The Anthropology and History of Medical Research in Africa*. edited by P. W. Geissler and C. Molyneux, 297–32. Oxford: Berghahn.

Geissler, Paul Wenzel. 2013. "Public Secrets in Public Health: Knowing Not to Know while Making Scientific Knowledge." *American Ethnologist* 40, no. 1: 13–34.

Geissler, P. Wenzel. 2013. "The Archipelago of Public Health: Comments on the Landscape of Medical Research in Twenty-First Century Africa." In *Making and Unmaking Public Health in Africa, Ethnographic and Historical Perspectives*, ed. R. Prince and R. Marsland, 231–56. Athens: Ohio University Press.

Geissler, Paul Wenzel, Ann Kelly, Robert Pool, and Babatunde Imoukhuede. 2008. "'He Is Now Like a Brother, I Can Even Give Him Some Blood'—Relational Ethics and Material Exchanges in a Malaria Vaccine 'Trial Community' in The Gambia." *Social Science and Medicine* 67, no. 5: 696–707.

Geissler, P. Wenzel, and Ferdinand Okwaro. 2014. "Discuss Inequality: Confront Economic Differences to Strengthen Global Research." *Nature* 513: 303.

Gieryn, Thomas F. 1983. "Boundary-Work and the Demarcation of Science from Non-Science: Strains and Interests in Professional Ideologies of Scientists." *American Sociological Review* 48, no. 6: 781–95.

Gilson, Lucy, and Di McIntyre. 2008. "The Interface between Research and Policy: Experience from South Africa." *Social Science and Medicine* 67, no. 5: 748–59.

Harrison, Mark. 2004. *Medicine and Victory: British Military Medicine in the Second World War*. Oxford: Oxford University Press.

Hayden, Cory. 2003. "From Market to Market: Bioprospecting's Idioms of Inclusion." *American Ethnologist* 30, no. 3: 359–71.

Hayden, Cory. 2007. "Taking as Giving: Bioscience, Exchange, and the Politics of Benefit-sharing." *Social Studies of Science* 37, no. 5: 729–58.

Hoppe, Kirk Arden. 2003. *Lords of the Fly: Sleeping Sickness Control in British East Africa, 1900–1960*. Westport, CT: Praeger.

Hunt, Nancy Rose. 1999. *A Colonial Lexicon: Of Birth Ritual, Medicalization, and Mobility in the Congo*. Durham, NC: Duke University Press.

Hutchinson, Lauren. Forthcoming. "Independence and Malaria Research in Kenya, 1977–1985." PhD diss., University of London.

Iliffe, John. 1998. *East African Doctors: A History of the Modern Profession*. Cambridge: Cambridge University Press.

Ishiguro, Kazuo. 2005. *Never Let Me Go*. London: Faber and Faber.

Kelly, Ann. 2011. "Will He Be There? Mediating Malaria, Immobilizing Science." *Journal of Cultural Economy* 4, no. 1: 65–79.

Kickbush, Ilona. 2003. "Global Health Governance: Some New Theoretical Considerations on the New Political Space." In *Globalization and Health*, edited by K. Lee, 192–203. London: Palgrave.

Lachenal, Guillaume. 2010. "Le médecin qui voulut être roi: Médicine coloniale et utopie au Cameroun." *Annales: Histoire, Sciences Sociales* 65, no. 1.

Langwick, Stacey A. 2011. *Bodies, Politics, and African Healing: The Matter of Maladies in Tanzania*. Bloomington: Indiana University Press.

Le Carré, John. 2000. *The Constant Gardener*. London: Hodder and Stoughton.

Livingston, Julie. 2012. *Improvising Medicine: An African Oncology Ward in an Emerging Cancer Epidemic*. Durham, NC: Duke University Press.

Lupton, Deborah. 1995. *The Imperative of Health: Public Health and the Regulated Body*. London: Sage.

Malowany, Maureen, Paul Wenzel Geissler, and Alfred Lwoba. 2011. "'Go Back to the Land!' Negotiating Space, Framing Governmentality in Lambwe Valley, Kenya 1954–75." *Canadian Journal of African Studies* 45, no. 3: 440–79.

Marjanovic, Sonja, Rebecca Hanlin, Stephanie Diepeveen, and Joanna Chataway. 2012. "Research Capacity-Building in Africa: Networks, Institutions and Local Ownership." *Journal of International Development* 25, no. 7: 936–40.

Marsland, Rebecca. 2014. "Who Are the Public in Public Health? Debating Crowds, Populations and Publics in Tanzania." In *Making and Unmaking Public Health in Africa: Ethnographic Perspectives*, ed. R. Marsland and R. Prince, 75–95. Athens: Ohio University Press.

Marsland, Rebecca, and Ruth Prince. 2012. "What Is Life Worth? Exploring Biomedical Interventions, Survival, and the Politics of Life." *Medical Anthropology Quarterly* 26, no. 4: 453–69.

Masquelier, Adeline. 2001. "Behind the Dispensary's Prosperous Façade: Imagining the State in Rural Niger." *Public Culture* 13, no. 2: 267–91.

Mbembe, Achille, and Janet Roitman. 1995. "Figures of the Subject in Times of Crisis." *Public Culture* 7: 323–52.

McGregor, JoAnn. 2005. "The Social Life of Ruins: Sites of Memory and the Politics of a Zimbabwean Periphery." *Journal of Historical Geography* 31, no. 2: 316–37.

Mol, Annemarie. 2008. *The Logic of Care: Health and the Problem of Patient Choice.* London: Routledge.

Molyneux, C. S., N. Peshu et al. 2005. "Trust and Informed Consent: Insights from Community Members on the Kenyan Coast." *Social Science and Medicine* 61, no. 7: 1463–73.

Nguyen, Vinh-Kim. 2005. "Antiretroviral Globalism, Biopolitics, and Therapeutic Citizenship." In *Global Assemblages: Technology, Politics, and Ethics as Anthropological Problems*, edited by A. Ong and S. J. Collier, 124–44. Oxford: Blackwell.

Nguyen, V. K. 2009. "Government-by-Exception: Enrollment and Experimentality in Mass HIV Treatment Programmes in Africa." *Social Theory and Health* 7: 196–217.

Nordling, Linda. 2012. "African Researchers Sue Flagship Programme for Discrimination: Conflict at Kenya Medical Research Institute Exposes Widespread Tensions." *Nature* 487, no. 7405: 17–18.

Nyairo, Joyce. 2005. "'Zilizopendwa': Kayamba Africa's Use of Cover Versions, Remix and Sampling in the (Re)Membering of Kenya." *African Studies* 64, no. 1: 29–54.

Nyamnjoh, F. B. 2004. "A Relevant Education for African Development—Some Epistemological Considerations." *Africa Development* 29, no 1: 161–84.

Oakley, Ann. 2004. *Private Complaints and Public Health: Richard Titmuss on the National Health Service*. Bristol, UK: Policy Press.

Okwaro, F., and P. Wenzel Geissler. 2015. "In/dependent Collaborations: Perceptions and Experiences of African Scientists in Transnational HIV research." *Medical Anthropology Quarterly*, forthcoming.

Ombongi, Kenneth. 2011. "The Historical Interface between the State and Medical Science in Africa: Kenya's Case." In *Evidence, Ethos and Ethnography: The Anthropology and History of Medical Research in Africa*, edited by Paul Wenzel Geissler and C. Molyneux, 353–72. Oxford: Berghahn.

Ong, Aihwa. 2006. *Neoliberalism as Exception: Mutations in Citizenship and Sovereignty*. Durham, NC: Duke University Press.

Packard, Randall. 1989. *White Plague, Black Labor: The Political Economy of Health and Diseases in South Africa*. Berkeley: University of California Press.

Patra, Prasanna Kumar, and Margaret Sleeboom-Faulkner. 2009. "Bionetworking: Experimental Stem Cell Therapy and Patient Recruitment in India." *Anthropology and Medicine* 16, no. 2: 147–63.

Petryna, Adriana. 2002. *Life Exposed: Biological Citizens after Chernobyl*. Princeton, NJ: Princeton University Press.

Petryna, Adriana. 2007. "Clinical Trials Offshored: On Private Sector Science and Public Health." *Biosocieties* 2: 21–40.

Petryna, Adriana. 2009. *When Experiments Travel: Clinical Trials and the Global Search for Human Subjects*. Princeton, NJ: Princeton University Press.

Prince, Ruth J. 2006. "'The World Is Finished': Ambiguities of Death and Love, Nostalgia and Morality in Contemporary Luo Popular Music." In *Youth in Contemporary Africa*, edited by C. Christiansen and H. Vigh, 117–52. Uppsala, Sweden: Nordic Africa Institute.

Prince, Ruth. 2012a. "HIV and the Moral Economy of Survival in an East African City." *Medical Anthropology Quarterly* 26, no. 4: 534–56.

Prince, Ruth J. 2012b. "The Politics and Anti-Politics of HIV: Healthcare and Welfare in Contemporary Kenya." In *Rethinking Biomedicine and Governance in Africa: Contributions from Anthropology*, edited by Paul Wenzel Geissler, R. Rottenburg, and J. Zenker, 97–118. Bielefeld, Germany: Transcript.

Prince, Ruth J. 2013. "Introduction: Situating Health and the Public in Africa Historical and Anthropological Perspectives." *Making and Unmaking Public Health in Africa*, edited by Ruth J. Prince and Rebecca Marsland, 1–54. Athens: Ohio University Press.

Prince, Ruth J., and Rebecca Marsland. 2013. "Making Public Health in Africa." *Ethnographic and Historical Perspectives*. Athens: Ohio University Press.

Rajan, Kaushik Sunder. 2006. *Biocapital: The Constitution of Postgenomic Life*. Durham, NC: Duke University Press.

Ranger, Terence O. 1992. "Godly Medicine: The Ambiguities of Medical Mission in Southeastern Tanzania." In *The Social Basis of Health and Healing in Africa*, edited by S. Feierman and J. M. Janzen, 256–83. Comparative Studies of Health Systems and Medical Care. Berkeley: University of California Press.

Redfield, Peter. 2012. "The Unbearable Lighness of Expats: Double Binds of Humanitarian Mobility." *Cultural Anthropology* 27, no. 2: 358–82.

Reubi, David. 2010. "Blood Donors, Development and Modernisation: Configurations of Biological Sociality and Citizenship in Post-Colonial Singapore." *Citizenship Studies* 14, no. 5: 473–93.

Reverby, Susan M. 2009. *Examining Tuskegee: The Infamous Syphilis Study and Its Legacy*. Chapel Hill: University of North Carolina Press.

Robbins, Steve. 2008. *From Revolution to Rights in South Africa: Social Movements, NGOs and Popular Politics*. Oxford: James Currey Publishers and University of KwaZulu Natal Press.

Roitman, Janet. 2004. *Fiscal Disobedience: An Anthropology of Economic Regulation in Central Africa*. Princeton, NJ: Princeton University Press.

Rose, Nikolas. 1996. "The Death of the Social? Re-figuring the Territory of Government." *Economy and Society* 25, no. 3: 327–56.

Rose, Nikolas. 2001. "The Politics of Life Itself." *Theory, Culture and Society* 18, no. 6: 1–30.

Rose, Nikolas, and Carlos Novas. 2005. "Biological Citizenship." In *Global Assemblages: Technology, Politics, and Ethics as Anthropological Problems*, edited by A. Ong and S. J. Collier, 439–63. Oxford: Blackwell.

Rottenburg, Richard. 2009. "Social and Public Experiments and New Figurations of Science and Politics in Postcolonial Africa." *Postcolonial Studies* 12, no. 4: 423–40.

Schumaker, Lyn. 2001. *Africanizing Anthropology: Fieldwork, Networks, and the Making of Cultural Knowledge in Central Africa*. Durham, NC: Duke University Press.

Schumaker, Lyn. 2011. "The Mosquito Taken at the Beerhall: Malaria Research and Control on Zambia's Copperbelt." In *Evidence, Ethos and Ethnography: The Anthropology and History of Medical Research in Africa*, edited by Paul Wenzel Geissler and C. Molyneux, 403–28. Oxford: Berghahn.

Scott, J. C. 1998. *Seeing Like a State: How Certain Schemes to Improve the Human Condition Have Failed*. New Haven, CT: Yale University Press.

Shapin, Steven. 1988. "The House of Experiment in Seventeenth-Century England." *Isis* 79, no. 3: 373–404.

Simpson, Anthony. 1998. "Memory and Becoming Chosen Other: Fundamentalist Elite-Making in a Zambian Catholic Mission School." In *Memory and the Postcolony*, edited by R. Werbner, 209–28. London: Zed Books.

Sleeboom-Faulkner, Margaret, and Prasanna Kumar Patra. 2011. "Experimental Stem Cell Therapy: Biohierarchies and Bionetworking in Japan and India." *Social Studies of Science* 41, no. 5: 645–66.

Tangri, Roger K. 2000. *The Politics of Patronage in Africa: Parastatals, Privatization, and Private Enterprise in Africa*. Trenton, NJ: Africa World Press.

Tilley, Helen. 2011. *Africa as a Living Laboratory: Empire, Development, and the Problem of Scientific Knowledge*. Chicago: University of Chicago Press.

Tousignant, Noemi. 2013. "Broken Tempos: Of Means and Memory in a Senegalese University Laboratory." *Social Studies of Science* 43, no. 5: 729–53.

Vaughan, Megan. 1991. *Curing Their Ills: Colonial Power and African Illness*. Cambridge: Polity Press.

Wendland, Claire. 2012. "Animating Biomedicine's Moral Order: The Crisis of Practice in Malawian Medical Training." *Current Anthropology* 53, no. 6: 755–88.

Werbner, Richard. 1998a. *Memory and the Postcolony: African Anthropology and the Critique of Power*. London: Zed Books.

Werbner, Richard. 1998b. "Smoke from the Barrel of a Gun: Postwars of the Dead, Memory and Reinscription in Zimbabwe." In *Memory and the Postcolony*, edited by R. Werbner, 71–102. London: Zed Books.

White, Luise. 2004. "Poisoned Food, Poisoned Uniforms, and Anthrax: Or, How Guerillas Die in War." *OSIRIS* 19: 220–33.

Yahya, Maryam. 2007. "Polio Vaccines—'No Thank You!' Barriers to Polio Eradication in Northern Nigeria." *African Affairs* 106, no. 423: 185–204.

PART I

Rupture, Continuity

CHAPTER 1

Treating to Prevent HIV: Population Trials and Experimental Societies

Vinh-Kim Nguyen

This chapter explores how Africa has emerged at the heart of global bio-politics in ways that drive biomedical research and the development of new health interventions. Novel approaches to intervening on human popula-tions are currently being fashioned through population-based experiments, with potentially remarkable biological and social results. The focus of this chapter is the emergence of a breakthrough in addressing HIV: the ability of mass treatment to potentially eradicate the epidemic. Treatment as pre-vention (TasP) is this new strategy. TasP was cobbled together from already existing science and is now the subject of over fifty large studies around the world and is the subject of this chapter (Granich et al. 2011). My sugges-tion is that these large trials of treating-to-prevent herald the birth of ex-perimental societies: large-scale forms of social organization assembled on biopolitical terrains left fallow by retreating states. This happens when ex-periments deploy a form of governmentality that leaks, through space and time, outside the trial. Under the right circumstances, residues of protocols, procedures, discursive practices, experimental biologies, and embodied ex-periences may congeal to constitute experimental societies. The para-state is visible as a kind of shadow of the experimental society: both cause (as a zone of abandonment [Biehl 2005]) and effect (as an assemblage of evidence-driven interventions, mobile governmentalities). Let me begin by setting the stage, before turning to examine the genesis and origins of TasP.

In July 2010, the Eighteenth International AIDS Conference was held in Vienna. Host cities are chosen by a complex calculus that includes geo-graphic representation, receptivity to the messages of the AIDS world, and a reading of which strategies must be given a boost.[1] Hence the slogans sported by each conference: in this case, "Rights Here Rights Now." Vienna was a geographical proxy for Eastern Europe, and the issue of human rights was a particularly timely one in this part of the world, where the AIDS epidemic was growing faster than anywhere else, largely driven by an epidemic of intravenous drug use fuelled by a toxic combination of postsocialist social breakdown and abundant, cheap heroin flowing out of post-Taliban Afghanistan (Beyrer 2010). The link between the epidemic and the historical geography of state failure in the postsocialist world contrasted with that in Africa, where arguably the state never had the same material presence. In Eastern Europe the tendency to criminalize drug use was viewed with concern by the organizers of the conference. They justifiably argued that fighting drug use with repression violates the rights of drug users, most notably their right to mitigate the deleterious effects of drug use through "harm reduction" such as methadone substitution therapy. Of considerable public health concern was the fact that, in this part of the world, prisons were in fact epidemiological pumps, concentrating those most vulnerable to HIV in one place and thereby facilitating the spread of HIV and its companion infections, such as tuberculosis. In this view drug use was a medical problem, not a legal issue, and human rights is the right treatment. While in Eastern Europe there was too much state, in Africa there was not enough.

The focus on "rights here" (that is, Eastern Europe) and "right now" (that is, as the epidemic explodes in this part of the world) blurred during the conference, which went noticeably off message from the get-go. The culprit: TasP, an idea that had been making the rounds over the past year in obscure epidemiological articles and had now burst into the limelight. The concept of TasP is simple. When people infected with HIV are administered powerful antiretroviral (ARV) drug cocktails, their "viral load" (the quantity of virus in the blood) drops to undetectable levels. As a result, they become much less infectious. In this view, if everyone who is HIV positive is treated, no more HIV transmission—and no more epidemic. (I will return to this supposition a bit later.) While many factors account for this shift, my discussions with scientists and policy makers at the time suggested that the global geopolitics of HIV was driving the push for TasP.

Because it bears the brunt of global HIV infections, it is in Africa that the success of the response to the epidemic is measured; it is where international donors have invested the most and correspondingly have the most at stake. This was not always the case: the epidemic was first recognized in the United States and rapidly described in Europe, where robust health systems were able to detect the epidemic early. Recognition of the epidemic's severity in

Africa lagged, partially because a patchy, poorly funded and equipped health system (a symptom of state weakness) was ill-equipped to differentiate AIDS from the common diseases that ravaged the continent. Until ten years ago, the technoscientific response was mainly driven by the needs for addressing the epidemic in the north, and it was possible to see—and denounce—a "two-track" approach to the epidemic: individualized prevention and treatment for the north, and collective prevention and palliative care for Africa. After the Durban conference, the two-track approach was officially abandoned, such that treatment was deemed a priority for the developing world too. In Africa massive treatment programs were scaled up and millions put on the antiretroviral drugs.

By 2008 concerns began to be raised that treatment was occurring at the expense of prevention programs (for an overview see Merson, O'Malley, Serwadda, and Apisuk 2008). These concerns were motivated by alarming reports that the incidence of HIV was increasing in some gay men in the north, where prevention had until then been a resounding success, and that it was not decreasing appreciably in the south. It would not be possible, we were ominously warned, to "treat our way out of the epidemic." Backstage, the concerns were more strongly worded. The lion's share of the funding was going to treatment: expensive but with easily measured results that could be marketed using the powerful metrics of "lives saved." Prevention was no longer appealing, and donors were no longer interested. Nowhere was this clearer than at the epicenter of the epidemic, where the human, financial, and geopolitical stakes were high. As some had feared, the biomedical lobby had "hijacked" the HIV train. The arrival of TasP, two years later, was an opportunity: prevention and treatment could be reconciled, and perhaps a breakthrough appeared where prevention alone had had only limited success.

Biomedical Prevention: New Technologies, Old Issues

TasP was but the latest salvo in the deployment of biomedical prevention, so-called because it involves the use of biomedical technologies to prevent HIV, rather than behavior change or condoms (Rosengarten et al. 2008 alerts to the challenges involved; for a recent review, see Padian et al. 2011). Such biomedical technologies include the use of drugs to prevent infection, either applied locally as microbicidal gels or taken prior to or after sexual exposure: respectively, pre-exposure prophylaxis (PrEP) and post-exposure prophylaxis (PEP). Circumcision of males has been shown to protect men against HIV and has joined the armamentarium of biomedical prevention as medical circumcision programs are ramped up. Within the AIDS industry, these approaches are referred to as the "new prevention technologies" (NPTs). It must be underlined that most of these NPTs have been developed mindful of the particular epidemiological realities of HIV in Africa, where it is widely accepted that HIV is largely heterosexually transmitted, gender norms make women particularly vulnerable and men resistant to older behavioral prevention approaches, and a generalized epidemic dictates measures targeting the entire population rather than focused "high-risk" groups. (It is also worth underlining that these assumptions themselves reveal a certain tendency to homogenize and stereotype a highly diverse continent and its social realities as a kind of mirror image of the West. The recent "discovery" that men who have sex with men are of epidemiological importance in Africa and that gender norms are in fact far more mutable than previously assumed are two examples that argue against this simplistic view.) Biomedical research in HIV had up until then largely focused on the north, but biomedical technologies are now being engineered specifically as a function of Africa's (perceived) epidemiological specificities—and tested there for eventual re-export back to the rest of the world.

Post-Vienna, the stress on TasP and other NPTs seemed to be redefining HIV as a purely medical problem best left in the hands of doctors and scientists. Backstage, it was possible to detect exasperation with the messy world of unruly subjects, refractory gender norms, unreasonable activists, and noncompliant states (see Lachenal's chapter on medical nihilism in this volume). That impatience reflected the difficulty in finding a simple, technical fix to the otherwise challenging problem of prevention, mired in issues of gender, power, and poverty.

Searching for a Magic Bullet: From Vaccination to Mass Treatment

A vaccine in contrast promised a simple, technical fix to the seemingly intractable issues that dogged HIV prevention—a magic bullet. There would be no need to change behavior, no need to target specific groups, no risk of incurring the wrath of activists. Vaccine trials, however, have not borne out these hopes. For instance, in the wake of the highly visible failure of the STEP trials in 2007, leading scientists and the NIH proclaimed that it was "back to the drawing board." An important point however is often glossed over, perhaps because of the pervasiveness of the idea of the vaccine as a magic bullet. Because of the way HIV, and the immune system, interact, it is highly unlikely that any vaccine would confer the kind of total immunity that we associate with usual vaccines—for mumps, measles, rubella, hepatitis, and the like. So if an HIV vaccine is not fully protective, that is, only reduces the risk by say 50 percent or so, this has several implications. The first is that a very large number of people will have to be vaccinated for the vaccine to have a notable effect at the population level. This is referred to as "herd immunity": once a certain threshold of the population is immunized, the infectious disease effectively dies out because not enough susceptible individuals are left in the population to ensure a chain of transmission. When vaccines are 100 percent effective, they will protect a population once 75 or 80 percent are immunized. This will not be the case for HIV unless an unforeseen breakthrough occurs.

The presumed weakness of HIV candidate vaccines has several implications. First, that the clinical trials needed to demonstrate their effectiveness will need to recruit comparatively larger numbers of subjects to prove—or disprove—efficacy. A second, related point is that should a marginally better vaccine come along, even larger numbers will be required to tease out the relatively small differences in efficacy between the vaccine candidates, driving up the cost of subsequent trials for ever-diminishing preventive returns. In other words, it is unlikely that an eventual HIV vaccine would actually be a magic bullet.

Given the paucity of promising results on the vaccine front, it is not surprising that other approaches have been tried. Early awareness that gender dynamics made condom use problematic, particularly in Africa's burgeoning heterosexual epidemic, spurred the search for female-controlled methods such as the female condom and microbicides (Hardon 2012). Microbicides were touted as the next best thing to a vaccine, but hope quickly gave way to pessimism as trial after trial showed disappointing results, with some even suggesting that microbicides could increase HIV transmission (e.g., Van Damme et al. 2002; Gawrylewski 2007; for a recent editorial overview, see Quiñones-Mateu and Vanham 2012). It was amid this global gloom that good news sprang seemingly out of nowhere in 2007. Male circumcision, it was convincingly showed, resulted in a striking decrease in HIV incidence—on the order of 50 percent—in men circumcised in three different randomized clinical trials, relative to those left "intact." The only problem was that male circumcision does not protect women, at least in the short term. Its protective effect is therefore much like a vaccine given only to men: it will only protect the women once enough of the "herd" is vaccinated (WHO 2007). Male circumcision too is a population approach that dispenses with the need to engage with the messy world of human behavior, gender identity, and social constraint. But no magic bullet here either.

Another approach, which has generated considerable interest since 2008 has been PrEP. Initial optimism that PrEP might furnish a new tool in HIV prevention began in the late 1990s with animal studies that showed that treated monkeys with the antiretroviral tenofovir seemed to protect them when they were "challenged" with HIV (Tsai et al. 1995). Further support came from clinical trials of the antiretroviral drugs AZT and nevirapine, which showed that both could protect infants from acquiring HIV from their mothers during labor and birth. Eventually, trials of tenofovir as PrEP were begun in 2004 in Cambodia, Cameroon, and Malawi, with female sex workers as experimental subjects, only to be aborted by concerns that appropriate ethical standards were not in place. Eventually the ethical concerns were apparently addressed, and twelve trials are currently under way testing various antiretroviral combinations as PrEP, with a combined enrollment of thousands of patients. The trials generated intense interest after the Vienna conference, where a South African trial of PrEP with a tenofovir gel was shown to reduce incidence of infection by up to 50 percent in the women who used it (Abdool-Karim et al. 2010). Yet PrEP remains particularly prone to scientific and ethical challenges in testing as earlier controversies show. It is difficult not to view those who are infected in the context of a prevention trial as "victims" of that trial. As a result, the specter of those "failed" by prevention haunts these trials.

TasP dodges these issues, shifting the focus to those who might transmit rather than those who might be contaminated. Because potential transmitters are offered the benefit of treatment, there appear to be no "losers" when testing this approach. TasP comprises two similar approaches that differ in one important respect. The first, called test-and-treat, represents a public health, or population-based, strategy for controlling the epidemic (Cambiano, Rodger, and Phillips 2010). The most effective strategy would require automatic treatment of *all* individuals with HIV in a population. Such an approach would entail compulsory systematic testing and treatment, posing ethical challenges in pitting individual and collective interests. A more palatable alternative is to maximize testing and treatment through vigorous campaigns to incite testing ("increase uptake"). Importantly, those who test positive would then be treated with antiretroviral drugs, *even if their condition does not warrant it.*

The more conventional approach seeks to maximize testing and treatment but only treat if clinically warranted; that is, according to standardized guidelines that recommend treatment once the CD4 count (a measure of the immune system) is below a specific amount (in mid-2013 this threshold was increased from 350 to 500 cells/mL). This approach encourages testing and treatment, but treatment only if clinically indicated, and has been called various things from "expanded access" to "treatment 2.0" (WHO 2011). In this chapter I refer to both these approaches as TasP, which highlights the emphasis given to the preventive benefits of expanding treatment that is common to efforts to expand and intensify treatment efforts.

TasP thus comprises two strategies: the more aggressive test-and-treat strategy and more conservative treatment 2.0, which relies on increasing treatment coverage to achieve preventive effects. The former represents a classic public health approach to population health whereby ARV drugs are used even if not clinically indicated and therefore of no benefit to the person treated (the benefit of decreased transmission registers at the population level), while the latter is a clinical approach: treat only if warranted for the patient's health. TasP is not a scientific discovery that came out of the blue; rather it results from the cobbling together of existing pieces of science. These scientific building blocks were in place long before TasP was actually formulated as a strategy, suggesting that TasP's arrival on the international stage was at least partially in response to political and social circumstances rather than compelling scientific evidence that was already evident from the early 2000s.

How It All Fell into Place

The idea that systematic treatment could serve as a powerful form of prevention and eventually eradicate HIV epidemics was not a preordained one, but it fell into place like pieces of a jigsaw puzzle at the close of the first decade of the twenty-first century. In this section I will explore three of the critical pieces that, once in place, served as cornerstones to the development of TasP. As hopes for a holy grail to the epidemic, an effective preventive vaccine, slowly faded from the 1990s, scientists and activists came together to search for other potential "magic bullets": simple, biomedical technologies that could prevent HIV transmission. In this there was already a precedent.

In 1994 a landmark Franco-American clinical trial (called ACTG 076, the acronym standing for aids clinical trials group) showed that giving a pregnant woman the antiretroviral drug AZT could dramatically reduce the chances of passing the infection on to the baby (Connor et al. 1994). The prevention of mother to child transmission, PMTCT, as it is commonly known, was the first time a biomedical technology proved effective in preventing HIV. The concept of PMTCT was based on early studies in monkeys that showed that an antiretroviral could block infection. The landmark ACTG 076 results were subsequently validated in Africa, although these trials generated controversy since they used a placebo arm (for a critical review of this controversy, see Wendland 2008; see Booth 2010 for a critique of PMTCT as a "magic bullet"). Even more encouraging was the discovery, also in 1994, that combining three or more ARV drugs resulted in a potent "cocktail"— dubbed highly active antiretroviral therapy, or HAART. HAART not only stopped viral replication in the bodies of those who took it but allowed immune systems to grow back and health to be restored.

A further, and powerful, boost to the concept of ARVs that could prevent HIV infection—and not just treat it—came from a study conducted also in rural Uganda in the mid-1990s (Quinn et al. 2000). The study had initially been designed to look at whether aggressive treatment of sexually transmitted infections or STIs—known to facilitate HIV infection—could reduce transmission of HIV. It involved following over 6,000 people to compare the rates of HIV incidence between those who received an STI control intervention and those who did not. Disappointingly, this proved not to be the case, contradicting results of another similar study conducted in Tanzania and leading to an intense scientific debate. The researchers had frozen blood samples from the study participants, and in order to better understand their contradictory results they thawed the samples and measured the quantity of virus present. They identified 415 couples who were in a "sero-discordant" relationship, where one member was HIV positive and the other not. The researchers found that there was no transmission when the infected partner had a low viral load. Since HAART decreases viral load, it could be assumed that treatment would have a preventive effect (see, e.g., Eyawo et al. 2010).

Gradually the idea that these drugs could be used in prevention took hold. Perhaps they could be taken *before* exposure to prevent infection? Yet many worried the drugs were too toxic for use by healthy individuals—that the risks of toxicity were greater than the potential benefit of protection. The concern dissipated somewhat when newer drugs began to appear that had been tailored specifically for HIV and as a result tended to have fewer side effects. One of these newer drugs was tenofovir, manufactured by Gilead. Indeed, very early studies done in the 1990s with the intent of preventing perinatal transmission had already shown that tenofovir had chemical and antiviral properties that made it particularly well suited and potentially effective (at least in monkeys) as a preventive agent. Tenofovir was a drug designed specifically to attack HIV, and it also had the benefit of having chemical properties that would allow it to be appropriate for local use. Moreover, unlike the antiretroviral drugs that preceded it, tenofovir was largely free of side effects. In the late 1990s animal studies showed that monkeys treated with the antiretroviral tenofovir had resisted infection. This led to the 2004 tenofovir PrEP trials, mentioned earlier, that were quickly halted because of ethical concerns. PrEP remains of considerable interest, with twelve trials currently under way testing various antiretroviral combinations as PrEP, with a combined enrollment of thousands of patients. The results that are trickling out from these studies are mitigated, suggesting that PrEP is unlikely to emerge as a magic bullet.

So by 2004 it was clear that traditional prevention approaches relying on behavior change and condoms had limitations, a vaccine was not forthcoming, PrEP was controversial, and microbicides were flawed. Breakthroughs had occurred in the treatment of HIV, such that it was known that HAART decreases viral load, transmission is highly unlikely at low viral loads, and ARVs could prevent HIV transmission in pregnant mothers. Yet discussion of the idea that treatment could serve to prevent HIV infection, introduced in the early 2000s (Velasco-Hernandez 2002), did not start to be discussed until the second half of the decade (Montaner et al. 2006). Two important milestones were reached in 2008 and 2009. The first was the publication of the controversial "Swiss statement": a declaration by Swiss HIV specialists that persons with HIV were not sexually infectious if they were consistently taking HAART, had undetectable viral loads, and were not suffering from a STI (Vernazza et al. 2008). The Swiss statement amounted to saying that for those meeting the criteria just described, it was no longer necessary to practice safe sex.

Though controversial, the Swiss statement validated what was in fact already being practiced. In North America and Europe, some HIV positive men saw in HAART—and the undetectable viral loads that resulted from their treatments—an opportunity to negotiate unprotected sex without risking transmitting HIV. While this may have been a reasonable strategy for preventing the spread of HIV by itself, increasing rates of other STIs demonstrated the downside. As HIV treatment programs scaled up in the developing world, and in Africa in particular, patients regained their health. The vast majority were heterosexual, and many dreamed of starting a family. In those years I was working with organizations of HIV positive people in West Africa. The assumption that being HIV positive meant one always had to have protected sex rapidly became a source of contention between those who wanted to have children and medical personnel who felt uncomfortable about "authorizing" unprotected sex. The Ugandan study (Quinn 2000) gradually became known and, with gentle pressure from activists, some medical personnel allowed that procreative sex might not be a risk for transmission, if the positive partner was treated. So, while the strategy of treating to prevent HIV was being pieced together from the relevant scientific studies from above, the preventive benefits of treatment were already being put to use and that experience was percolating from below.

The second milestone was the publication in 2009 of a mathematical modeling study that showed that universal screening and treatment could *eradicate* an HIV epidemic (Granich et al. 2009). In other words, if everyone was tested for HIV and enough went on treatment, it would be possible to halt transmission entirely. The biological and epidemiological rationale for TasP was now in place, and the next step would be to test the intervention to see if it would really work. Already, studies were being done to see if there was a correlation between increasing the numbers of patients treated and the number of new infections. Some studies suggested that the two were inversely correlated (that is, more treatment appeared to prevent new infections) while some did not. The jury was still out, and so the next step would be to test TasP. But doing so would require experimenting on entire populations.

Enthusiasm and Hesitation about Biomedical Prevention

This account so far shows how the search for a magic bullet for HIV prevention drove the development of biomedical prevention technologies. The enthusiasm for male circumcision came from impressive results from three randomized controlled trials (RCTs) that showed a remarkable protective effect. These results were front-page news and generated a wave of optimism. These striking results emerged against a bleak landscape of disappointing results on the prevention front, an elusive vaccine, and a relentless epidemic. As many policy makers and global health experts emphasized repeatedly to me, the protective effect demonstrated in the male circumcision trials was by the far the most dramatic figure they had ever seen. It was as good as a vaccine, they noted.

Yet these impressive numbers were an artifact of the study design and the intervention. Randomized controlled trials can only reliably measure simple interventions over short periods of time under controlled circumstances. Simply put, the numbers are not a measure of what might actually happen *outside* the laboratory of the trial (epidemiologists refer to this as the problem of "generalizability"). Second, more complex interventions—for instance, economic and social empowerment of women—are very difficult to turn into a standard package that can be randomly allotted in an RCT.[2] Lack of evidence of efficacy of many interventions doesn't mean that they don't work—just that they have never been subjected to an RCT, either because this is methodologically impossible or pointless. Just as there has been no RCT demonstrating the efficacy of parachutes in preventing death when jumping from airplanes, there has been no RCT of condom use.

Despite the powerful evidence for male circumcision, hurdles remained. The bulk of the critique focused on the "social acceptability" of male circumcision (e.g., Aggleton 2007). African specificities resurfaced in discussions where concerns were voiced that male circumcision may not be "culturally appropriate" in certain settings, and that in settings where circumcision is practiced in the setting of male initiation into adulthood its medicalization may in fact be counterproductive because it removed a "traditional" site where sexual responsibility is taught. Stigma was also often mentioned as a concern; that is, that both users and nonusers of NPTs (in this case, circumcised and uncircumcised men) could be stigmatized, either because they might appear as "promiscuous" or because they would be blamed for the ongoing spread of HIV. More broadly, there was worry that the focus on biomedical prevention would draw attention, energy, and most importantly financial resources away from "standard" prevention approaches that relied on education, behavior change, partner reduction, and condom use. Finally, there was worry that such biomedical prevention strategies marked a return to the early days of the epidemic, when it was considered a strictly medical problem amenable to technical solutions (Nguyen et al. 2011). From the point of view of skeptics, TasP was a particularly radical option, in effect "carpet bombing" the entire population with pharmaceuticals.

Nonetheless, at the 2010 International AIDS Conference, Myron Cohen, a leading AIDS prevention researcher and proponent of new prevention technologies, voiced what he called "uncomfortable truths" about TasP (Cohen 2010; see also Padian et al. 2011) as follows. The notion that treatment is prevention may be seductive, but the observation that increased treatment coverage led to decreased incidence (in British Columbia and San Francisco) has not been replicated in other studies. Indeed, public health experts worldwide point out that HIV incidence has not decreased (and in some cases is even increasing) in many jurisdictions where HAART is widely available and free. While some studies have shown that treatment reduces transmission among sero-discordant couples (where one individual is HIV positive and the other not), others have not. Finally, molecular studies suggest that up to half of HIV transmission occurs from individuals who have themselves just been infected, have not yet developed an antibody response to the infection, and therefore are not yet diagnosable as HIV positive by standard testing, which measures anitbodies to HIV—and therefore would not be "caught" in time for treatment to work. These concerns are particularly relevant in Africa, in light of the challenge of achieving sufficient population "coverage" to achieve a "herd immunity" effect given the weakness of health systems—particularly when even the powerful health systems of the north are unable to achieve these levels of treatment coverage![3]

Despite these reservations and the absence of RCT evidence, TasP was greeted with enthusiasm. The mathematical modeling study, a WHO informant told me, was a "breath of fresh air": here was an exciting new idea that could be used to breathe life into flagging prevention efforts! Others expressed similar views. Moreover, TasP was "elegant," proposing a single, simple solution solving two major problems: meeting growing treatment needs in the context of a global economic crisis that threatened to dry up flows of funds for drugs, and preventing future infections. Two birds with one stone. Some activists saw a third bird falling to TasP's single stone: casting in benign humanitarian light a pharmaceutical logic of market expansion—visible in how the pharmaceuticals industry has consistently pushed studies that favor earlier treatment over later.

Behind these pragmatic concerns lay a philosophical difference. Many activists were concerned that, in the quest for a magic bullet, a fundamentally social problem was being turned into a medical one. The spectrum of those who view HIV as a social issue—an epidemic driven by social forces—is wide and spans HIV dissidents such as former South African President Thabo Mbeki, who infamously called into question the causal role of HIV, to medical professionals (Paul Farmer and Didier Fassin being the best known), who argue that social inequalities and the "structural violence" of racism and other extreme forms of social exclusion drive the biology of the epidemic. This broad front of unease with, and critique of, new biomedical prevention approaches rallies those wary of medicalizing the response to the epidemic. Struggles over medicalization have been at the heart of the epidemic since its very beginning. Classical public health approaches that sought to contain the epidemic through "exclusion and control" (i.e., by shutting down gay bathhouses in the United States) caused the first battles that led, eventually, to framing HIV rather in terms of human rights and empowerment (Seidel 1993). Arguments were marshaled for consideration of HIV as a "social problem," requiring social solutions that materialized in the shape of multisectoral development approaches, gender education, and so on. Practically, activists wrested control (to an extent) of the response to the epidemic from doctors and in the process "empowered" (some) social scientists to deploy their expertise. So today, interventions that promise a biomedical, technical fix to the apparently intractable social challenge of prevention appear to mark a worrisome remedicalization of the epidemic (e.g., Nguyen et al. 2010). But is this really the case?

Revisiting Medicalization

Social scientists have, since the 1960s, pointed to medicalization as a central tendency in modern society. *Medicalization* refers to how social conditions are transformed into medical problems and are therefore managed through interventions that target individuals and populations in the name of health.[4] The concept of medicalization, at least in the way it is used in claims that NPTs are "medicalizing" prevention, presumes that there is a social sphere to medicalize. What is medicalized is that which was social in the first place: gender relations, economic inequality, poverty, and exclusion, for instance. In this view, HIV, attention deficit disorder, lead poisoning, obesity, and so on are the embodied end result of a cascade of social processes. So, the argument goes, treating these conditions as purely medical ones is a Band-Aid solution. Rather, social policy is required to address these upstream social determinants. Underlying this approach is a normative view of the social, borne of the rise of the European nation-state and the mechanisms that forged a social bond between anonymous members of the "imagined community" of the nation.

But if the social is to be understood as a tissue of social relations moored to the state, which acts as a guarantor of a stable future, as sociologists claim,[5] this might not neatly correspond to the "social" that is to be found throughout much of Africa. Of course, there are vibrant social relations and a vigorous "civil society" of community and religious groups and nongovernmental organizations. The notion of a "strong society" taking the place of a "weak state" expresses this idea. But as the chapters in this volume show, this is a somewhat optimistic formulation. Society is a fragile thing where life is about struggling from day to day in a state of perpetual uncertainty, where systemic poverty corrodes social ties. Terms such as *failed state, postcolony* (Mbembe 2001), *necropolitics* (Mbembe 2003), and the *politics of the belly* (Bayart 2006) have tried to capture a reality that can be characterized by the absence of a "social" in the sense of a tissue of social solidarity that binds people together in a common national project (see also Ferguson 2006).

On those terrains left fallow by the state, opposing what is "social" to what is "biomedical" may obscure more than it reveals. Medicalization therefore is unlikely to be the same process in societies structured through state action. To put it another way, biomedical intervention is often viewed as desocializing because it targets individuals, isolating them from the social relations in which they are embedded. These social relations span friends and family to embrace a wider society structured along economic gradients and symbolic systems. When poverty and dysfunctional institutions make it difficult to envisage the future, as is the case for many Africans, it is not difficult to imagine that one is already "individualized," alone with one's fate, rather than being embraced by the collective security that comes from belonging to a social body forged through the state. Demands for solidarity can overwhelm kinship and community ties. This is certainly the picture that emerged from my fieldwork with people living with HIV in Africa and from ethnography of contemporary Africa. Adding biomedical intervention into the mix does not really change this fundamental reality. The concept of *pharmaceuticalization*, as elaborated by sociologists (see Abraham 2010) and anthropologists (for foundational work, see Whyte, Van der Geest, and Hardon 2003; a more recent elaboration is Biehl 2007), captures succinctly what happens when pills are introduced to manage complex health problems without the apparatus of a functioning health system and, more generally, social security net.

So, to recap: new prevention strategies rely on biomedical technologies such as microbicides or pharmaceuticals (as in PrEP and TasP) that target individuals rather than known determinants of health (e.g., gender or economic inequality). Because they shift the focus to the individual, rather than the social, they are seen as returning to a biomedical rather than social approach: they are "remedicalizing" the epidemic. My point, in line with others in this volume and elsewhere, is that the "social" in many African contexts is not the same "social" as in countries where a robust fabric of social connectedness has been woven through state action: fiscal policy, social programs, and so on. (Once again, this is not to say that there is not a "social" sutured together from kinship relations, school friendships, village connections, communities of worship, and so on; but this is not a "social" that systematically links together strangers' fates through social insurance and that can withstand demands placed on it for health and security when the bulk of the population is economically and biologically precarious.)

So if not medicalization, then what? To answer this question, I propose to marshal three findings from social studies of biomedical research in Africa. The first finding comes from published ethnographies of biomedical research institutions in Africa. It is that biomedical research only "works" in the context of complicated and unstable forms of exchange—for example, blood for access to health care—that in effect enact the figure of a para-state. The second finding comes from historical work that shows how traces of early biomedical experiments persist as traces, embodiments, and material residues. Even after the memory of the experiment has faded, tangible configurations of social organization persist: entire communities woven together around a long-forgotten clinical experiment. This may be another figure, in retrospect, of the para-state. Third, I introduce ethnographic evidence from trials of life-giving antiretroviral drugs in Africa. I then consider an emerging ethnographic field, to which this volume contributes: that of population trials. I consider population trials of TasP to show how these trials cannot be conducted without an infrastructure that allows a population to be mapped, enrolled, and monitored—a para-state of sorts.

Ethnographies of Biomedical Research

Medical research in developing countries necessarily often involves the exchange of blood and bodily substances for medical care. Participants and even researchers have viewed the social relationships that develop and sustain such medical research as a kind of economy, as the following quote obtained by the anthropologists James Fairhead and Melissa Leach shows:

"The Medical Research Council takes blood from healthy people and sells it. . . . When one joins the . . . study, they will take much blood and if you are not lucky the child may die" (Fairhead, Leach, and Small 2006, 1118). Fairhead and Leach were investigating a clinical trial of a vaccine to protect against pneumonia that had been conducted in this poor West African country by the British Medical Research Council (MRC), which has research stations in seven Gambian towns. The MRC has conducted research in the Gambia for over sixty years, and its base in Fajara is an impressive complex that houses a hospital, gleaming laboratories, a computer center, as well as offices, training rooms, and housing. In the course of their study, Fairhead and Leach observed how the research practices of MRC workers intersected with local understandings of blood and vitality—what the authors called an "economy of blood." Their reports echo similar observations reported by other researchers—medical and anthropological—in many other parts of the world. Writing about East Africa, the historian Luise White noted "vampire rumours" that locate Western origin biomedical practices within a broader economy of extraction and exploitation (White 2000). As we shall see shortly, a veritable global economy in blood and body parts does indeed exist, making such rumors even more trenchant.

In the Gambia, what Leach and Fairhead showed however is that these observations are just surface manifestations of a deeper way of life, whereby entire communities have settled into an uneasy coexistence with a research apparatus that gives jobs and economic incentives even as it collects blood, body parts, and snatches of narrative. The MRC complex is dedicated to the study of tropical diseases such as malaria as well as nontropical diseases that are found in the Gambia—most notably HIV. Its base in Fajara is a gleaming icon of modernity in a desperately poor country, complete with the most advanced laboratories and computer technology, the whole secured by a barbed wire fence and top-level security. While the rest of the town is often plunged into darkness because of a tenuous power supply, even in the middle of the night the research complex glows brightly. The MRC complex resembles other research facilities that constitute far-flung outposts of biomedical research run by public health agencies and universities: the American CDC; Canadian, French, and Swiss development agencies; wealthy universities such as Harvard, Columbia, Pennsylvania, and so on. It must be underlined that such research has made, and continues to make, significant progress in understanding diseases of the poor, and that critical ethnographic studies—such as that of Fairhead and Leach—are often embraced by research institutes and agencies whose staff is all too aware of the ethical challenges posed by research in developing countries. Research institutes pass unnoticed in wealthier countries, where the ambient poverty is not as striking; in places like Fajara, however, the contrast can at first glance be unsettling.

Leach and Fairhead were among the first to make use of ethnography to examine the impact of this medical research apparatus on the lives of those with whom it interacts. They interviewed research subjects and field staff of malaria research programs and vaccine trials, as well as those who live in the communities from which research subjects were recruited. The MRC was widely appreciated for the quality of the health care it provided. This was not surprising because the contrast between MRC medicine and local facilities was as starkly visible as that between the brightly lit facility and the surrounding villages. The MRC facility was older than most of those who were interviewed and, in many ways, provided them with more services than did the Gambian government. While the scientists at the center came and went, as did the trials and experiments, the facilities stayed. Only that of the church exceeded the temporal stability of the MRC. Leach and Fairhead describe how "being with MRC" (Fairhead, Leach, and Small 2005) anchored a set of pragmatic calculations by which local people weighed the dangers of participating in the blood economy of the researchers against the benefits that could accrue from letting one's blood be taken and presumably sold to strangers in faraway places.

The anthropologist Paul Wenzel Geissler studied a malaria vaccine trial conducted by the MRC in the Gambia. In this trial, field staff was drawn from the same communities from which research subjects—called "volunteers" in this experiment—were recruited. Two aspects of the trial stood out in the minds of those associated with the trial: the requirement to carry out regular blood drawing to check for malarial parasites, and the provision of free medical care to all the "volunteers." Moreover, "if the volunteer was young and unmarried, his parents were entitled to share his benefits, whereas if he was married, his wife and children were," a situation where Geissler's informants described the regular provision of blood samples as "a high but necessary price for family health care," with the result that "the exchange of blood specimens and medicines was the defining feature of research" for these "volunteers" (Geissler et al. 2008, 699).

Research staff referred to research subjects as "brothers" or "sisters" to express the sense of relatedness that grew during the two-year-long study, constituting what Geissler called a "trial community." This idiom of kinship ended up being crucial to the trial's remarkable success at recruiting, and retaining, research subjects. Geissler notes that "staff and villagers . . . underlined this kinship to underscore that no harmful or selfish intentions could enter the trial community, e.g., to counter the suspicion that the MRC represented Europeans' interests" (Geissler et al. 2008, 701). Staff were able to draw on the metaphor of kinship to reassure villagers they could be trusted and, by extension, the foreign researchers with whom the staff worked. Kinship also played an important role in deciding how to allocate health care, a complicated process that highlights the unstable forms of exchange engendered through trial communities:

> Because the biogenetic rules of entitlement mixed kinship and economic transactions in ways that did not always coincide with villagers' lives and understandings of kinship, fieldworkers found it difficult to apply them. Distributing medicines broadly, irrespective of the sick people's link to the trial, quickly exhausted scarce resources; yet, limiting benefits to active volunteers caused conflicts with the communities. Fieldworkers had to balance their diverging responsibilities towards the people they lived with and the trial management. They took decisions in face-to-face interactions, responding to particular requests rather than realizing formal prescriptions, and variously made and erased boundaries and emphasized or ignored connections in more fluid ways than the rules of health care entitlement, even after their field-based adaptations, foresaw. (Geissler et al. 2008, 702)

These ethnographic studies point to another paradox associated with this kind of human experimentation. While the authority of the evidence that accrues from clinical trials derives from procedures to ensure "objectivity" (such as randomization and blinding researchers to the results for the course of the trial), creating such conditions is not possible without a tissue of social ties, reciprocal obligations, and material and symbolic exchanges already in place. Two apparently irreconcilable moral economies intersect during such trials: that of science and the objectivity that it prizes and those of "trial communities" that bind both commodified and noncommodified forms of exchange (see also Geissler and Molyneux 2011).

For many people, such as poor Gambians, the existence of ethical differences from the standards of medical research conducted in the West in local research protocols is the lesser of two evils—the choice is no medical care at all or medical care that comes from participating in a clinical trial. Neither altruistic nor brute exploitation, these trials are simply another form of exchange between the powerful, their intermediaries, and the powerless. The anthropologist Kris Peterson argues that ethical practice requires recognition that trials may have important social consequences that transform the lives of both research subjects and those around them, and that researchers should act accordingly. But such consequences are often "misrecognized" because they occur long after the trial has ended and outside the frame within which the research is conducted.

The Gambian example shows that the global apparatus of biomedical research, particularly clinical trials and other experiments that enroll populations, relies on highly localized and unstable forms of exchange. These enable an economy of the gifting of blood specimens necessary for the production of evidence. The social relations reworked through this economy of research nonetheless persist after experiments end. Importantly these social relations condition access to biomedical care and other resources that may in fact produce biological differences between those they enfold and those they exclude. The MRC and other medical research organizations are now heavily involved in trialing and rolling NPTs. Will the unstable forms of exchange and working misunderstandings needed to make these trials work provide a beachhead for more enduring social relations? And in so doing, will they enact a formation akin to the para-state that is the subject of this volume? Let us now examine these propositions by turning to an example that affords the historical hindsight not yet afforded by these ethnographic studies of the MRC.

In the 1920s a leper colony was established by the French colonial physician Emil Marchoux on the outskirts of Bamako in the colony of French West Africa. Marchoux was a Pasteurian, having trained in the emerging science of microbiology at the Institut Pasteur of Indochina. Subsequently, he was charged with founding the first African microbiology laboratory in Saint-Louis, in what is today Senegal. His interests eventually turned to leprosy and he founded the Institut Central de la Lèpre some twenty kilometers from Bamako, capital of the French Sudan. Marchoux was a humanist and did not seek to control the ravages of leprosy by forcibly rounding up and quarantining lepers. Rather, he sought to attract lepers to the *lazaret*, as leper colonies were called, with the promise of humane treatment. Marchoux's approach was a successful one, drawing in many who had been ostracized from their communities. However, treatment at the time was largely ineffective, and those who flocked to the institute for relief became a willing group of experimental subjects when the institute's scientists tried out new treatments in a quest for a cure for the stigmatized disease. The leprosarium was renamed the Institut Marchoux in 1935 and continued to experiment with new agents. The historian Eric Silla has chronicled how a community of lepers and their families grew up around the institute, when patients intermarried and settled around the grounds of the facility. Gradually this community became the small town of Djikoroni, which has since been swallowed up by sprawling Bamako, becoming one neighborhood among many in the city, but distinguished by this particular biomedical history (Silla 1998).

HIV Research on African Terrains

Seventy years later in the same part of West Africa, in the mid 1990s, two large clinical trials of AZT for the prevention of mother to child transmission of HIV were carried out, one sponsored by the French National AIDS Research Agency (ANRS) and the other by the rival American CDC. Even though these trials were placebo controlled, they did not attract the same scrutiny as the Ugandan trial, probably because they took place in French-speaking countries. The French study tested 14,385 women in Bobo-Dioulasso (Burkina Faso) and Abidjan, while the U.S. study tested 12,668 women in Abidjan. All the women received state-of-the-art pretest counseling in connection with HIV. Of the total of over 27,000 women tested, 3,424 were found to be positive. However, in the U.S. study 618 HIV positive women never returned for their results and the post-test counseling; in the French study the figure was 648. Researchers told me that the rate of dropout was lower in HIV negative women, suggesting that women suspected their diagnosis and decided not to return for results. Of the HIV positive women who returned for their results, only 711 were included in the actual trials; the remaining 1,447 women were either excluded for reasons described below or simply did not consent (Dabis et al. 1999; Wiktor et al. 1999).

The trials had an enormous impact in shaping the early response by the local population to the epidemic simply because of the sheer number tested at a time when HIV testing was not routinely offered elsewhere. Based on my fieldwork with HIV prevention and care programs in both countries in the mid-1990s, the majority of people who knew their HIV status had found this out by having been recruited into the trials. Of course, only a small minority of women were actually enrolled in the trials, although a very large number had been screened in order to ensure a significant pool from which to enroll a necessarily smaller number of selected, eligible study subjects. There were numerous reasons that disqualified women, most usually not presenting themselves early enough in pregnancy to receive AZT or suffering from anemia, which could be dangerously worsened if they received AZT. Women who had tested positive but were not eligible to enroll in the trials complained bitterly that they had been "discarded." They resented the lack of access to what they perceived to be a panoply of services for women who had been included in the trials, and therefore had been randomized to receive either placebo or AZT.

Indeed, the women who were included in the trial did receive medical care and social services that were not available to others. After having been tested, many of them found their way into community groups in search of material and social support; some even set up organizations for their fellow would-be trial subjects. The ethical requirements that informed the "inclusion criteria" that determined who was accepted into the trial generated a perception of injustice that ironically laid the groundwork for a shared solidarity that, over time, would resurface when women enrolled in the trials were prioritized to receive antiretroviral drugs in the French government's first HIV treatment program. Nonetheless, over time, as drug access broadened and health returned to the women, the groups that grew out of the trial flourished. Some of the widows remarried, and many of the younger women went on to find husbands—some of whom they met in the groups—and to have children. Like the Bamako leper colony that became a village that later on would blend into an expanding city, these clinical trials spawned community groups whose members' access to treatment has kept illness at bay, attenuating many of the differences that set them apart from the expanding cities in which they now go about their everyday lives unnoticed.

Testing Treatment as Prevention in Populations

What will be the social impact of experiments with TasP? The ethnography of clinical trials in Africa show how the moral economies of clinical trials, and the unstable forms of exchange they generate, pattern social relations. The historical example of the leprosarium suggests that these relations can endure as traces long after the experiment is forgotten. When we turn to HIV trials in West Africa, we see again how these experiments produce new forms of subjectivity, trigger unstable forms of exchange, and generate novel social forms. Rather than medicalization, perhaps we should speak about the production of a kind of social or even an "experimental society." The state is the absent counterpart to this sociality; perhaps then it might be better to explore how a para-state (taking the form of the MRC, CDC, or Harvard University) tills the soil left fallow by existing states, and how the social forms that emerge reflect back another para-state.

TasP appears as a potentially powerful generator of the para-state because it shifts the paradigm from the clinical trials described above. This is because TasP will be tested on entire populations, rather than individuals drawn from those populations. *Cluster randomization* refers to experiments that require randomization and comparison of *groups* of people rather than *individuals*; they are as a result also known as cluster randomized trials, group randomized trials, or place randomized trials. Cluster randomized trials in Africa are central to the genesis and future of TasP. This strategy entails mass population screening and treatment of all those who are found to be HIV positive. Importantly, this is being done in settings where the functions of mapping and describing populations are not carried out by the state. Rather, private organizations are charged with surveying and intervening.

It is in South Africa that the first population-based trial of TasP is scheduled to begin. The trial involves comparing HIV incidence rates in communities chosen randomly to either receive a TasP intervention or not. The TasP intervention involves aggressive measures to test and treat all those found to be HIV positive in the selected communities, in order to achieve sufficient ARV coverage rates to be able to impact transmission and, therefore, HIV incidence. The trial is conducted in a rural part of KwaZula Natal that was formerly a Bantustan, where a considerable research infrastructure exists that notably has used modern demographic surveillance techniques, including GPS, to comprehensively map the entire population and gather reams of data on demographic and behavioral aspects of individuals there.

My point here is not to criticize this important trial on ethical grounds, although that is certainly a relevant issue. It is rather to think about what would happen should the trial prove the intervention effective in reducing HIV incidence, as is its goal. It is reasonable to think that the intervention's effectiveness is as much due to the quasi-military organization of the intervention strategy (systematic surveillance and testing of the population) as the actual ingestion of drugs by bodies. The implication is that, to "generalize" the findings of the trial to the "real world," it will be necessary in fact to make the world correspond to the laboratory of the trial. We are back to Latour's classic reading of Pasteur. Test-and-treat, as it is now called, is a Pasteurian strategy par excellence. Give me a laboratory, and I will raise the world (Latour 1988; see also Dozon 1991, for a historical view on Pasteurians in French Africa).

The metaphor of the laboratory has been used to underline how the colonial period gave birth to forms of experimentation—intentional or not (e.g., Tilley 2011; Lachenal 2010). The notion of the laboratory can be used to point to ruptures and continuities with the colonial past. Although this could be a useful exercise, that is not my point here. As Nikola Bagic (2012) has pointed out, the use of the laboratory in anthropology and indeed historiography has been more metaphoric, with slightly pejorative undertones. I take inspiration from Bagic to extend the notion of the laboratory from metaphor to analytic concept. Bagic cites a recent paper by Michael Guggenheim that draws on sociological studies of science and experimentation to define the laboratory as

> the result of a procedure that separates between an outside, an environment that is considered negligible for some epistemic claim or technological invention, and an inside, a (partly) controlled environment that is considered relevant for this claim or invention. The lab is not so much a closed space, but a procedure that often results in a space with the properties to separate controlled inside from uncontrolled outside. Control means not necessarily physical control but a procedure whereby data and objects are managed to behave in a way the scientist wishes. The separation between inside and outside allows for the two central features of the lab, placelessness and consequence-free research. (Guggenheim 2012, 101)

Guggenheim's definition points to how the cluster-randomized controlled trials imagine the population as a laboratory. Of course, a population is not a laboratory in the common sense we imagine of a gleaming, tiled room with shiny machines. But in the sense of Guggenheim's definition, cluster randomized trials are procedures that group populations into clusters and allow the data emitted to be managed so as to generate meaningful comparisons between clusters or groups within the trial. The results may then be applied to the populations outside the trial. Yet ethnographic findings from the present-day Burkina Faso, the Gambia, or colonial Mali, presented above suggest that the experiment is not a closed space, that it leaks people, practices, and commodities. This is perhaps not surprising, after all we are not talking about a "real" bricks and mortar lab (although sociologists of science and technology would make the same argument about even that kind of lab). But the more salient point is that these leakages remain as fragments and traces, available for reassembly. Recall how trials comprise technologies that enroll bodies, complicate moral economies, and network exchange. These elements display a degree of autonomy where there is not a robust state to provide health services, ensure social security, and regulate human relationships. What is reassembled is therefore more than just another experiment; it is a complex of social relations, what we can refer to as a kind of para-state.

In the face of an intractable public health problem (HIV, in this case), our post-ideological, evidence-based age increasingly demands interventions be "trialed" on subject populations and proven before applied. This may seem innocuous, or even a welcome development, until the following points are considered. First, only certain kinds of interventions may be evaluated in this manner, with the result that other—largely more complex—forms of intervention are neglected. Second, the technology of the clinical trial—whose scope is now expanding to include development economics, for instance—is hardly a neutral one. New prevention technologies are particularly amenable to large-scale population trials: they are simple to implement, and their effect is equally simple to measure. The population trials needed to validate their use differ significantly from the clinical trials we have discussed because they enroll entire populations.

The globalization of the clinical trial has been chronicled by anthropologists such as Adriana Petryna and Robert Abadie, who have pointed to the (predictably) "dark underside" of human experiments. My point here is not to reiterate these critiques but to underscore how the multisited clinical trial has in fact escaped the confines of pharmaceutical research to become a globalized biosocial form. The work we have examined above shows how these trials become an important site of mediation between a global biopolitical apparatus and local ways of life. I would argue that this site is more than just an intersection where two different social worlds collide: it is an "interzone," a borderland where social forms and moral economies bleed across borders and entangle with unanticipated consequences. The population-laboratory can never be truly dismantled, living on long after the experiment as traces in bodies and as an unseen armature of social relations: an experimental society (Kachur 2010). I would define an *experimental society* as the social relations that span trial populations and expand and mutate beyond the original experiments that gave birth to them, at times recombining into forms no longer recognizable in terms of the goals of the original research. At this point, let me conjugate this hypothesis further, while apologizing for the speculative nature of my writings henceforth.

From Trial Communities to Experimental Societies

We have seen how globalized efforts to produce biomedical knowledge have a number of unforeseen consequences. The first is that biomedical experiments—clinical trials, cohort studies, or population trials—produce unintended and unique forms of social relations. These forms of sociality are particularly salient in settings where they are directly linked to individual and collective vitality, notably in settings where nonexistent public health infrastructure and poverty means that participating in research becomes a survival strategy. The anthropologist Paul Rabinow first proposed the idea of "biosociality"—new forms of social relations organized on the basis of biological conditions or common genetic makeup—over a decade ago. Today, we see a kind of research-driven sociality as people gather together with the intent to participate in clinical trials. The consequences of such forms of sociality will be a crucial field site for future medical anthropological investigation, particularly with a view to capturing the biosocial differentiation of those who are included and those who are excluded from clinical research.

Elsewhere I have argued that the response to the HIV epidemic has resulted in the humanitarian assemblage of populations that, in turn, materialize a global biopolitical laboratory that allows a full range of novel technologies (ranging from highly individualized biomedical interventions to policies to juridical systems) to be trialed (Nguyen 2009). This allows these technologies to be redeployed and their effects reproduced. The conjugation of this biopolitical "machine for producing the future" with a closed epistemological loop is what I called *experimentality*. This of course draws on Foucault's notion of *governmentality*, which refers to the proliferation of mechanisms, or technologies, that individuals take up to govern their biological existence. I use the term *experimentality* to advance the hypothesis that the experiment has become a new biopolitical form. More specifically, that the clinical trial has become a technology of rule, a method by which individuals come to constitute themselves as subject to government.

Experimentality constitutes a curious inversion of the orthodox model of scientific discovery and knowledge transfer, whereby evidence of efficacy permits intervention. In contrast, the urgency of intervention drives the need for self-validating evidence (i.e., that the intervention was effective). The conjugation of these standardized humanitarian problems and populations with the production of post-facto, self-validating knowledge (most often described as "lessons learned" or "best practices") leverages the deployment of these interventions across the globe. The old epidemiological problem of "generalizability" refers to the "gap" that makes it difficult to translate clinical trials results into real-world results. My hypothesis here is that the deployment of clinical trial–validated interventions—such as male circumcision—will drive downstream efforts to bridging the gap. More specifically, the deployment of evidence validated in clinical trials necessarily leads to the dissemination of social relations that seek to reproduce the conditions of the trial.

In her well-known book *The Shock Doctrine*, Naomi Klein argues that neoliberal capitalism takes advantage of—or even provokes—disasters in order to administer the "shock therapy" of neoliberalism. Kris Peterson (2012) has made a similar, though more subtle and ethnographically researched argument in her consideration of how the AIDS "disaster" leveraged neoliberal market reforms in Nigeria and elsewhere. Peterson's work points to a third hypothesis. In the case of treatment as prevention, the threat of AIDS is being used to promote a preventive intervention that leverages highly coercive measures that include a remarkably intimate degree of surveillance. TasP mobilizes highly individualized technologies of adherence and monitoring, launched from the platform of mass HIV treatment programs, to deploy them to entire "at risk" populations.[6] It thus furnishes a model for how global health programs may be able to use current disease-specific programs to launch population-wide forms of biopolitical regulation and surveillance.

These then are three possible post-experimental para-states. Drawing on the existing ethnographies and histories of medical research in African terrains, we find the residue of long-finished experiments that persist in expectations of biotherapeutic (that is, blood for care) exchange such as those documented by Fairhead, Leach, and Geissler, or in the traces of a long-forgotten leprosarium in Bamako. This is the para-state sedimented from unstable forms of exchange that happen in a moral economy without a future. Or we might ponder the para-state that emerges, cobbled together by NGOs, philanthropies, national governments, and therapeutic entrepreneurs to bend the "real world" to conform to expected results. This is a para-state that results from the authorizing center of evidence-based medicine, driven by results generated in population trials. Finally, we might worry that the para-state is no accident. Rather, it is the intentional consequence of a drive to shape the world according to an inexorable logic of disciplining unruly populations and strengthening surveillance. Whatever the case, we might worry that the para-state is here to stay and consider that it may even be the shape of the state to come.

Notes

1 It was the conference in 2000, held in Durban, that put Africa on the map for many AIDS researchers who had, despite the fact that the continent bears the brunt of the global burden of the disease, until then largely ignored it.

2 A solution, to which we will turn shortly, is the *population* randomized trial — but such trials raise other issues, as we shall see.

3 The Granich (2009) mathematical modeling study assumed 90 percent treatment rates to reduce incidence sufficiently to lead to HIV eradication; in the United States this rate is 28 percent (Garnett, Becker, and Bertozze 2012, 159).

4 A review of this concept, which has been a central theme of medical anthropology and sociology, is beyond the scope of our discussion. For a recent review, please see Clarke and Shim (2011).

5 This is in fact the central tenet of classical sociology, as founded by Émil Durkheim. For two succinct and more contemporary formulations, see Éwald (1986) and Wittrock (2000).

6 I was recently at a meeting in Amsterdam where this was made abundantly clear in presentations of ramped-up treatment programs in a number of African countries. Smart cards and databases had been developed to track patients' adherence to treatment as well as clinical outcomes.

References

Abdool-Karim, Q., et al. 2010. "Effectiveness and Safety of Tenofovir Gel, an Anti-retroviral Microbicide, for the Prevention of HIV Infection in Women." *Science* 329, no. 5996: 1168–74.

Abraham, J. 2010. "Pharmaceuticalization of Society in Context: Theoretrical, Empirical and Health Dimensions." *Sociology* 44: 603–22.

Aggleton, P. 2007. "'Just a Snip?' A Social History of Male Circumcision." *Reproductive Health Matters* 15, no. 29: 15–21.

Bagic, N. Unpublished. Towards a critique of the colonial laboratory. Universität Zürich.

Bayart, J. F. 2006. *L'État en Afrique: La politique du ventre*. Paris: Fayard.

Beyrer, Chris, A. Wirtz, S. Baral, A. Peryskina, and F. Sifakis. 2010. "Epidemiologic Links between Drug Use and HIV Epidemics: An International Perspective." *Journal of Acquired Immune Deficiency Syndromes* 55: S10–S16.

Biehl, J. 2005. *Vita: Life in a Zone of Abandonment*. Berkeley: University of California Press.

Biehl, J. 2007. "Pharmaceuticalization: AIDS Treatment and Global Health Politics." *Anthropological Quarterly* 80, no. 4: 1083–126.

Booth, K. M. 2010. "A Magic Bullet for the 'African' Mother? Neo-imperial Reproductive Futurism and the Pharmaceutical 'Solution' to the HIV/AIDS Crisis." *Social Politics* 17, no. 3: 349–78.

Cambiano, V., A. J. Rodger, and A. N. Phillips. 2010. "'Test-and-treat': The End of the HIV Epidemic?" *Current Opinion in Infectious Diseases* 24: 19–26.

Clarke, A. E., and J. Shim. 2011. "Medicalization and Biomedicalization Revisited: Technoscience and Transformations of Health, Illness and American Medicine." In *Handbook of the Sociology of Health, Illness, and Healing: A Blueprint for the 21st Century*, edited by B. A. Pescosolido et al., 173–99, DOI: 10.1007/978-1-4419-7261-3_10.

Cohen, M. S. 2010. "ART and HIV: Treatment as Prevention." Eighteenth International AIDS Conference, Vienna, Austria.

Connolly, M. 2008. *Fatal Misconception: The Struggle to Control World Population*. Cambridge, MA: Harvard University Press.

Connor, E. M., R. S. Sperling, R. Gelber et al. 1994. "Reduction of Maternal-Infant Transmission of Human Immunodeficiency Virus Type 1 with Zidovudine Treatment: Pediatric AIDS Clinical Trials Group Protocol 076 Study Group." *New England Journal of Medicine* 331, no. 18: 1173–80. DOI:10.1056/NEJM199411033311801. PMID 7935654.

Dabis, François, Philippe Msellati, Nicolas Meda et al. for the DITRAME Study Group. 1999. "6-Month Efficacy, Tolerance, and Acceptability of a Short Regimen of Oral Zidovudine to Reduce Vertical Transmission of HIV in Breast-fed Children in Côte-d'Ivoire and Burkina Faso: A Double-Blind Placebo-Controlled Multicentre Trial." *Lancet* 353, no. 6: 786–93.

Dozon, Jean-Pierre. 1991. "D'un tombeau l'autre." *Cahiers d'études africaines* 31, no. 121: 135–57.

Éwald, F. 1986. *L'État Providence*. Paris: Grasset.

Fairhead, J., M. Leach, and M. Small. 2005. "Public Engagement with Science: Local Understandings of a Vaccine Trial in the Gambia." *Journal of Biosocial Science* 38: 103–16.

Fairhead, J., M. Leach, and M. Small. 2006. "Where Techno-Science Meets Poverty: Medical Research and the Economy of Blood in the Gambia, West Africa." *Social Science and Medicine* 63: 1118.

Ferguson, J. 2006. *Global Shadows: Africa in the Neoliberal World Order*. Durham, NC: Duke University Press.

Forsyth, A., and R. O. Valdiserri. 2012. "Reaping the Prevention Benefits of Highly Active Antiretroviral Treatment: Policy Implications of HIV Prevention Trials Network 052." *Current Opinion in HIV Research* 7, no. 2: 111–16.

Garnett, G. P., S. Becker, and S. Bertozzi. 2012. "Treatment as Prevention: Translating Efficacy Trial Results to Population Effectiveness." *Current Opinion in HIV Research* 7: 157–63.

Gawrylewski, A. 2007. "Failure of HIV Microbicide Raises Concerns." *Scientist*, February 21. Accessed March 8, 2012. http://classic.the-scientist.com/news/display/52861/.

Geissler, Paul Wenzel, and C. Molyneux. 2011. *Evidence, Ethos and Experiment: The Anthropology and History of Medical Research in Africa*. London: Berghahn.

Geissler, Paul Wenzel, A. Kelly, B. Imoukhuede, and R. Pool. 2008. "'He Is Now Like a Brother, I Can Even Give Him Some Blood'—Relation Ethics and Material Exchanges in a Malaria Vaccine 'Trial Community' in the Gambia." *Social Science and Medicine* 67: 696–707.

Granich, R. M., et al. 2011. "ART in Prevention of HIV and TB: Update on Current Research Efforts." *Current HIV Research* 9, no. 6: 446–69.

Granich, R. M., C. F. Gilks, C. Dye, K. M. De Cock, and B. G. Williams. 2009. "Universal Voluntary HIV Testing with Immediate Antiretroviral Therapy as a Strategy for Elimination of HIV Transmission: A Mathematical Model." *Lancet* 373, no. 9657: 48–57.

Guggenheim, Michael. 2012. "Laboratizing and De-laboratizing the World: Changing Sociological Concepts for Places of Knowledge Production." *History of the Human Sciences* 25, no. 1: 99–118.

Hardon, A. 2012. "The Turn to Female Controlled Safe Sex Technologies." In *Technologies of Sexuality, Identity and Sexual Health*, edited by L. Manderson, 55–72. London: Routledge.

Karim, S. A. 2010. "Understanding HIV Transmission Mechanisms: Microbicides and PrEP." Eighteenth International AIDS Conference. Vienna, Austria.

Lachenal, Guillaume. 2010. "Le médecin qui voulut être roi: Médecine coloniale et utopie au Cameroun." *Annales, Histoire, Sciences Sociales* 65, no. 1: 121–56.

Lange, J. M. A. 2005. "We Must Not Let Protestors Derail Trials of Pre-Exposure Prophylaxis for HIV." *PLoS Med* 2, no. 9: e248. DOI:10.1371/journal.pmed.0020248.

Latour, Bruno. 1988. *The Pasteurization of France*. Cambridge, MA: Harvard University Press.

Mbembe, A. 2001. *On the Postcolony*. Berkeley: University of California Press.

Mbembe, A. 2003. "Necropolitics." *Public Culture* 15, no. 1: 11–40.

Merson, M. H., J. O'Malley, D. Serwadda, and C. Apisuk. 2008. "The History and Challenge of HIV Prevention." *Lancet* 372, no. 9637: 475–88.

Montaner, J. S. G., V. D. Lima, R. Barrios et al. 2010. "Association of Highly Active Antiretroviral Therapy Coverage, Population Viral Load, and Yearly New HIV Diagnoses in British Columbia, Canada: A Population-Based Study." *Lancet* 376: 532–39.

Montaner, J. S. G., R. Hogg, E. Wood et al. 2006. "The Case for Expanding Access to Highly Active Antiretroviral Therapy to Curb the Growth of the HIV Epidemic." *Lancet* 368, no. 9534: 531–36.

Nguyen V.-K. 2009. "Government-by-Exception: Enrollment and Experimentality in Mass HIV Treatment Programs in Africa." *Social Theory and Health* 7, no. 3: 196–222.

Nguyen, V.-K., N. Bajos, F. Dubois-Arber, J. O'Malley, and C. M. Pirkle. 2011. "Remedicalising an Epidemic: From HIV Treatment as Prevention to HIV Treatment Is Prevention." *AIDS* 25, no. 3: 291–93.

Padian, N. S., S. I. McCoy, S. S. Abdool Karim et al. 2011. "HIV Prevention Transformed: The New Prevention Research Agenda." *Lancet* 378: 269–78.

Peterson, K. 2012. "AIDS Policies for Markets and Warriors: Dispossession, Capital, and Pharmaceuticals in Nigeria." In *Lively Capital: Biotechnologies, Ethics and Governance in Global Markets*, edited by Kaushik Sunder Rajan. Durham, NC: Duke University Press.

Quinn, T. C., M. J. Wawer, N. Sewankambo et al. 2000. "Viral Load and Heterosexual Transmission of Human Immunodeficiency Virus Type 1: Rakai Project Study Group." *New England Journal of Medicine* 342, no. 13: 921–29.

Quiñones-Mateu, M., and G. Vanham. 2012. "HIV Microbicides: Where Are We Now?" *Current HIV Research* 10: 1–2.

Rabinow, Paul. 1992. "Artificiality and Enlightenment: From Sociobiology to Biosociality." In *Incorporations*, edited by Jonathan Crary and Sanford Kwiner, 234–52. New York: Zone Books.

Rosengarten, Marsha, Mike Michael, Eric Mykhalovskiy, and J. Imrie. 2008. "The Challenges of Technological Innovation in HIV." *Lancet* 372, no. 9636: 357–58.

Seidel, Gill. 1993. "The Competing Discourses of HIV/AIDS in Sub-Saharan Africa: Discourses of Rights and Empowerment vs. Discourses of Control and Exclusion." *Social Science and Medicine* 36, no. 3: 175.

Silla, E. 1998. *People Are Not the Same: Leprosy and Identity in Twentieth-Century Mali*. London: Heineman.

Singh, J. A., and E. J. Mills. 2005. "The Abandoned Trials of Pre-Exposure Prophylaxis for HIV: What Went Wrong?" *PLoS Medicine* 2, no. 9: e234.

Tilley, H. 2011. *Africa as a Living Laboratory: Empire, Development, and the Problem of Scientific Knowledge, 1870–1950*. Cambridge: Cambridge University Press.

Tsai, C. C., et al. 1995. "Prevention of SIV Infection in Macaques by (R)-9-(2-phosphonylmethoxyproyl)adenine." *Science* 270, no. 5239: 1197–99.

Van Damme, Lut, Gita Ramjee, Michel Alary et al. 2002. "Effectiveness of COL-1492, a Nonoxynol-9 Vaginal Gel, on HIV-1 Transmission in Female Sex Workers: A Randomised Controlled Trial." *Lancet* 360, no. 9338: 971–77.

Velasco-Hernandez, J. X., H. B. Gershengorn, and S. M. Blower. 2002. "Could Widespread Use of Combination Antiretroviral Therapy Eradicate HIV Epidemics?" *Lancet Infectious Diseases* 2: 487–93.

Vernazza, P., et al. 2008. "Les personnes séropositives ne souffrant d'aucune autre

MST et suivant un traitement antirétroviral efficace ne transmettent pas le VIH par voie sexuelle." *Bulletin des médecins suisses* 89, no. 5. English translation, including translator's affidavit, available at http://tinyurl.com/cpyt5n.

Wendland, Claire L. 2008. "Research, Therapy, and Bioethical Hegemony: The Controversy over Perinatal AZT Trials in Africa." *African Studies Review* 51, no. 3: 1–23.

White, L. 2000. *Speaking with Vampires: Rumor and History in Colonial Africa*. Berkeley: University of California Press.

WHO. 2007. *New Data on Male Circumcision for HIV Prevention: Policy and Programme Implications*. Geneva: World Health Organization. http://www.who.int/hiv/pub/malecircumcision/research_implications/en/index.html.

WHO. 2011. *The Treatment 2.0 Framework for Action: Catalysing the Next Phase of Treatment, Care and Support*. Geneva: World Health Organization.

Whyte, S., S. Van der Geest, and A. Hardon. 2003. *Social Lives of Medicines*. Cambridge: Cambridge University Press.

Wiktor, S. Z., I. Ikpini, J. M. Karon, J. Nkengason, C. Maurice, S. T. Severin, T. H. Roels et al. 1999. "Short-Course Oral Zidovudine for Prevention of Mother-to-Child Transmission of HIV-1 in Abidjan, Côte-d'Ivoire: A Randomised Trial." *Lancet* 35, no. 6: 781–85.

Wittrock, Björn. 2000. "Modernity: One, None or Many? Europeans' Origins and Modernity as a Global Condition." *Daedalus* 129, no. 1: 31–60.

CHAPTER 2

Trialing Drugs, Creating Publics:

Medical Research, Leprosy Control,

and the Construction of a Public Health

Sphere in Post-1945 Nigeria

John Manton

Visiting Uzuakoli, 2006

Between 1948 and 1967, the Leprosy Research Unit for Nigeria was stationed at the leprosy hospital and one-time colony at Uzuakoli, and some of the most important research on the chemotherapy of leprosy was carried out there, beginning with the standardization of dapsone in 1949 through 1951 and concluding with the trials of clofazimine in 1961 through 1966. The safe dose for dapsone was determined here, marking the first reliable treatment for leprosy. Clofazimine, a compound initially formulated in a university-sector research lab in Ireland and developed and refined by Geigy in Switzerland, was trialed at Uzuakoli as a treatment for complications and reactions in leprosy, and it was shown markedly to reduce the incidence and severity of some of the more disabling aspects of the human immune response to the disease. These were among the most significant advances in medicine to have taken place in Nigeria at the time, and though they were published by non-Nigerian scientists, the contribution of Nigerian lab workers, technicians, health professionals, and patients was critical to the whole enterprise. It stood to reason that the patient records at Uzuakoli would therefore comprise one of the most significant archives of medical work in Nigeria, but I doubted their existence, as I had been told that the hospital was largely destroyed during the Nigerian Civil War. I couldn't be certain until I went to see for myself.

On arrival, we went first to the medical department, where the patient records were generated, used, and stored. I asked to meet some people whose names I had been given and did my best to explain what I was looking for. The notion that anyone would be interested in closed files, useless records, defunct material elicited the usual mixture of incomprehension and disdain, and, as regularly happened, I was shown some recently closed files from the mid-1980s—the coming of multidrug therapy (MDT) for leprosy in the early 1980s is the absolute horizon for even the most historically minded leprosy control officer currently working. Another angle of attack was clearly needed. I crossed to the ostensibly more active and better-appointed welfare department and was introduced to the current director. He was very pleased to have a visitor and to hear of my project. He told me of the hospital's ongoing rehabilitation and resettlement program, which had returned four long-term residents to their communities of origin the Sunday before my visit, complete with housing, the sensitization and support of their compatriots, and the means for their own support (mostly in the form of garri mills for the processing of cassava, which they could use to offer a service to their neighbors).

We spoke of Ikoli Harcourt Whyte, a prominent "inmate" and patient organizer at Uzuakoli who had become an important composer of church and Christian music. The hospital was making plans to celebrate the thirtieth anniversary of his death later in 2006 with the opening of a music school, to go with the computer center (now up and running, with the assistance of UK Volunteer Service Overseas [VSO]), palm-oil mill, and piggery, all of which I toured en route to the camps where the permanent residents lived. We passed a water pump, where I was told that the entire complex had no running water, and all water used across the hospital had to be hand pumped from this one well. This was to be the first of many alarming notes sounded about the running of the hospital over the course of a long day of revelations and surprises.

This alarm was soon to be made aggressively manifest back at the medical department. I returned there with the welfare director and his associate, also with an American missionary we had encountered while touring the hospital, and the German Leprosy Relief Association (GLRA) welfare officer, who was currently inspecting work at Uzuakoli. I had met the woman from the GLRA in November 2000, and she felt sure that she could get the records staff to find something for me. She asked the same questions I had and found that all of the old records were in a building to the rear, but the key had been lost. She suggested they break into it, and a man and a woman went off to see what they could do. Before I had managed to figure out what was going on, they came back with a small bundle of old files, which they lay down on the table and began to examine. They appeared relatively intact.

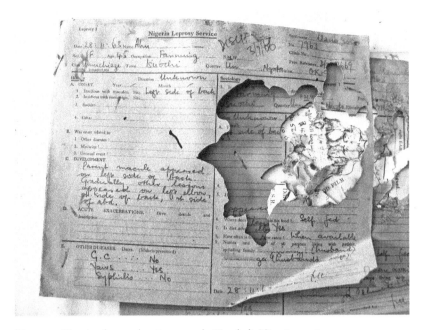

Figure 2.1. Termite-damaged patient records, Uzuakoli, Nigeria, 2006.
Photograph by author.

"1961," the woman announced, and passed a file over to me to have a look. "Clofazimine," I thought, and turned the first page. I saw first the network of holes, whose startling extent became apparent as I turned page after page, gaping, shedding dirt, and termites onto the table and floor. My heart sank. File after file was passed to me. The files for 1954, 1965, and 1973 were all in the same condition. I asked to see where they had found the files. I was led around the back of the building in question, to a broken window, where a bunch of files sat exposed to the elements. I climbed through the narrow gap, inside, where stacks of records were heaped along a wall under two open windows, a haul stretching back to the 1940s if not further. Each bound bundle I examined was hollowed out by termites, stuck together at the corners, in such a parlous and fragile state that I dared not disturb them. Bundles began to crumble to the touch. I stood back, scared to breathe.

The patients at Uzuakoli had fled the advancing front of the civil war between Nigerian Federal Forces and the Biafran Army sometime toward the end of 1967 or early 1968. Whether the records had remained at the hospital or travelled with a conscientious member of staff, they had certainly survived the Nigerian Civil War, one of the most vicious conflicts in modern

Africa. Many patients survived and had returned to Uzuakoli by 1971, where some semblance of care seems to have been resumed. Thirty-five years later, visited by the depredations of successive civilian and military governments, the continual degradation of hospital and staff conditions, and the deprioritization of almost all of a state's specific welfare responsibilities for its citizens, histories and memories that survived a catastrophic war had been eviscerated by the mundane action of accumulated neglect.

The integrity of records provides only the weakest register of this malaise—the historian's particular sensitivity to this register is cold and inhumane if it cannot respond to and illuminate the appalling corrosion of social provision that accompanies the action of termites on the human past. Alongside a hard-working welfare department sat a largely nonfunctioning hospital. The management of the hospital was in dispute between the church and the government, with the government hesitant about implementing its hand-over plan. Patients cured of leprosy, clamoring to return home, were stuck in Uzuakoli because they couldn't receive treatment for open ulcers.

The fate of former "dreams of modernity," of state-mandated programs in public health, disease control, and related medical research, of attendant bureaucracies, which materialized the bilateral relations between the colonial state—and its immediate successor developmentalist state—and subject populations, are commented on elsewhere in this volume and form a backdrop to contributions on issues of more directly contemporary import. This chapter complements a shared skepticism about the disappearance of the state, in this case querying the centrality of the state, in any of its colonial, developmental, or neoliberal forms, to the prosecution of the totality of medical research taking place within its territorial remit.

It presents a case that prefigures the coarticulation of the humanitarian, the emergency, and the experimental, which Richard Rottenburg has described as a hallmark of postmodern modalities of scientific research in Africa, and yet seems not only to draw on many of the same rhetorical strategies of emergency and experiment visible in more recent humanitarian actions considered by Rottenburg but also presents a surprisingly similar collage of nonstate actors involved in producing and standardizing materia medica and generating research reputations, careers, protocols, and results (Rottenburg 2009, 423–24). In assessing what has disappeared, and what has transformed over the past half-century of medical research in Africa, I suggest that it is configurations and forms such as are indicated in this chapter that need to be recuperated to our narratives.

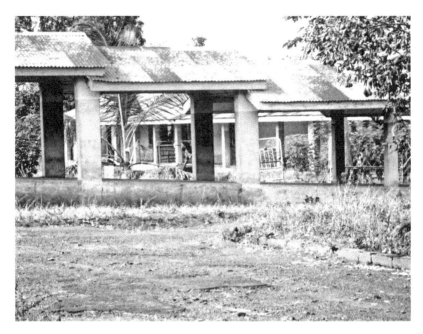

Figure 2.2. Walkway between wards, Oji River, Nigeria, 2006. Photograph by author.

Uzuakoli, Leprology, and the "Developmentalist State," 1962

In 1962 *Leprosy Review* published a report on the use of a new drug for the treatment of leprosy, a compound known as B.663. The clinical trial on which the report was based, carried out with a small number of patients at the Uzuakoli Leprosy Settlement in eastern Nigeria, headlined the process of integrating the Leprosy Research Units at Uzuakoli and in London with the spatially extensive and resource-intensive Nigeria Leprosy Service, founded in response to the exceptionally high prevalence of leprosy in colonial eastern Nigeria and its high profile as a public health problem. Over the preceding fifteen years, drugs tested and standardized at Uzuakoli were circulated in semiformal networks among Nigerian leprosy workers and their patients in exchange for data on the administration and efficacy of new doses, combinations, and compounds.

Practical difficulties in researching leprosy outside the human host and under laboratory or controlled conditions forced the rapid dissemination of emerging drug technologies into areas where leprosy control was among the few existing government services. This took place against the backdrop of an increasing reluctance on the part of public health officials to contemplate the segregation of leprosy patients. This chapter explores transformations in the political economy of health care in Nigeria in the 1950s and 1960s, using as its lens the spatial, social, policy, and technological ramifications of leprosy control and, specifically, the instance of the clinical trial in the context of developing and rapidly differentiating medical services.

The discussion focuses on a portrayal of the ad hoc evolution of a research capacity in eastern Nigeria's leprosy control institutions between the end of the Second World War and the outbreak of the Biafran War in 1967. In doing so, it positions the clinical trial amid constructions of expertise in twentieth-century leprosy control, suggesting avenues toward a political economy of scientific knowledge. It considers the construction of prestige and renown through the means of research and the clinical trial, contrasting the outcomes and presentation of two sets of clinical trials carried out in the early 1950s and early 1960s.

Helen Tilley (2004, 30–32, 38) has noted the relation between scientific responses to epidemic disease and the growth of African medical departments, describing a proliferation of disease ecological niches in close dialogue with particularistic visions of empire held by the various European powers with a stake in early twentieth-century African life. The emphasis on variability and the need for scientific fieldwork in order to stabilize the conditions for the exploitation of colonial human and productive resources were key in the application of the scientific method to problems in African life prior to World War II.

The adaptation of these varied practices to aspects of colonial development and hence of governance is a significant feature of late colonial science and its public presentation, as discerned by Christophe Bonneuil. Bonneuil's vision of a "development regime," which straddles the ends of empire and characterizes the scientific practice of what he terms the "developmentalist state," captures an important dynamic that suffused state-level and nongovernmental planning in science, technology, agronomy, and welfare, as well as encoding the aspirations of Africans, ranging from men and women aspiring to leadership in new late colonial and independent political dispensations to workers, farmers, schoolchildren, and therapy seekers throughout African urban and rural societies (Bonneuil 2000, 259–61, 280–81).

The British Empire in Africa is generally held to have paid minimal heed to the material and welfare needs of the great majority of its African subjects. Similarly, the reliance of British colonial states on Christian missionaries for the rural extension of health services is well attested (Vaughan 1991,

56; Etherington 2005, 283; Hardiman 2006, 5). But while leprosy work was seen as "a field that [the missions had] made peculiarly their own" (Phillipson 1949, 34), the emerging architectonics of scientific publication and correspondence in leprosy control, epitomized in the sequence of International Leprosy Congresses, the proliferation of journals in the field—notably *Leprosy Review* and the *International Journal of Leprosy*—and consistent correspondence on leprosy in mainstream medical journals brought leprosy control work more in line with the forms of scientific fieldwork described by Tilley.

By the mid-twentieth century this field of inquiry, characterized by the scientific and bureaucratic practice of leprosy control, had become known as *leprology* and was anchored by the figure of the *leprologist*. The leprologist was at once a noble paramount of the medical mission, and a combination of scientist, researcher, public health planner, and colonial administrator. He or she harried district officers, badgered pharmaceutical and medical ordnance firms, entreated with customs officials, wrote for and to medical journals, religious papers, and the popular press, made films and took photos, and circulated among an international professional coterie.

A would-be social engineer and welfare evangelist, the autonomy of the leprologist was constrained by material poverty, resource shortages, administrative deficits, and community unconcern or skepticism. In significant ways, notably through the troubled legal and moral discourse on segregation of leprosy patients, the epidemiological terrain and the minutiae of social interaction in medical institutional settings produced both leprology and leprologists. This process was at its most intense in the period from the late 1930s through the mid-1960s, when the classification of leprosy was subject to constant revision in dialogue with new data emerging from clinician-supervised leprosaria across the colonial and developing world.

The unusual heritage of the leprologist ensured that the new resonance between leprosy control and imperial field sciences was not an unproblematic convergence. As the outlines of the "developmentalist state" began to take shape in the forge of late colonial Africa, the continent's public health problems came into clearer view. In post-1945 leprosy control, global allegiances based on support for research and treatment yoked together colonial and national governments, missionary foundations and institutions, leprosy charities and research organizations such as the British Empire Leprosy Relief Association (BELRA), postwar NGOs such as Oxfam, and global health and welfare agencies such as WHO and UNICEF. While greater resources were focused on leprosy control than ever before in the history of human-kind's relationship with the disease, the relationships and pressures emerging around research and treatment were often at odds with long-standing clinical emphases on local forms and expressions of the disease. The ability of individual leprologists to manage clinical, therapeutic, and research obligations was undermined by their placement in poorly resourced institutions, without the support structures available in metropolitan centers. In this atmosphere, semiformal networks among researchers took on an added significance, with ingenuity at a premium, acting as the glue that held the community of researchers together.

In the last quarter century of colonial rule in Nigeria, and through its first decade of independence, the control of leprosy became increasingly entangled with the reproduction of colonial and expatriate control and the production of development expertise. While African aspirations had yet to founder on neoliberal shores, trajectories in the globalization of health care, medicine, and pharmaceutical research and marketing had already begun to transform international traffic in medical knowledge and expertise, setting the scene for the processes whereby "humanitarian and relief agencies [in Africa . . . became] increasingly reliant on extra-state mechanisms to establish patchworks of political order where states have become non-governmental" (Ferguson 2006, 47). In the period under scrutiny, the nature and extent of this traffic remains frustratingly opaque. Pointedly, though, the bland ascription to state power of any degree of successful integration of research and public health is already problematized in the late colonial era, as this discussion will show, by discerning linkages between the history of science and medicine and histories of welfare, community, and governance.

Refining Research Priorities in Nigerian Leprology

By the middle of the twentieth century, the scientist with an interest in leprosy was greeted with an abundance of new data on the clinical progress and therapeutic responsiveness of the disease. It was, of course, the increasing bureaucracy of leprosy control that elicited this data, as leprosy control institutions sought to cleave more tightly to community structures, an evolving apparatus for public health, and the contours of leprosy's prevalence. In the eastern Nigerian case, this bureaucracy elicited a clear sense of a prevalent emergency in the period from 1936 to 1948, with the newly surveyed incidence of leprosy described as "phenomenal" and "formidable"

(Davey et al. 1956, 65–68). The hybridization of colonial government technical, missionary humanitarian, and local administrative responses to this emergency, and the harnessing of experimental insights and resources amid evolving structures for the management of health and debility among leprosy sufferers, gave rise to a powerful articulation of medicine and development, which was crucially able to operate in areas beyond the reach and remit of state action.

Amid the resulting institutional and experimental fusion, a rich epidemiology emerged, sensitive to the vast array of presentations of leprosy, its mildness or severity, its epidemicity or endemicity, and its relation to conditions of housing, sanitation, and nutrition. As this process intensified, developments in chemotherapy and clinical research from the mid-1940s promised intriguing avenues of research for leprosy workers. Since testing on leprosy could not be carried out in the laboratory and needed human subjects, the clinicians in charge of leprosy control institutions became crucial research gatekeepers caught up in the adventure of global public health in the era of decolonization.

Leprosy, bacteriologically similar to tuberculosis, could not be cultivated in vitro. Thus, the practice had arisen of assaying in leprosy any compound that had exhibited antitubercular activity in humans, on the grounds that the bacilli were of the same family. The state of knowledge regarding the disease and its treatment had been set out at Rio de Janeiro in 1946 and at the International Leprosy Congress in Havana, Cuba, in April 1948. The congress was able to present new sulphone drugs proving effective in treating leprosy, and for the first time, with dapsone, to unreservedly recommend a treatment for leprosy.

In order to develop a system of clinical safeguards, given that all experimentation was necessarily carried out on human subjects, the Havana congress proposed minimum therapeutic requirements for clinical tests, centering on evidence of antibacterial action, absence of toxic effects or irreversible physiological changes, freedom from undue discomfort, and visible clinical and bacteriological evidence of suppression or regression of leprosy within twelve months (International Leprosy Congress 1949, 68–69). These requirements were predicated on classifications proposing a polar opposition of recognizably lepromatous (malignant) and tuberculoid (benign) leprosy, each internally differentiated according to measure of severity, bridged by a class of indeterminate (undifferentiated) cases. The congress recommended that tuberculoid and indeterminate cases, held to be non-infective, should not be included in the evaluation of chemotherapeutic trial results (International Leprosy Congress 1949, 69). The notion that tuberculoid and indeterminate cases were non-infectious was vigorously contested and proved a controversial issue in Nigerian leprosy research over the following years, especially in the Eastern Region, where the tuberculoid and indeterminate forms vastly predominated over the lepromatous.

Institutional capacity for leprosy control in Nigeria had developed greatly since the foundation of Itu and Uburu leprosy settlements in the late 1920s. A provincial scheme with extensive outreach facilities was developed following the 1936 visit of Ernest Muir, an India-based British leprologist. From 1945 the government took over a number of these facilities formerly run by missionaries. The new Nigeria Leprosy Service developed training and research at two eastern Nigerian facilities, Oji River and Uzuakoli, respectively, bringing leprosy control into the heart of public health and disease control through the era of decolonization. One effect of government cherry-picking of the most advanced missionary medical facilities was the evolution of marked spatial inequalities in funding, expertise, and research capacity.

Further, the government service continued to rely on the cordial relations with missionaries, indeed retaining a significant missionary staff on government contracts, while relying on the fundraising clout of the nongovernmental BELRA for the extension of leprosy work in areas outside the catchment of its facilities at Uzuakoli and Oji River. Given the intimate relations between innovations in treatment and patient care in dapsone-era leprosy, this had important implications for the management of leprosy control in 1950s and 1960s Nigeria.

In the late 1940s, however, continued problems in supervising the administration of dapsone in the following years ran alongside an increasingly active search for alternative drugs. It was not until 1948 that the Nigeria Leprosy Service Research Unit at Uzuakoli came into operation, and much later in the 1950s before it came into its own. Research continued to be decentralized and disarticulated through to the mid-1950s. Relations built around research reflected both the organizational shortcomings of the relatively new Nigeria Leprosy Service and the relative infancy of the immunology and epidemiology of leprosy in comparison with tuberculosis. This can be shown with reference to one group of compounds with evident potential for the treatment of leprosy developed at the laboratories of the Medical Research Council of Ireland (MRCI) through the 1940s and 1950s, leading to the synthesis of clofazimine.[1] This compound, trialed in Nigeria in the early 1960s, is still an effective component of the multidrug regimen used to treat leprosy today.

Building Contraptions for Medical Research

In rhetoric, and increasingly in terms of employment opportunities for British scientists, health workers, and educators, 1940 witnessed a transformation in the developmental aims of the British Empire. For its part, the Colonial Office saw itself as a key institution in facilitating the emergence of what Sabine Clarke terms "a technocratic imperial state" (Clarke 2007, 455, 479–80). From the viewpoint of the Nigerian leprologist, the output and impact of this technocracy was limited in relation to medical governance in rural eastern Nigeria. Indeed, the persistent reliance on missionary resources and reach and on non-state transnational networks in sourcing new compounds and adequate therapeutic materials to secure and stabilize medical practice in the region remained a striking feature of late colonial leprosy control. In this respect, the conduct and integration of medical research in the context of leprosy therapy owed as much to personal resources, networks, affections, and technical skills (or their absence), and to good fortune and careful rhetoric, as it did to carefully elaborated and well-funded research under the aegis of colonial development. The case of clofazimine and its trajectories through Irish, British, and Nigerian research and therapeutic regimes is an important and illustrative case in point.

In the early 1940s, with the incidence of tuberculosis in Ireland experiencing an alarming spike in contrast to much of the rest of Europe, there was as yet no specific treatment for the disease. In light of this, it was decided to focus Ireland's meager research resources on setting up a laboratory in Dublin to investigate the chemotherapy of tuberculosis, to be run by the MRCI.[2] In early 1944 Vincent Barry was chosen to lead the MRCI investigations, originally located at University College, Dublin (UCD). Barry was a systematic and rigorous organic chemist with significant research experience, which he brought to the identification, development, and testing of compounds for the treatment of tuberculosis: the MRCI laboratory, in its various guises, published copiously on its syntheses and processes until its demise in 1990.

Barry's theoretical focus on interrupting the metabolism of *Mycobacterium tuberculosis*, and his emphasis on in vitro testing of all promising compounds derived in the MRCI laboratories, streamlined the rapid development of compounds for animal and human trials, which had traditionally been bogged down in extensive guinea pig trials (Barry 1997, 45). Barry's first enterprise was to examine a series of branched-chain fatty acids derived from the remnants of an earlier UCD study on lichen by-products and, by iteration, determine what modifications would inhibit the growth in vitro of *M. tuberculosis*. Going on to look at diploicin, Barry's team decided to simplify the structures being examined, so that the physical characteristics of the molecules could be altered more readily and in repeatable fashion (Barry 1997, 47).

One unsuccessful compound, the hydrochloride of 2-aminodiphenylamine, was inadvertently not discarded and was left in storage for a number of months (Twomey 1986, 11). It demonstrated striking antitubercular properties upon its retrieval. It had also oxidized from near colorless to dark red, and a series of similar phenazine dyes was subsequently examined by Barry and his team. Among them, one in particular maintained its effectiveness as an antitubercular agent both in serum and in mouse and guinea pig tuberculosis, and it was as such one of the few investigated compounds to retain its activity beyond the in vitro stage (Barry 1951b, 453).[3] This compound, 2-anilino-3-imino-5-phenyl-phenazine, known by Barry's team as B.283, was subject to encouraging animal trials (Barry 1951b, 470), was taken orally by Barry and his associates to demonstrate its low toxicity (Lane 1951, 163),[4] and was later applied in clinical assessments on human subjects in the Meath Hospital (Lane 1951) (urogenital tuberculosis) and Rialto Chest Hospital (pulmonary tuberculosis) in Dublin.

Barry's work came to the attention of Joe Barnes, an Irish doctor on leave from the Catholic Mission Leprosy Scheme in Ogoja Province. While on leave, Barnes married Elizabeth Allday, an English doctor, and he and his wife traveled to Ogoja in July 1949. There they set about trialing new chemotherapeutic agents in the leprosy settlements. Barnes was unconvinced by the use of dapsone in treating leprosy, as he objected to what he saw as its excess toxicity in the doses administered in the late 1940s. Barnes and Allday compared the toxicity of sulphetrone, dapsone, and thiosemicarbazone—the most significant drugs in terms of worldwide research in leprosy chemotherapy at the time—and the results produced at Ogoja, some of which were highlighted in the *Lancet*, contributed to attempts to refine and standardize the administration of these drugs (Allday et al. 1951, 205–6; Barnes 1951a, 268; Barnes 1951b, 595).

In the case of B.283, however, the experimental work carried out in Ogoja was both novel and somewhat exotic. The initial trial begun in January 1951 was with ten patients, and, consistent with the recommendations of the Havana congress, all ten had been diagnosed with lepromatous leprosy (All-day et al. 1952, 422). No reports were yet available on the success of the drug in treatment of tuberculosis in Ireland, although concurrent human trials were in progress. Alongside the trial in lepromatous leprosy, a report on which was published in the *Irish Journal of Medical Science*, ten patients with tuberculoid leprosy were also treated with B.283 under the supervision of Dr. Denis Freeman, Barnes's replacement at Ogoja from mid-1951. This dual trial, in contradiction to the recommendations of the Havana congress, reflected new research trends occurring in eastern Nigeria at the time, where the predominance of tuberculoid and "indeterminate" rather than lepromatous leprosy seemed to render internationally conceived and agreed experimental strictures worthless (International Leprosy Congress 1949, 75).

Robert Cochrane, among the most eminent working leprologists, based by this time in Britain, had visited Freeman in Ogoja and had queried some of Barnes's diagnoses on which case selection for the B.283 trial was based. Commenting on the resulting disagreements, Barnes wrote that they may have arisen

> because you had only an abbreviated summary history of the cases and none of the original photographs . . . from these photoes [*sic*] and descriptions you may classify for yourself these cases, but it is not likely many will disagree for as you know there is a variety of classifications for leprosy. It must have been difficult for Cochrane who never saw these cases if he had not all the data I have now given you, as well as a missing lepromin reaction and tissue section which from your letter I understand he requires for the complete diagnosis of such cases.[5]

Barnes queried the accuracy of the term *atypical*, applied to the diagnosis of a presentation of leprosy he had classed as *pre-lepromatous*, noting infiltrations on the nose and ears, giving positive smears, as evidence of the case having crossed a border to lepromatous.

Coupled with diagnostic difficulties were a series of technical issues that obviated the validity of some of the eventual conclusions of the trial. The nearest pathology lab was in Lagos, and at the time of the jointly conducted trial on B.283, Barnes and Freeman relied on black-and-white photography to document their diagnoses. Neither doctor was confident in his documentary abilities with a camera, and the results, some of which have entered the published record, satisfied none of the investigators.

Unusually, the patient notes and published report on the trial were not anonymized; Barnes inquired on the physical and material progress of a number of patients in his correspondence with Freeman,[6] and his notes contain remarks such as "Wona's physique is, like his character, tough and lean," "Dick presents a most striking picture in his red jersey, cast-off battle dress and navy shorts." Indeed, for Barnes, the distinction between trial and treatment, key to the specifications outlined in Havana, was at best distracting, and possibly spurious, as evidenced by his report that "we have been unable to employ an untreated control group as our patients would not remain isolated without the inducement of treatment" (Allday et al. 1952, 422). The diagnostic tensions experienced between Barnes, Freeman, and Cochrane, together with Barnes's personal interest in his patients, epitomize transitions experienced across the world of leprosy control during the early 1950s, where nascent and as yet poorly defined international standards of ethical order in medical research are continually and dynamically in tension with the clinical context evolving around the doctor's familiarity with individual patients.

The changing state of knowledge with regard to treating tuberculoid leprosy, signaled in the recommendation of the Havana congress that clinical trials be carried out on lepromatous cases, impacted on the validity of the results of many trials being carried out in Nigeria in the early 1950s. Freeman's second trial on B.283 in tuberculoid leprosy seems, for instance, to have disappeared without a trace. At the same time, Cochrane and others continued to assent to the utility of B.283 in the treatment of both tuberculoid and lepromatous leprosy, even as it became clear that other compounds were both cheaper and more effective.[7] Significantly, the seeds of various research relations, with both BELRA and the new Leprosy Research Fund in London via Cochrane, between Ogoja and the Leprosy Research Unit at Uzuakoli in Nigeria, and between the MRCI chemotherapy labs and leprosy research, were all sown in the conduct of the trials in Ogoja and the publication of the results.

Another positive result of the Ogoja trial, and one that perpetuated its reputation over the next decade, was that Barry was able to demonstrate some success in the treatment both of tuberculosis and of leprosy by the time of Barry's 1951 Dublin colloquium on the chemotherapy of tuberculosis, thanks in part to a series of photographs exhibited by Barnes, relating to promising interim results of the first Ogoja trial of B.283 (Barry 1951a, 540). In a testament to the complementarity of clinical and laboratory-based studies at this particular conjuncture in the history of chemotherapy, the scientific team based around Barry saw Barnes's desire to trial B.283 in the treatment of lepromatous leprosy as promising "fresh clues to guide synthetic work," and it was noted that "the activity *in vivo* of these basic fatty substances is of especial interest, as it provides some justification for the long preoccupation of workers in the field with compounds of a fatty character." Meanwhile, for Barry and his team, the seeds of a long association with the treatment of leprosy had been definitively sown.

Harnessing Research Capacity in Public Health

The synthesis, evaluation, and production of B.663 (G 30 320, clofazimine) was the result of a growing collaboration between the MRCI laboratory and the Swiss drug company Geigy. The compound, first of a family named rimino-compounds, or rimino-phenazines, was originally synthesized at the MRCI laboratory in 1954 (Yawalkar 2002, 121) by means of a fortuitous catalytic reduction of a glyoxalino-phenazine (Barry 1969, 157–58).[8] While less active in vitro than the family of compounds from which B.283 had emerged, it proved prodigiously active in murine tuberculosis. The exceptional difficulties of synthesizing many of the compounds developed by Barry's team on site in Dublin, B.663 among them, lent great importance to the collaboration with Geigy, who could provide facilities for production, toxicology, and coordination of animal and human trials on a scale to which the MRCI could never aspire. While the resulting partnership was at times fraught, exemplifying a growing distinction between university-led and pharmaceutical industry research,[9] it enabled Barry's team to be more productive and refined in their exploratory and experimental methods and strengthened the international profile and accessibility of their work.

From Geigy's perspective, preliminary investigations on clofazimine in human tuberculosis had not been encouraging. Further assessment was almost abandoned (Yawalkar 2002, 121), but interim results in murine leprosy trials conducted by Y. T. Chang,[10] a previous collaborator of Barry's at the U.S. National Institutes of Health (Barry 1969, 159), evidently persuaded Geigy to reconsider, and at a 1960 London meeting between Barry, Vischer, and R. G. Cochrane, by now director of the Leprosy Research Unit in London, it was suggested that Browne trial B.663 in leprosy at Uzuakoli, Nigeria (Yawalkar 2002, 121). Having been appointed director of the Leprosy Research Unit at Uzuakoli in 1959, Stanley Browne returned there to begin the trial in September 1960 in collaboration with Lykle Hogerzeil.[11] By the time of his arrival in Nigeria, Browne had earned a notable reputation as a leprologist as a result of work carried out in the Belgian Congo, where he had begun as a missionary surgeon in 1936 (Hunt 1999, 209, 228). His structured way of working, and of organizing, reporting, and publicizing his investigations,[12] and his dedication to bolstering research competence and linking clinical capacity in leprosy control across eastern Nigeria in the early years of Nigerian independence (e.g., Browne et al. 1961) were important in developing outpatient leprosy control as a template for public health in the region in the years before the civil war in 1967.

This structured approach also underlined the contrast between his trials in B.663, and the earlier trials of B.283 carried out in Ogoja. Already at the time of Barnes's trials, the unit at Uzuakoli was at the forefront of systematic evaluation of chemotherapy in leprosy, with the scale and facilities to carry out complex series of investigations such as those needed to standardize the dosage of dapsone in the treatment of leprosy, research carried on at Uzuakoli in the early 1950s. By the time of Nigerian independence in October 1960, it had a worldwide reputation for the quality of its research. Together with the leprosy training facility at Oji River, Uzuakoli had spearheaded the standardization of leprosy control structures in Nigeria, focusing increasingly on outpatient treatment of leprosy. The theoretical distinction between treatment and research, unworkable for Barnes, seemed acceptable, if not routine, to Browne.

However, the pilot trial of B.663 was very small in scale, three patients receiving B.663 in combination with dapsone, and three receiving B.663 alone.[13] All had lepromatous leprosy of comparable severity. There seem to have been four other patients receiving B.663, in an exercise that was not recorded in the published results of the trial (Browne and Hogerzeil 1962a). Further, Browne sought to observe the effects of clofazimine in selected patients as consultant at other leprosy schemes in eastern Nigeria, a process that does not seem to have been closely documented.[14] The trial determined that B.663 improved the clinical state of the patient with lepromatous leprosy, leading to a fall in the bacterial index, an effect enhanced in combination with dapsone. A supplementary report noted a form of drug resistance and discounted B.663 as a serious rival to dapsone, due to its high cost (Browne et al. 1962b).

———————

The definitive terms in which this trial was reported contrasts with the potentially tendentious nature of the data and the manner in which it was elicited. However, the presentation of striking effects by noted researchers based at high-profile institutions, together with further studies by Browne and by F. Imkamp at Liteta Leprosarium, Zambia, which demonstrated anti-inflammatory properties of B.663 and lessened the dependence of an important cohort of leprosy patients on corticosteroids, proved a crucial boost to the reputation of the drug, which was introduced under the trademark Lamprene in 1969.

Stanley Browne derived significant acclamation from his role as director of the Leprosy Research Unit, first at Uzuakoli, and later in London, and from his early success with B.663. This acclamation enabled him to act as arbiter with respect to later trials of the compound and signaled a sea change in the relation of the research institute to the treatment of leprosy. Much of this change was due to the existence of successful chemotherapeutic agents, starting with dapsone in the late 1940s, but developments in the conduct, reporting, and reception of clinical trials in the postwar decades are clearly discernible in the contrast between the trials of B.283 in Ogoja and B.663 in Uzuakoli.

Whatever the validity of Barnes's methods and diagnoses, publication in the *Irish Journal of Medical Science* gave this work a currency, and gave the relation of Barry's work on tuberculosis chemotherapy to leprosy a continuing identity, which emerged as vital in the development of clofazimine, from Barry's work, and in the Nigerian research center at Uzuakoli in the 1960s. More to the point, at a time when the balance in medical research was shifting ever more decisively from the clinical to the laboratory-based, and the clinical trial took its place as an ancillary of healing, among the range of technical operations performed in expanding colonial health care institutions, the trial of B.283 at Ogoja provided an especially eloquent index of the plans, aspirations, and capacities of even the most remote of medical enterprises. Indeed, the less than ideal physical and geographical circumstances of most leprosy research, the impossibility of cultivating leprosy outside a living human host, and the persistent privileging of local clinical knowledge — at times promoted in the most willful terms—all help us understand the experimental clinical setting of Ogoja as characteristic rather than anomalous.

With the burden of leprosy in Nigeria so heavily skewed toward the tuberculoid, the strictures elaborated at Havana in 1948 seemed to impoverish the context for leprosy research in Nigeria. The technical capacity to sustain a successful clinical trial and to firmly ground the results of a clinical research intervention did not exist in Ogoja in the early 1950s: Barnes's counterarguments to objections to the conduct of the trial of B.283 in lepromatous leprosy, based on notions of personal practice and individual clinical expertise, exposes a moment of transition in clinical research in leprosy. Over the next decade, leprosy work in Nigeria contributed to an enriching of the classificatory and diagnostic contexts elaborated in Havana, enabling a more robust circulation between the local instance and the global phenomenon of leprosy and its control, and providing a more systematic grounding for the appreciation of research results in clinical leprosy trials.

Indeed, the intervening years wrought infrastructural and capacity changes so great that it is difficult to consider the trial of B.663 at Uzuakoli as linked in any more than a circumstantial way to the Ogoja trials. The startling success, from a scientific point of view, of a trial hardly larger or more ambitious than that carried out at Ogoja testifies to a shift in attitudes to local clinical knowledge even regarding a condition as experimentally intractable as leprosy. The methodological developments separating the trials in Ogoja and Uzuakoli, contingent as much on infrastructural capacity as on growth in knowledge, affected the work of the MRCI laboratory in other ways. As the main link between the two trials, and the foremost locus of Irish medical research from the 1940s through the 1980s, the fate of the MRCI laboratory reflected the development of experimental chemotherapy in the twentieth century.[15] Increasingly unable to replicate the success of large pharmaceutical companies, the laboratory was seen to represent a diminishing return on investment: the MRCI was folded into the new Health Research Board in 1986, and the laboratory followed its parent organization into oblivion in 1990, much to the consternation of the international leprosy medical fraternity.

By this stage, multidrug therapy for leprosy had been standardized by the WHO, combining dapsone, clofazimine, and rifampicin and involving pharmaceutical companies in charitable contracts for the provision of a series of outpatient control programs administered by developing country state health systems together with international leprosy foundations. Yet in already close relation to formally and informally brokered research networks by the 1950s and 1960s, the spatial reach of leprosy control in eastern Nigeria, coercive and segregatory in its initial impulses, had yielded a wide-ranging public health apparatus capable of delivering outpatient leprosy control alongside a variety of other health services.

Investigating the periodization of the research and therapeutic networks invoked in post-1945 Nigerian leprosy control, we can see that the weak reach of state power was continually bolstered by nongovernmental action in both public health and medical research. Such research was not always predicated on a stable and manageable constituting of the experimental subject and often took on what we might describe as an entrepreneurial aspect. Similarly, rural public health frequently relied on missionary resources, which varied with levels of donor interest and engagement. While one cannot trace a continuous logic of experimentality based solely on this series of interventions—across a quarter-century period spanning the late colonial and early postcolonial era and prefiguring Rottenburg's new (and emphatically "postmodern") figurations—there is visible here a dominant and recurrent fabrication and refurbishment of transnational (and not merely colonial) research and treatment partnerships that both construct and respond to experimental opportunities in relation to perceived medical emergency.

This chapter has highlighted some of the more unpromising and tentative roots of this process, with a view to capturing in its infancy the elaboration of new global research relationships and capacities, and researching, producing, and consuming publics in an exciting and optimistic period in the evolution of international public health. In this way, it imagines an ambiguous and evocative prehistory of postmodernity, where the evidence for a shift from bilateral (colonial or developmentalist-state) models of development toward multilateral and unaccountable models is uncertain and where the reach of the state is seen to have always relied on the arms of missionaries, adventurers, and capitalists. Finally it registers a discomfort with the ascription of novelty to recent forms of interaction between bodies concerned with medical research in Africa and the inscription of an epochal shift into narratives of these relations that, on closer investigation, may not fully bear this weight of interpretation. It may well be time to revisit our figurations of postcolonial science in the light of a much longer and more strikingly familiar prehistory.

Notes

1   I routinely use the standard name *clofazimine* to refer to the drug synthesised by the MRCI as B.663 (Dublin), produced by Geigy as G 30 320 (Basle), and marketed as Lamprene. In the main set of clinical trials to which I refer, the compound was known as B.663, and I will adopt this usage in reference to these trials and to its original synthesis in Dublin.

2   National Archives, Ireland (NAI), TAOIS/S 13025 A, Medical Research. T. S. Wheeler and R. A. Q. O'Meara, Memorandum for An Taoiseach in regard to the organisation in Eire of research on the chemotherapy of tuberculosis, dated November 12, 1942.

3   Intriguingly, of the compounds listed by Barry that retained antitubercular activity in the guinea pig, the three that had some measure of success in treatment of leprosy—dapsone (diaminodiphenylsulphone), Conteben (thiosemicarbazone), and B.283 (2-anilino-3-imino-5-phenyl-phenazine)—were noted as having "one property in common: they all contain a basic nitrogenous group," while seemingly sharing no other obvious relationship.

4   Lane's note is the only reference I have seen to self-administration of compounds at the MRCI laboratory; Barry (1969, 156) later claimed that B.283 "toxicity was considerable."

5   Ogoja Convent Files. A letter dated September 29, 1951, from J. Barnes (Dublin) to D. Freeman (Ogoja) mentions the two sets of cases.

6   Ogoja Convent Files. Letters from Barnes to Freeman, dated "last Sunday in Sept. [1951]" and April 2, 1952.

7   Ogoja Convent Files. Letter from Barnes to Freeman, postmarked June 14, 1952. This letter mentions a trial carried out in England by Cochrane on a number of patients with tuberculoid leprosy.

8   Barry notes here that it was later discovered that the rimino-compounds could be derived from the anilinoaposafranines, of which B.283 was one.

9   Personal correspondence with Stanley McElhinney, Trinity College, Dublin.

10 References to murine leprosy in the medical literature acknowledge the development by the 1960s of an experimental model for assaying toxicity in chemotherapeutic agents for leprosy on the mouse footpad successfully inoculated with *M. leprae.*

11 Wellcome Library Archives, WTI/SGB/C.1/4/1—B.663 in leprosy. This date is given in a handwritten note dated "Aug. 1960."

12 Wellcome Library Archives, WTI/SGB/C.1/4/1—B.663 in leprosy. Browne's notes for F. Inkamp's trial of B.663 in corticosteroid-dependent patients give some idea of the rigor of his observations regarding patient history, type, and degree of side effects observed, degree of neuritis and lepra reaction observed, psychological effects of treatment, method of drug administration, and toxic effects observed.

13 Wellcome Library Archives, WTI/SGB/C.1/4/1—B.663 in leprosy. Note headed

"B 663 — Uzuakoli patients," detailing the timing and labeling of biopsies taken from the patients in the trial subject group.

14 Conversation with Dr. Esther Davis, formerly of Ekpene Obom Leprosy Scheme, June 23, 2006.

15 Personal correspondence with Stanley McElhinney, Trinity College, Dublin.

References

Allday, E. J., and J. Barnes. 1951. "Toxic Effects of Diaminodiphenyl-sulphone in Treatment of Leprosy." *Lancet* 258, no. 6675: 205–6.

Allday, E. J., and J. Barnes. 1952. "Treatment of Leprosy with B.283." *Irish Journal of Medical Science* 6th series, no. 322: 421–25.

Barnes, J. 1951a. "Treatment of Leprosy with Thiosemicarbazone." *Lancet* 258, no. 6676: 268.

Barnes, J. 1951b. "Diaminodiphenylsulphone in Leprosy." *Lancet* 258, no. 6683: 595.

Barry, V. C. 1951a. "Chemotherapy of Tuberculosis." *Nature* 168, no. 4274: 539–41.

Barry, V. C. 1951b. "An Organic Chemist's Approach to the Chemotherapy of Tuberculosis." *Irish Journal of Medical Science*, 6th series, no. 310: 453–73.

Barry, V. C. 1969. "Boyle Medal Lecture: Synthetic Phenazine Derivatives and Mycobacterial Disease, a Twenty Year Investigation." *Scientific Proceedings of the Royal Dublin Society* 3, no. 16: 153–71.

Barry, V. C. 1997. "Antitubercular Compounds: Presidential Address" [reprint of 1946 address to the Irish Chemical Association]. *Irish Chemical News* (winter): 44–50.

Bonneuil, C. 2000. "Development as Experiment: Science and State Building in Late Colonial and Postcolonial Africa, 1930–1970." *Osiris* 15: 258–81.

Browne, S. G., and L. M. Hogerzeil. 1962a. "'B 663' in the Treatment of Leprosy: Preliminary Report of a Pilot Trial." *Leprosy Review* 33: 6–10.

Browne, S. G., and L. M. Hogerzeil. 1962b. "'B 663' in the Treatment of Leprosy: Supplementary Report." *Leprosy Review* 33: 182–84.

Browne, S. G., and E. Ridge. 1961. "Toxic Epidermal Necrolysis." *British Medical Journal* 1, no. 5225: 550–53.

Clarke, S. 2007. "A Technocratic Imperial State? The Colonial Office and Scientific Research, 1940–1960." *Twentieth Century British History* 18, no. 4: 453–80.

Davey, T. F., C. M. Ross, and B. Nicholson. 1956. "Leprosy: A Changing Situation in Eastern Nigeria." *British Medical Journal* 2, no. 4984: 65–68.

Etherington, N. 2005. "Education and Medicine." In *Missions and Empire*, edited by N. Etherington, 261–84. Oxford: Oxford University Press.

Ferguson, J. 2006. *Global Shadows: Africa in the Neoliberal World Order*. Durham, NC: Duke University Press.

Hardiman, D. 2006. "Introduction." In *Healing Bodies, Saving Souls: Medical Missions in Asia and Africa*, edited by D. Hardiman, 5–57. Amsterdam: Rodopi.

Hunt, N. R. 1999. *A Colonial Lexicon of Birth Ritual, Medicalization, and Mobility in the Congo*. Durham, NC: Duke University Press.

International Leprosy Congress. 1949. *Memoria del V Congreso Internacional de la Lepra: Celebrado en La Habana, Cuba del 3 al 11 de Abril de 1948/organizado por el Gobierno de la República de Cuba con la colaboración de la Asociación Internacional de la Lepra*. Havana: Editorial Cenit.

Lane, T. D. J. 1951. "Chemotherapy in Urinary Tuberculosis." In *Proceedings of the Colloquium on the Chemotherapy of Tuberculosis*, edited by Medical Research Council of Ireland, 155–75. Dublin: MRCI.

Phillipson, S. S. 1949. *Grants in Aid of the Medical and Health Services Provided by Voluntary Agencies in Nigeria*. Lagos: Govt. Printer. Accessed March 12, 2010. http://openlibrary.org/b/OL21866951M/Grants_in_aid_of_the_medical_and _health_services_provided_by_voluntary_agencies_in_Nigeria.

Rottenburg, R. 2009. "Social and Public Experiments and New Figurations of Science and Politics in Postcolonial Africa." *Postcolonial Studies* 12, no. 4: 423–40.

Tilley, H. 2004. "Ecologies of Complexity: Tropical Environments, African Trypanosomiasis, and the Science of Disease Control in British Colonial Africa, 1900–1940." *Osiris* 19: 21–38.

Twomey, D. 1986. "An Irish Solution for a Non-Irish Problem." *Irish Chemical News* (spring): 10–12.

Vaughan, M. 1991. *Curing Their Ills: Colonial Power and African Illness*. Oxford: Polity Press.

Yawalkar, S. J. 2002. *Leprosy for Medical Practitioners and Paramedical Workers*. 7th ed. Basel: Novartis Foundation.

PART II

Pasts, Futures

CHAPTER 3

Lessons in Medical Nihilism:

Virus Hunters, Neoliberalism, and

the AIDS Pandemic in Cameroon

Guillaume Lachenal

When I met Nathan Wolfe in 2003, he was a postdoc from Johns Hopkins University (JHU) expatriated in Yaoundé, the capital of Cameroon. There, he led a team of U.S. and Cameroonian researchers and technicians, who studied the circulation of retroviruses in rural areas of the country. His lab—benches with basic HIV testing tools and a couple of freezers—was situated in the decayed premises of Yaoundé's military camp. I interviewed Dr. Wolfe about his work and career. I found him sharp and enthusiastic and was impressed by the way he dramatized the importance of his task—he allowed me to interview him for "15 minutes" and refused to be recorded, which rarely happened in this fieldwork. I was also impressed by the relative luxury of Johns Hopkins' outpost: I remember that I saw there for the first time ever wireless connections at a time when checking email from Cameroon was still a challenge.

Five years later, Nathan Wolfe was full professor of epidemiology at UCLA. He headed a big research project, funded by a multimillion dollar grant from the NIH, which aimed to replicate his Cameroonian experience in several sites in the world. First named the "Wolfelab," the project was later known as the Global Viral Forecast Initiative.[1] Its goal was simple: "to prevent the next pandemic before it starts,"[2] by establishing a global network of surveillance of viral infections in selected human populations.

Retroviruses were the main targets: "to stop the next HIV in its tracks,"[3] the program focused on some communities of Central Africa in contact with apes, such as the hunters of the so-called bushmeat,[4] the channel through which novel, unknown simian retroviruses could provoke another AIDS-like pandemic in humans. Presenting itself as a renewal in the fight against emerging viruses, the "forecast initiative" earned Nathan Wolfe wide press

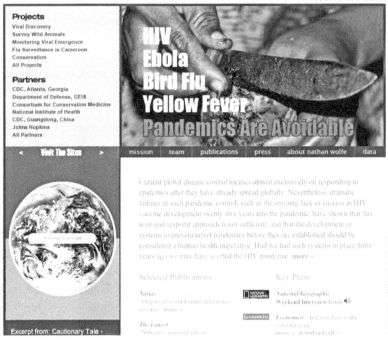

Figure 3.1. Homepage of the website of the "Wolfelab" (California), presenting the rationale of viral forecasting (www.wolfelab.com, accessed on September 16, 2008).

coverage, from the *Economist* to *Scientific American*, and, so far, academic and fundraising success.

This chapter puts this exemplar (though unexceptional) trajectory in a wider historical context. During the 1990s, Cameroon became a hot spot for retrovirology. Following the discovery of unidentified AIDS-causing viruses among Cameroonian patients, Western research institutions and pharmaceutical firms rushed to Yaoundé, with the hope of finding the HIV-3—only two major types of AIDS viruses, HIV-1 and HIV-2, were then (and are still) known. The virus hunt, driven by scientific as well as commercial interests coincided with the neoliberal transformation of biomedical research in Cameroon. While local hospitals and research institutions were weakened by the economic crisis and structural adjustment reforms, a handful of doctors organized transnational collaborations—often limited to sampling and shipping to the north of biological materials from local patients. Minimalist projects multiplied; high-profile virological discoveries followed one another; a new pattern of extractive, privatized, and internationalized research emerged in the local landscape. In a first part, I will describe how the study of HIV in Cameroon channeled new forms and norms of scientific work, in a context of neoliberal reforms and economic collapse. From this perspective, the JHU enclave will seem quite representative—as yet another success story in times of crisis.

In a second part, I will discuss how the study of retroviruses in Cameroon became framed as a global "biosecurity" issue. From the mid-1990s, the research on Cameroonian viruses took part in "emerging infectious diseases'" narratives and interventions. Not only because the local strains of HIV threatened to spread worldwide but also because virologists warned that HIV-3 or HIV-4, if not already in circulation, could appear at any moment in the country. Most projects based in Yaoundé studied, in addition to HIV, the simian immunodeficiency virus (SIV), which circulated among local monkeys and apes. After the discovery of a dozen new SIVs in Cameroon, virologists announced that the simian viruses could pass to humans through the hunting and eating of bushmeat by Cameroonian populations and produce new, unknown HIVs. The "bushmeat crisis," as conservationists termed it, could lead to a new AIDS pandemic. I will analyze how virologists constructed this viral risk, and how they elaborated responses to it. Here also, Professor Wolfe's "forecasting project," brought back from Cameroon to California, will appear as a typical example of the way unknown viruses became objects of surveillance and menaces to global security.

In the last part, I will focus on the public display, understanding, and critiques of the research on emerging HIVs in Cameroon. While the research projects themselves had a discreet material presence in Yaoundé, the narratives on bushmeat viruses inspired ambitious and well-publicized forms of public health interventions. These interventions were the target of specific criticisms, which contrasted with the usual denunciations, in Cameroon as elsewhere, of transnational research as a form of exploitation and extraction (see Le Carré 2001; Shah 2006). What became the focus of the criticism was the strong affinity of the fight against emerging HIVs with absurdity, hubris, and pretense. As unknown, nonexistent viruses were turned into public health priorities and became the targets of elaborate (and unmaterialized) programs of control, the virologists were portrayed as figures of impotence and ridicule. I will draw inspiration from this specific critique to propose, as a heuristic hypothesis, that the practices, theories, and debates associated with the bushmeat viruses participated in a *nihilistic* regime of scientific knowledge, intervention, and critique.

Though a complex concept, the notion of nihilism may help problematize the recent transformation of the landscape of medical research and public health in Africa. The effects of neoliberal globalization on biomedicine in Africa have recently received much attention. A triple transformation has been described. First, historians and anthropologists have described how the advent of the "emerging diseases worldview" in the 1990s shifted the priorities of international health and biomedical research toward the surveillance of unknown pathogens in the name of global health security and relegated in the background more classical views of public health centered on the nation-state and welfare (King 2002, 2004; Lakoff and Collier 2008; Dry and Leach 2010). More radically, neoliberalization has sometimes been described as an "antigovernemental" turn: a "collapse of public health," as Laurie Garret put it, organized through the privatization and the "shrinking" of health systems, especially in Africa where it conflated with a more general "collapse of the state" (Garrett 2000). Third, some scholars have associated neoliberal globalization with the advent of quite fascinating forms of biopolitical interventions in Africa, such as transnational clinical trials or large-scale therapeutic programs, which fashioned specific types of political rationalities, moralities, and communities (Nguyen 2010, 2005).

Yet taken together these interpretations of the neoliberal turn are not fully satisfactory, for they tend to take for granted the material effects of the global, private, and transnational biopolitics they see emerging in Africa and, therefore, tend to exaggerate the retreat of the nation-state, which is supposed to have prepared their rise. An alternative approach to examine what has changed in African biomedicine since AIDS, structural adjustment, and the advent of "global health" may be to look at what bioscientists and governments *do not do*. Attention, for example, to the way biomedical interventions in Africa were framed as "minimalist biopolitics" (Redfield 2005, 345): not in the sense of the rationalization *a minima* of the state as a "security apparatus," which characterized, according to Foucault (2004), neoliberalism, but in the sense, developed by Peter Redfield, of a politics of life *reduced* to the witnessing and measurement of suffering—one that leaves aside past ambitions to deal with its causes. In Cameroon we will see that the paradigm of emerging viruses advocated typically *noninterventionist interventions* (the sampling and shipping abroad of biomaterials and the surveillance of fictive pathogens), while the material capacity of the "adjusted" Cameroo-nian state to care for real public health seemed anyhow uncertain.

Nihilism, in the sense of a renunciation to action (the idea that "nothing can be done"), has been a major motif in the history of medicine, both as a dominant institutional discourse (defining medical science as a natural his-tory of diseases and medical practice as an art of diagnosis) and as a regime of critique (defining medicine as nothing but a farce) (Porter 1997, 680–81; Porter 2001, 24–25). The AIDS epidemic, as was noted during the early years of the epidemic, revived explicit forms of therapeutic nihilism: when no treatment existed, of course, but also during the (long) 1990s, when access to efficient therapy was denied to African patients (Oppenheimer and Bayer 2007). As Paul Farmer (1999) and Didier Fassin (2007) have reminded us, nonintervention was not, in that case, an option by default: it was *positively* endorsed and theorized by many doctors, experts, and policy makers, as the most "cost-efficient" and even "ethical" way to fight AIDS in Africa.[5] I pro-pose to term as nihilistic this acceptance, rationalization as necessary, orga-nization, and moral valuation of inaction.[6] In this sense, this chapter will explore the nihilistic dimension of AIDS research in Cameroon where, until the recent expansion of antiretroviral delivery programs, research projects prioritized de facto the detection of new viruses over clinical interven-tion, by providing simultaneously (and in the name of good science) "first world diagnostics" and "third world therapeutics" to their research subjects (Farmer 1999, xxiv).

In addition, nihilism accounts for the well-known affinity between public health hubris and failure. The coupling between the hopes of social medicine and discourses of renunciation and reaction responding to them has been pivotal in the history of public health (Fassin 2001). The hygienist ambi-tions of "colonial governmentality" not only systematically failed, as colo-nial studies scholars have demonstrated (Stoler and Cooper 1997; Anderson 2006), but also this failure had a part of *positivity*: it shaped politics, prac-tices, and subjectivities. The literature on colonial medicine, from Céline to Sartre,[7] offers series of examples of such aesthetics of faith and failure and as many stories reminding that "a doctor is not immune from 'the long despair of doing nothing well,'" as Graham Greene (1961, ii) put it. How-ever, scholars have hitherto poorly accounted for the nihilistic possibility contained in the greatest hopes of colonial hygienists, virus hunters, and international technocrats—be they the postwar dreams of disease eradica-tion or the present hype about the "prevention of pandemics." In southeast

Cameroon especially, the history of public health in the twentieth century is haunted by charismatic colonial doctors turning into unfortunate heroes, whose stories remind us that the line is thin between utopia and megalomania and great hopes and lost illusions (Lachenal 2010). Perhaps here also, Nathan Wolfe could appear as a familiar case.

Lastly, the hypothesis of nihilism allows us to confront the question of *absurdity* and of its uses in contemporary Africa. This theme has been central in the recent scholarship, political critique, and artistic creation in and about Cameroon (Monga 2009). Thinking through the Cameroonian experience of democratization and neoliberalization, Achille Mbembe (2001, 114) has described African postcolonies as regimes of powerlessness, where the core of government is obviously not "security" but an "unusual and grotesque art of representation." Drawing from Mbembe's depiction of absurdity and obscenity as the logics and aesthetics of state power, I will try to make sense of an emerging regime of bioscientific interventions and critiques of bioscience, which existing literature has little considered. It pictures global biomedicine in Africa not so much in terms of greed, extraction, and surveillance but rather as a world of inaction and impotence—of scientists not doing much, promising a lot, and telling stories to themselves.

To make it clear, this chapter does not draw a representative panorama of the AIDS field in Cameroon during the last two decades.[8] All the more so, since changes had been tremendous between 2005 and 2008, with the implementation of nationwide programs of free antiretroviral treatment: in times of "AIDS exceptionalism," my point on nihilism may seem outdated or unfair and fortunately so. Still, by bringing to the fore nonintervention, hubris, and absurdity, this chapter intends to identify a fundamental pattern in the articulation between biomedical knowledge and public health interventions, which played a long-lasting role in the history of biopolitics in Africa and which fashions in part the current, and strange, para-states of science on the continent.

Appropriating Viruses, Privatizing Science: A Brief
History of Research on HIV in Cameroon

"The welfare state is long dead," proclaimed the Ministry of Public Health of Cameroon, giving an appropriate conclusion in a 1994 interview in the daily *Cameroon Tribune* to the nation's annus horribilis.[9] Within a couple of months, structural adjustment measures and the devaluation of the CFA franc hastened the slump in the population's purchasing power, while many public institutions, including hospitals and research centers, went bankrupt (Courade 2000).[10]

That moment of breakdown coincided with a scientific success story. In May 1994 the *Journal of Virology* announced that a new strain of the AIDS virus, the HIV-1 O, had been isolated from Cameroonian patients (Gurtler et al. 1994). The publication was of major significance: the new virus caused AIDS but remained undetectable by the tests routinely used for HIV screening; its genetic structure puzzled specialists; its origin was mysterious. The discovery of that "highly divergent African HIV isolate" (Vanden Haesevelde et al. 1994), named *O* for *Outlier*, hit the news during the summer. A special session was organized to discuss it at the International AIDS Conference in Yokahoma; from Atlanta to Paris, virologists, public health authorities, and test manufacturers looked toward Cameroon. In Yaoundé two researchers, who worked at the blood bank of the university hospital, were associated with the discovery: Professor Lazare Kaptue, a hematologist trained in France in the 1960s and one of the most prominent medical figures in Cameroon, and his assistant Dr. Leopold Zekeng, a medical biologist trained in Dakar and in Paris. Their names were not, however, mentioned in the local press. At the moment of the publication, the university hospital was literally running on empty. Staff salaries had not been paid for the first nine months of the year, reagents were missing, and the entire hospital was on stoppage (*débrayage*).[11]

HIV-1 O: THE MAKING OF AN EMERGING VIRUS

The work on the atypical virus began in 1990, when Zekeng received a twenty-six-year-old woman for a consultation at the blood bank. Though she presented signs of full-blown AIDS, the woman tested negative with the screening tests. The interest of the case was clear: it was well known that such anomalies could indicate the presence of unidentified, AIDS-causing retroviruses. For that reason Kaptue was in regular contact, since 1989, with Lütz Gurtler, a German virologist from the Max Von Pettenkofer Institute in Munich, who wished to investigate Cameroonian retroviruses. With a grant from the German Cooperation Agency (GTZ), Zekeng flew to Munich, bringing with him the patient's biological samples.[12] The German and Cameroonian team showed that the patient's lymphocytes hosted an unknown type of HIV-1, which provoked atypical immunological reactions. With the help of the German firm Behring Laboratories, a leading manufacturer of HIV tests, the team characterized the virus and devised "home-made" tests to detect it. Announced in 1994, the discovery rewarded an original north-south public-private collaboration. Seen from Cameroon, it had almost invisible but vital consequences: in exchange for the access to the blood samples, Behring furnished the university hospital with HIV tests to secure blood transfusions.

Most surprising about the discovery was, perhaps, who had *not* made it. Since independence in 1960, the local field of medical research had been dominated by the Centre Pasteur du Cameroun (CPC), a large medical analysis and research laboratory located in downtown Yaoundé. Headed by French expatriates since the late colonial period, the CPC was linked to the Pasteur Institute in Paris and, at the same time, owned by the Cameroonian state as an integral part of the Ministry of Health. For three decades, it had been a symbol of Cameroon's ongoing development: it proved the nation's modernity, by the high standards of expertise and services it provided; it signaled, at the same time, that this modernization was still in process, as it depended on France's science and benevolence (Lachenal 2009, 2011). Things changed after 1988. The Pasteurian outpost, where the French doctors had initiated research on AIDS in the mid-1980s, vanished from the scientific scene. The CPC was paralyzed by the economic crisis, for it was funded by (cut) state subsidies and by (unaffordable) commercial medical services. The CPC also had to deal with the competition of a generation of local "AIDS doctors,"[13] including Lazare Kaptue, who in 1987 became the first director of the National Program to Fight AIDS (PNLS). While the WHO Global Program on AIDS, which patronized the PNLS, sought to promote African responses to the epidemic, the French experts had become anachronistic. The mobilization against AIDS thus accompanied a symbolic turn: while the monopoly of an emblematic state institution and its postcolonial tutelage were contested, a redefinition of the local forms of biomedical research was under way.

EMERGING VIRUSES AND EMERGING MARKETS

HIV-1 O was isolated just when the "emerging infectious diseases" world-view became established as the new paradigm of international health. It was offered worldwide coverage, as a prototype of a viral menace from Africa, from the *New York Times* to *Le Monde* (Pollack 1994). Health agencies, from the Center for Disease Control (CDC) in Atlanta to the French National Agency for Aids Research (ANRS) announced upcoming programs to study it. Before the end of 1994, dozens of HIV-1 O infected patients in Cameroon and in Europe were identified; two other specimens of HIV-1 O viruses were already isolated in Europe (Charneau et al. 1994).

The virus frightened international health authorities because it spread globally, but above all because its carriers could pass as seronegative—which was, a virologist later recalled, "a nightmare for those who managed blood transfusions."[14] A team of Parisian clinicians rang the alarm bell in June 1994, with a publication in the *Lancet*: it reported cases of "HIV-1/HIV-2 *seronegativity* in HIV-1 subtype O infected patients" (Loussert-Ajaka et al. 1994). In the United States the CDC confirmed a few months later "that the adaptation of current tests [was] urgently needed" to detect the new AIDS virus (Schable et al. 1994); the Food and Drug Administration (FDA) decided to exclude from blood donation any person "linked to Cameroon and its adjacent countries."[15]

The detection of HIV-1 O was not only a matter of health security; it also had obvious commercial implications. Since the early 1980s, the development of immunological diagnostic techniques (such as Elisa tests) had given a huge economic importance to patents on viral proteins used as antigens. The controversy between France and the United States over the first isolation of HIV and the disputed race to isolate HIV-2 in West Africa had confirmed that viruses, regardless of their epidemic potential, were also a matter of royalties (Grmek 1995, 146).

In that context the study of the atypical immunological reactions of certain Cameroonian AIDS patients had started well before 1994. As early as 1988, the virology unit of the Institute of Tropical Medicine in Antwerp, the former Belgian institute for colonial medicine and one of the leading institutions in the African AIDS field,[16] had found a strange virus infecting a Cameroonian couple living in Belgium. A patent was filed in collaboration with Innogenetics, a newly created biotech firm neighboring the institute (Vanderborght, DeLeys, and Van Geel 1988): it officially named the virus HIV-3, although the virus was not characterized well enough to deserve the appellation in scientific publications.[17] By 1993, the team realized that their virus was genetically close to the divergent HIV-1 under study at the same time in Munich, and, after discussions with the German and Cameroonian team, published its full characterization in the same May 1994 issue of the *Journal of Virology* (Vanden Haesevelde et al. 1994; Gurtler et al. 1994). Behring and Innogenetics patented their respective viruses and settled a cross-licensing agreement to share the intellectual propriety of the discovery. No

Cameroonian institution was associated with either patent, but Zekeng and Kaptue, as individual inventors, were entitled to royalties. HIV-1 O—if not HIV-3—was invented.

HIV-1 O made a significant impact in the AIDS diagnostic industry.[18] In 2002 the licensing rights of HIV-1 O proteins still brought in to Innogenetics and Behring a low estimate of one million euros per year.[19] Put in the words of biotech investors, the emerging virus opened an emerging market.

THE SCRAMBLE FOR CAMEROON

In 1994 commentators in the *Lancet* hoped that "the intense hunt [that] has already begun to collect other isolates of the O sub-type" in Cameroon would "be more coordinated then the unbelievable scramble for HIV-2 which, in 1985, saw research teams, institutions of public health and industry squabble over opportunities to collect blood samples and the specimens themselves" (Dondero, Hu, and George 1994). The following years would prove that they were underestimating Yaoundé's potential.

Transnational arrangements, linking public research teams and private firms in the north with Cameroonian personalities, multiplied in Yaoundé between 1994 and 2000; all aimed at studying the local HIVs. Zekeng and Kaptue got engaged with additional collaborators, including Abott Laboratories, the CDC, the FDA, and the University of Kyoto in Japan. In parallel the Belgian codiscoverers of HIV-1 O partnered with another outstanding Cameroonian medical figure, Peter Ndumbe, a colleague of Kaptue at the Faculty of Medicine in Yaoundé.[20] Another set of transnational connections was established around Eitel Mpudi-Ngolle, a Cameroonian military doctor trained in France. In 1995 he began to collaborate with Dr. Eric Delaporte and his wife, Martine Peeters, two rising figures in the field of retrovirology, who were based at the ORSTOM (now IRD, the Institut de Recherche pour le Développement) in Montpellier, the former French agency for colonial research. Mpudi-Ngolle built on that link to organize other collaborations: at the CRESAR, his small installation at the military camp in downtown Yaoundé, he set up laboratories and offices for two other partners, the JHU and the CDC. The CDC project, named IRECAM (Investigations of Retroviruses in Cameroon) was led from Atlanta by Dr. Thomas Folks, also a specialist in the epidemiology of HIV. Sponsored by the Military HIV Research Program, the Johns Hopkins project was managed in the field by an American expatriate, Nathan Wolfe, a young biologist who had recently completed a doctorate at Harvard on infectious diseases among primate populations in Borneo. Professor Donald Burke, a U.S. Army colonel, professor of epidemiology at JHU, and a well-established figure of the HIV field, supervised it from the United States. Starting gradually from 1999 to 2000, the project called itself EICAM for Emerging Infections in Cameroon.

Housed in the same corridor, the two American projects remained low-tech, just like the other virological projects mentioned. Studies were limited to blood testing and administrative work, and arrangements were made with customs and air companies for the transportation of samples to the north, where the proper virology was done. In all projects, the pivotal task was the access to local blood samples, which were essential to search for new viruses, but also to obtain serums (a synonym of plasma, that is, the acellular fraction of blood containing antibodies) from patients infected by atypical viruses, which were needed in quantity to assess the sensitivity of diagnostic kits—to test the tests.[21]

That economy shaped research practices in Yaoundé. Being based in a blood bank, the university hospital team had "absolutely no problem to get raw material," as Kaptue frankly acknowledged.[22] The IRD project set up a large cohort of patients, who were provided with opportunistic infections treatment (at that time antiretroviral treatments were deemed inaccessible). The American EICAM project had to combine rural surveys throughout the country with the samples from the blood bank of the Central Hospital of Yaoundé, for they "didn't get enough positives, [because] there is low prevalence" in rural areas, a project employee explained to me.[23]

The value taken by blood samples contributed to the revival of the Centre Pasteur, where French expatriates resumed research on AIDS viruses. The biggest medical analysis lab in the country, the CPC, also received, as the National Reference Laboratory for AIDS, thousands of samples from the entire country for confirmation tests of positive cases and could screen them for atypical infections. The CPC also benefited from a "deal" with Sanofi-Diagnostics Pasteur (one of the commercial branches of the Pasteur Institute in Paris and a world leader in the HIV diagnostic industry): in exchange for samples from Cameroon, the firm provided, for free, the CPC with their diagnostic kits. The bargain was timely: the devaluation of the CFA franc currency on January 1, 1994, doubled the cost of imported goods, while the Centre Pasteur was unable to pay most of its suppliers. Here the privatization of research was instrumental to scientific success and even institutional renaissance (Lachenal 2002, 2005).

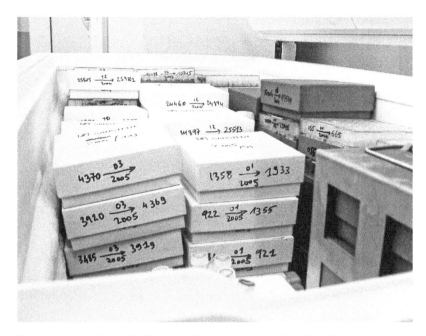

Figure 3.2. Serum bank (*sérothèque*). A refrigerator at the virology lab of the Centre Pasteur du Cameroun, storing several years of seras sampled in local populations using the medical analysis lab. The retrospective screening of the bank was instrumental in the identification of infections with atypical HIV (Lachenal, 2006).

The research on Cameroonian viruses made tangible a change of era: a shift from the welfarist public health of the late colonial and postindependence period to the transnational interventions against emerging diseases of the neoliberal times. The transition took the form of a historical short circuit in Yaoundé. To take one example, one of the latest projects studying Cameroonian HIVs was arranged for the American FDA in the abandoned wings of the Service d'Hygiene Mobile et de Prophylaxie, the very service that used to be in charge of the national mass medical campaigns (from vaccination to DDT spraying) until their disruption in the 1980s. The vestige of the Cameroonian welfare state kept its name, "Hygiene Mobile"; its walls were simply whitened, and freezers installed to store the HIV-positive blood samples before their transatlantic shipment to the FDA.

It would be misleading, however, to interpret this change as the mere manifestation of a "collapse of the state." In spite of its minimalism, the research was never clandestine or fully externalized: it was always funded as formal "projects" associated with centennial public (or para-public) institutions of tropical medical research in the north and always firmly linked to Cameroonian state institutions. Therefore the "scramble for Cameroon" initiated by the discovery of HIV-1 O was rather a sign, in the realm of science, of what Jean-François Bayart and Béatrice Hibou termed the "privatization of the state"—that is, the appropriation by local elites of positions within the formal state apparatus to select, control, and monopolize connections with the international and/or private sector (Hibou 1998, 1999, 2004). The "scramble" was not so much a product of Western greed but rather an episode in the wider political history of Cameroon's extraversion (Bayart 2000). As Fred Eboko (1999) has shown, Cameroonian AIDS doctors have never been passive objects manipulated by Western actors and interests: as they negotiated blood samples, official authorizations, and PhD grants for local students, they rather capitalized on, and sometimes actively constructed, their unequal connection with the external realm of global health institutions.

More Viruses to Come: "Bushmeat" and
the Simian Reservoir of HIV

By the end of the 1990s, the results of a few years of research were both sensational and disappointing. A series of new viruses—meaning patents, papers, research grants, and keynote lectures—were found in Cameroon. As judged by auto-referential criterions, the scientific output approached perfection. For instance, six of the ten most cited papers ever published in or about Cameroon in biomedical sciences are works on HIV variants.[24]

The most important was the isolation of a new group of HIV-1, the HIV-1 group N. Starting from 1993 the large-scale work done by the CPC, with the help of Sanofi Diagnostics, led to the identification of dozens of cases of group O infections, but it also led to "indeterminate" cases. Among these, a woman showed clinical signs of full blown AIDS but gave strange results in blood tests. Philippe Mauclere, the French military doctor in charge of virology at the CPC, elucidated the puzzle with the help of top-level virologists based in Paris. The patient was infected with a new atypical virus, different from all known strains and original enough to be patented by Sanofi. The discovery of the HIV-1 group N, for "Non M, Non O," was featured in 1998 in *Nature Medicine* (Simon et al. 1998). In another coincidence, the publication of the "biggest" paper ever published at the CPC came only weeks after a layoff of half of the staff, and a 50 percent pay cut for the remaining employees, as part of the "structural adjustment" of the institution.

Despite these successes, the search for patients infected with HIV-1 O or other atypical viruses proved unrewarding. O-infected patients were rare. After tens of thousands of tests, the CPC identified less than one hundred cases. In total, HIV-1 O infections accounted for fewer than 2 percent of all HIV infections in Cameroon. Even better, that prevalence rate actually decreased between 1989 and 1998 (Ayouba et al. 2001). In other words, there were no emerging viruses in sight.

The isolation of HIV-1 N in 1998 confirmed the low epidemicity of HIV variants. Only five cases, after more than 20,000 specific tests, were identified in Cameroon in the next years (Roques et al. 2004; Yamaguchi, Coffey et al. 2006; Yamaguchi, McArthur et al. 2006) — "a rare bird," as a commentator had foreseen in *Nature Medicine* (Wain-Hobson 1998). In addition, most standard tests easily detected HIV-1 N infections, which rendered useless the patent owned by the Pasteur Institute in Paris and Sanofi — and less explosive the fact that no Cameroonian institutions or individuals had signed it. In sum, the scenario of the emergence worldwide of undetectable human HIVs originating from Cameroon lost its efficiency. The emerging viruses did not emerge.

TALES OF ORIGIN

In their publications, researchers in the field turned toward another register of communication, more contemplative but not less efficient. It was centered on the evolutionary history of HIV or, for the lay public, on the "origin of AIDS." The discovery of HIV-2 and HIV-1 O had brought important clues, since both viruses were found to be genetically close to SIVs infecting, respectively, various West African monkeys and the Central African chimpanzees (SIVcpz). In 1994 it was hoped that the study of HIV-1 O in comparison with the SIVcpz found in Cameroon could "lead to the origin of HIV-1," the virus causing the AIDS pandemic (Vanden Haesevelde et al. 1994). The "aberrant virus" pointed out that the country could be "the birthplace of HIV-1" (Goudsmit 1997, 177). The discovery of HIV-1 N reinforced that view: though anecdotic from a public health perspective, it featured as the closest parent of the known specimens of SIVcpz.

The issue of the origin of AIDS had gained a considerable public importance in 1999 with the release of *The River*, the 1,000-page-long book by the

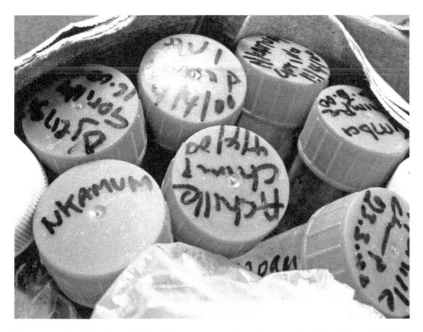

Figure 3.3. Samples (serum) from chimpanzees and gorillas stored at the virology lab of the Centre Pasteur du Cameroun (Lachenal, 2006).

British journalist Ed Hooper (1999), which claimed that HIV-1 had been transmitted from chimpanzees to humans through contaminated oral polio vaccines distributed in the Belgian Congo in the late 1950s. The controversy caused by *The River* stimulated investigations on the evolutionary history of HIV and a quest for samples from Central African chimpanzees and humans. More important, the origin of AIDS debate offered a tribune to the teams working in Yaoundé.[25]

This was an additional enticement to launch surveys of SIV infection in Cameroonian "nonhuman primates." From 1997, most teams working in Yaoundé had begun to collect samples from local monkeys and apes. The few animals living in zoos, primate sanctuaries, or kept as pets were immediately targeted (and keenly contested). But the most extensive studies used another source: blood sampled from the meat of apes and monkeys sold on markets, as part of the well-established trade of wild game meat—the so-called bushmeat (*viande de brousse*). A couple of years later in 2002, most teams began to use noninvasive methods, extracting viral RNA from wild animal feces. The hunt was successful. Dozens of new SIVs were identified in Cameroonian primates. The breakthrough, however, did not come from Cameroon's forests. In February 1999 a team led by Beatrice Hahn (certainly the most prominent retrovirologist in the United States)[26] at the University of Alabama announced that they had "solved the puzzle of HIV origins" in a *Nature* article, relayed by CNN coverage and a plenary lecture at the Conference on Retroviruses and Opportunistic Infections, the major yearly conference in retrovirology (Gao et al. 1999). Hahn (1999) presented the analysis of a new SIVcpz isolated from a U.S. chimpanzee of unknown origin, compared it to existing HIVs and SIVs genetic sequences, and concluded that chimpanzees, especially those found in Cameroon and other areas of west equatorial Africa, were the "host and reservoir" of HIV-1, which was transmitted to humans on three occasions, creating the three known groups of HIV-1: the Main group M and the "Cameroonians," N and O.

TALES OF EMERGENCE

The evolutionary puzzle being officially "solved," another genre of scientific narratives came out by 2001 and 2002. It extended the scenario of the origin of HIV to draw the perspective of imminent catastrophes for public health. It was mainly put forward by Beatrice Hahn, who collaborated with the Franco-Cameroonian team of the IRD (Hahn et al. 2000). It consisted of a synthesis between the early warnings on emerging HIVs and the "narratives of origin" dominant afterward. The message did not consist of new virological scoops but in a reconsideration of existing data to claim that the AIDS epidemic was a "zoonosis"—that is, a disease caused by animal-to-human transmission in the past (planting HIV-1 and HIV-2 in human populations) *but also in the present and future*. There were "more viruses to come" (Schoofs 1999).[27] What mattered was the "risk to human health from a plethora of SIV in primate bushmeat" found in Cameroon, as Hahn's group abruptly titled a paper in *Emerging Infectious Diseases*, the high-profile journal edited by the CDC (Peeters et al. 2002). Contamination by retroviruses during the butchery and eating of bushmeat might cause, the team warned, the pandemic emergence of HIV-3 or HIV-4.[28]

Fundamental to the argument—and to its success with Western media—was visual evidence of slaughtered ape and monkey carcasses sold for meat (Hahn et al. 2000). In 1998 Beatrice Hahn had contacted a Swiss photographer based in Kenya named Karl Amman, asking him to provide her with expertise on bushmeat (cited in Peterson 2003, 97–98). Amman, who had spent several years campaigning against bushmeat hunting, sent her photos and notes, which later made Hahn audiences "groan with disgust" (Schoofs

1999). The pictures, regularly used from 2001, assured Hahn unexpected media coverage. They sealed a coalition between conservationists and sociologists: "I am today convinced that the virus angle is our last and best hope to turn the bushmeat issue into a crisis scenario as far as the public in the west is concerned," Amman predicted once when proposing his pictures to the *National Geographic* (cited in Peterson 2003, 100). On the other hand, the virologists got their "story": according to their scenario, Cameroon was this special (and insecure) place where HIV originated and where HIV-3 could appear. They became entitled to propose their own development policy for the sake of human health: "it is in all our interests to put into place economic alternatives to help people move away from hunting and eating these animals," said Nathan Wolfe, who competed with Hahn and her French collaborators in the domain of bushmeat catastrophism, to *CBS News* in March 2004.

The EICAM project led by Wolfe gave a new dimension to these scientific narratives. Published from 2004 in first-class journals (Wolfe, Prosser et al. 2004; Wolfe, Switzer et al. 2004; Kalish et al. 2005; Wolfe, Daszak et al. 2005; Wolfe, Heneine et al. 2005), the results were groundbreaking. The study of hundreds of hunters, butchers, and consumers of bushmeat demonstrated, for the first time, an ongoing exchange of retroviruses between apes and humans. That these retroviruses (SFV and STLV) were actually not related to HIVs was not put forward (Wolfe, Switzer et al. 2004; Wolfe, Heneine et al. 2005): the results of Wolfe's group brought precision and a touch of finesse to the bushmeat hypothesis; by comparison, earlier warnings by Hahn's group appeared as rough speculations. The success not only confirmed the international significance of the research done in Cameroon; it also served as a bench test for Wolfe's global project of "viral forecasting" aiming to prevent, from California, the next pandemics before they start.

Emerging Viruses and Their Public: Nihilism as
a Regime of Intervention and Critique

Although it mostly took the quiet form of small projects, the research on Cameroonian viruses had a public significance: it inspired publicized scientifico-cultural narratives and specific public health interventions and became the target of ad hoc criticisms, voiced by scientists, health workers, artists, journalists, as well as lay observers.

Research practices were especially exposed to criticisms denouncing their extractive nature. Very frequently in interviews, researchers were pejoratively termed "DHL researches," limited to the express shipping to the north of biological samples, without a fair repartition of benefits for local scientists, health workers, patients, and communities. All the researchers in the field—be they Cameroonian or expatriates—were very familiar with this criticism and very keen on addressing it with rival teams.

Conflicts between the teams were regular, and the spiciest ones were publicized in the local press. Stories (unproven) are still told of patients needing to be "protected" by one team from the others to avoid repeated blood sampling,[29] or of atypical serums stolen in one group's fridge to be sold to another group. The depiction of a neocolonial "scramble for Cameroon" was hard to avoid, with more than ten international teams competing for blood samples in the same city of Yaoundé, making huge symbolic and financial profits and leaving very few benefits to local communities. Act-Up Paris, for example, denounced in 2002 the French project of the IRD. Following investigations in Yaoundé, the activists accused the French "researchers of self-congratulating in international meetings about the great discoveries [done in Cameroon]," while "feeling authorized to repatriate in the West the blood of the patients, without any regard for the life of the persons they vampirize." The reference to colonialism and exploitation appeared explicitly in the local press, on the occasion of rumors following conflicts between teams, for example when three teams, two of them French, fought for the exclusive use of the same zoo chimpanzee.[30] Similarly, a few journalists and researchers pointed out the stigmatizing overtone of the bushmeat stories.[31] Virologists liked to describe their work as the quest for the "missing link" (e.g., Muller-Trutwin et al. 2000), apparently ignoring the racist history of the nineteenth-century evolutionist metaphor.

Yet most projects could easily disarm such criticisms. The projects not only complied with the international ethical guidelines for research but also they pioneered the importation in Cameroon of the new norms of global ethicism. Surprising as it may seem, virus hunters—be they Cameroonian "big men" or expatriate "bush doctors"—were forerunners in the ethical normalization of research in Cameroon. The paradigmatic illustration was the role of Lazare Kaptue, who created in 1987 the National Ethics Committee of Cameroon and became its first (and so far, its only) president. Just as the Cameroonian archetype of the medical "patron" became the official critique of "medical paternalism" in local bioethics gigs, AIDS specialists in Cameroon led the way in the appropriation of the latest jargons of ethics and human rights activism. This innovative role had material effects, as virological studies became increasingly coupled, from 2001, with pilot schemes for antiretroviral treatment or the prevention of mother-to-child transmission. In addition, the value of patients carrying atypical viruses had sometimes positive effects: in the IRD project, they were included in priority in the treatment cohort, even after the recruitment was officially closed—their atypical infection was a life-saving detail in a context where no other possibility for treatment existed.[32] But as the virus hunters set the values as the vanguard of transnational ethical modernity (Dodier 2003, 2005), for the moral evaluation of research, possibilities for political debates, for example, about the intellectual property of viruses were scarce.[33]

The projects were also designed as exemplary collaborations—*capacity building* and other keywords were never forgotten in their presentations. The coauthorship of discoveries enacted the equity between individual partners but marginalized claims for compensations at the national scale. The projects were also exemplary of a new managerial style and spirit,[34] in rupture with an austere past of "neocolonialism." No white-coat gangsters à la John Le Carré in Yaoundé: as the media coverage made clear, research partners from the north and the south were *friends*, local populations laughed with them, Nathan Wolfe was *cool*, and all were committed to cutting-edge science.[35] In this context the denunciations of virus hunters as "FedEx researchers" were both omnipresent and inoffensive.

SCIENTIFIC NIHILISM EXPOSED

Such an impasse may explain the emergence of an alternative regime of critique. It derided virologists not for their greed but rather for their impotence, for their inaction and, at the same time, their theatricalized commitment to fight fictive viruses. What surfaced here, although in veiled form, is a radical critique of the nihilistic turn of research on HIV.

Seen from Yaoundé, the avalanche of discoveries had baroque manifestations. "A New Retrovirus Discovered in Cameroon" became a recurring headline of local newspapers. When the discovery of the HIV-1 O was announced "people on the streets were afraid," recalled a Cameroonian nurse, "when it is said that another virus has been discovered one more time, people says 'look, [AIDS] is going to augment again, there is one more virus.'"[36] The discovery of HIV-1 N was equally worrying. Published on a "fast-track" process in *Nature Medicine* in August 1998, the discovery scooped everybody, including its own French authors who were all on holiday break in France. The local press and the Ministry of Health were informed through French newspapers. At the CPC, the embarrassing task of speaking to local journalists was left to a junior Cameroonian researcher who was not associated with the paper. The next day, the national daily *Cameroon Tribune* wrongly proclaimed, in full front page, the discovery of HIV-3 in Cameroon.[37]

Later, when it was announced that Cameroon was the "birthplace of HIV," most local commentators underlined that there were more urgent issues in the field of AIDS research. Yet this was a rather heavy contribution to the world's health to bear, at the moment when the head of the state, represented by the First Lady Chantal Biya, aimed to lead Pan-African responses to AIDS.[38] It was not without irony that the inauguration of Chantal Biya's international humanitarian program to fight AIDS, Synergies Africaines, brought to Yaoundé the two enemies, "fathers" of HIV Luc Montagnier and Robert Gallo, for two days of ceremonies. Although both of them were fading lights in the AIDS academy, the theatricalization of their reconciliation was meant to catch the attention of the local and African press: twenty years of dispute on the virus paternity ended in public celebrations, under Biya's patronage. Did the reconciled fathers agree on the "birthplace" location? Pressed by journalists to take a position, Montagnier, who was accustomed to prophetic declarations (he frequently announced in the 1980s and 1990s the imminence of an AIDS vaccine), asserted that "AIDS does not come from Cameroon."[39] By denying a decade of virological findings, Montagnier reassured everybody. Maybe against his will, he suggested the absurd potential of his own science.

Such ceremonials did not leave the public passive and silent. Counternarratives on the iatrogenic origin of AIDS, reinforced by the wide impact of Hooper's book, never ceased to circulate in Cameroon and responded to bushmeat theories—which were anyhow, in spite of their broadcast on CNN, often ignored in Cameroon. Addressed to virus hunters, a critique of medical hubris and impotence resurfaced. The old Professor Montagnier, for example, was acclaimed in Yaoundé; yet his association with the Biya couple backfired. He was also derided, just as his presidential host, as an incarnation of aging masculinity and nihilism: "When that Professor, the one who discovered the HIV, came here, Montagnier, people said: 'Yes, he discovered the virus, but has he discovered the medicine?' People would acclaim

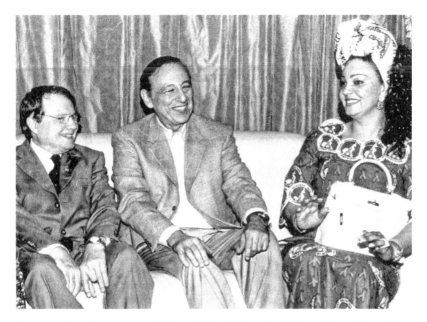

Figure 3.4. Luc Montagnier and Robert Gallo with First Lady Chantal Biya during their visit in 2002. According to Vincent Hugeux, the event was arranged by Paul Biya's French spin doctors and involved important cash remunerations for Montagnier and Gallo (Hugeux 2007). Photograph published in the pan-African journal *Afrique Education* 121 (December 1–15, 2002): 14–17.

him because he discovered the virus . . . then what? Because if economists do research, the crisis has to finish. If doctors and researchers on health do research, disease has to finish."[40]

FIGHTING HIV-3: PUBLIC HEALTH AS PRETENSE

The critiques evoked here might seem anecdotal, if absurdity and inaction had not constituted the core of public health interventions against emerging HIVs in Cameroon.

Two major types of intervention were imagined to fight HIV-3. The first was a surveillance network to monitor the transmission of retroviruses from apes to humans, so as to detect and contain emerging pathogens before they reached the general population—that is, the rest (West) of the world. The most impressive project, organized with the support of the U.S. military and the NIH, screened "sentinel populations" in Cameroon to detect emerging retroviral infections (curiously the "sentinels" were often recruited among captive populations, such as plantation workers and the military, which were easy for the project team to follow up). As explained above, the "viral forecasting" idea has met with massive success and enabled its charismatic leader to raise millions of dollars.

The second type of intervention was more modest: a health education campaign. To avoid the apparition of HIV-3 and HIV-4, Cameroonians had to be educated about the risks of bushmeat consumption. A brochure was prepared and printed by the Cameroon Ministry of Environment, with the support of the French scientists of the IRD. Explicit drawings and pedagogic texts sought to translate the viral hazards of bushmeat to the lay public. Obviously, not mentioned in the leaflet was the absence of scientific consensus about the risk of seeing a new pandemic HIV emerging from bushmeat—the works presenting "AIDS as zoonosis" were indeed criticized by major specialists in the field as entirely speculative, not to say dishonest (Apetrei, Robertson, and Marx 2004; Marx, Apetrei, and Drucker 2004). On the contrary, the campaign was mentioned by virologists in interviews and conferences as the "prevention campaign," which concluded and retrospectively justified "basic research"—in other words, the warnings brought HIV-3 into existence before it was even detected; the significance of the bushmeat crisis for global health was, at the same time, constructed and demonstrated. As the science studies have well shown in other cases, the public communication on the risk was a crucial step to stabilize it as a fact, all the more so that the scientific data supporting it was uncertain (Wynne 1996; Latour 2005).

The key point here is that the brochure was circulated very discreetly—my impression is that it was never distributed.[41] The actual intervention seems to have never occurred in practice; it remained fictive, existing only as a document printed, stockpiled, and forgotten, as a story told by scientists and authorities to themselves. The nondistribution might have been caused by bureaucratic obstacles, or by the conversion of scientists to less incendiary, and maybe more relevant, public health interventions. Still I would like to suggest that the nonintervention was not accidental, that it revealed a problematic relationship between research and intervention—a relationship that I propose to term *nihilistic*.

First, because scientists themselves assumed that it was impossible to act, their expertise constructed and named major obstacles to their action. They not only acknowledged but *stressed* the "complexity" of the bushmeat issue, depicted as the redeployment of a "traditional" practice in the middle of economic crisis, corruption, and the extension of logging concessions in south-

Le lien entre les singes et nous

Les singes et les Hommes sont apparentés.
Ensemble, nous formons un groupe connu sous
le nom de *primates*.

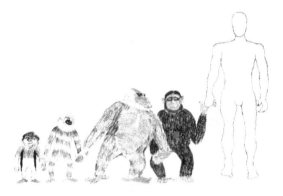

Quelle est l'une des conséquences majeures d'être apparentés aux singes ?

Les hommes et les singes étant apparentés,
certaines maladies peuvent nous être
transmises lors de contacts étroits entre eux et
nous.

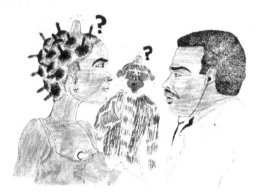

Figures 3.5 and 3.6. Educational leaflet "We and the apes," edited by the project PRESICA (IRD, France). The brochure explains the proximity of humans with apes and monkeys and the various diseases, including SIV infections, which may be transmitted from them. It gives recommendations for the better care of animals kept as pets and the avoidance of bushmeat.

Que peut-on faire pour éviter la transmission de ces maladies :

Nous pouvons réduire les contacts entre nous
et les singes en *évitant* :

- De chasser, manipuler, voir consommer de
  la viande de brousse

east Cameroon. Combined with "African culture," these were rather strong enemies to overcome for "public health prevention." Virologists' politico-cultural ambitions shrank, reflecting the more general move inherent to the "emerging diseases worldview": a shift from the colonial ideals of "conversion" (of Africans to modern public health through education) to programs of "integration" of irremediably different localities into techno-scientific circulations and surveillance networks (King 2002). Implicit to that turn were essentialist approaches to "culture" (no one seriously hoped to reform African habits anymore) and a nihilistic approach to public health. In the world constructed by bushmeat narratives, biomedicine *cannot* intervene, just measure and map global hazards. Not only that: it *must not* intervene. Field scientists, indeed, recommended nonintervention (and sometimes the dissimulation of the research aims), because they considered that educative messages on bushmeat, and even any public communication on "simian AIDS," could lead to "misunderstandings" and incidents with local populations and eventually undermine the whole scientific enterprise.

An additional nihilistic trait is that, according to the bushmeat hypothesis, biomedicine *never* intervened in the history of AIDS. Presenting AIDS as a zoonosis silenced the role of medical interventions (such as blood transfusions) in the emergence of the epidemic during the colonial period, by preferring irrefutable explanations based on the "disorders of decolonization."[42] According to Jacques Leibowitch, an iconoclastic figure in the French AIDS academy, the bushmeat hypothesis defined an "ecological-chic" paradigm.[43] *Ecological* because it naturalized the origin of AIDS by giving the first role to (implicitly abnormal) contacts between apes and humans; *chic*, because it ensured distinguished media coverage and a "clean" role to the medical profession as virus hunters and sentinels of global public health, but not as decisive historical factors for the expansion of the epidemic.

Another nihilistic trait is that scientists came to disavow their own statements. Several researchers based in Yaoundé, whether expatriates or Cameroonians, were very critical toward the "bushmeat angle" defended by senior American and French authors,[44] but the structure of collaborations silenced their voices. The task of writing papers indeed fell to junior scientists trained in phylogeny or molecular virology and to the heads of teams in the north, who mastered the art of "taking the maximum out of the data" to publish in the best journals. The other members of multinational teams often softened their criticisms, if they had some, given the sensational potential of the publications. What is problematic here is not the apparent overdetermination of scientific discourses by publishing strategies—what Edward Hooper called the "Hollywooding of science" when criticizing what he called the "bushmeat group," not without contradiction given his own success with storytelling.[45] It is rather the acknowledged ignorance and unaccountability of scientists about their own arguments. An insider glance at the coauthors' list leads to this remark: those who write acknowledge that they "know nothing" about Cameroon; those who (may) know acknowledge that they write nothing.[46]

Although the "viral forecasting" project refined the tone of the first works on bushmeat viruses, a similar criticism may be addressed to it. In its official presentations the project illustrates, rather brutally, the logics of triage inherent to global biosecurity visions: it contrasts the prevention of viral emergence, presented as a methodological breakthrough, with "current interventions" presented as failures and pejoratively described as "wait-and-respond" approaches—health workers in Africa will appreciate the compliment.[47] As the prose of viral forecasting draws a clear opposition between the prevention of future diseases and the care for present ones, the classic critique of the "biosecurity paradigm" can be recalled here: the talk on the "*next* pandemic" implies present and problematic choices in resource allocations, possibly at the expense of the mobilization against present catastrophes; it orders the values of present lives; it participates, in more general terms, in a fiction that devaluates the care for real life—the Nieztschean definition of nihilism (Deleuze 1962, 169–70).[48]

In its hubris and absurdity—how to recognize a "pandemic" when it has been stopped before it started?—the forecasting project points toward another general issue. The efforts made in Cameroon to define HIV-3—a nonexistent virus—as a public health priority epitomize, rather than a "securitization" of public health, the turn toward a regime of largely *fictive* interventions. Although any prevention act implies fictions about the future, the remark is not trivial. In the case of simian viruses, the neoliberal "reforms" prevented the state from enforcing the very policies its experts prescribed: the control of bushmeat trade was made illusory, not only by the always lamented "corruption" but also by the initial dismantlement—under the guidance of international authorities—of the state's capacity to police anything. The eradication of a thriving sector of Cameroon's informal economy seemed at odds with the latest principles of international development.[49] These double binds, and the paralysis they provoke when it comes to *acting*, suggest to us not to overestimate the practical effects of great projects of surveillance. Public health policy seems to be more about performance and pretense than discipline and control.

EPILOGUE: FROM SIMIAN AIDS TO AVIAN FLU

In recent years in Cameroon, other zoogenic menaces surpassed "simian AIDS" in terms of politico-scientific mobilization and public amazement.

The avian flu hit Cameroon in March 2006, when two domestic ducks were found dead and infected with the H5N1 virus in the north of the country. The reaction of the state was immediate and impressive. A large interministerial committee was created, and it imposed a ban on the exportation of eggs and chicken in and out of the country—which proved effective in ruining small producers of poultry and generating widespread anxiety. The scientific mobilization was equally impressive. It saw most institutions involved in the research on emerging HIVs reconvert to seize the many opportunities for funding offered as part of international efforts to monitor the global spread of H5N1. For example, the virology lab of CPC became the WHO national reference center for influenza in Cameroon, while the EICAM project led by Nathan Wolfe added influenza among the "emerging infectious diseases" placed under its surveillance and, furthermore, tried to secure its local position as the main local expert in "pandemic preparedness."

The continuity with the mobilization against emerging HIVs had more profound manifestations. As elsewhere in the world, the avian flu crisis saw the generalization of a new public health technique: the *simulation exercise*, which by definition consisted of fighting fictive threats with fictive means. The first one was organized on October 13, 2008, in the gardens of the Sawa Hotel, one of the most prestigious hotels of Douala. Sponsored by the USAID and the FAO (Food and Agriculture Organization), the workshop brought together representatives of the health and veterinary services, as well as delegates of various local authorities, international organizations, and development agencies based in Cameroon.

Gathered during four days in a seminar room, the attendees simulated the response to the imaginary detection of cases of avian flu among chickens in Cameroon and played their own role in the outbreak scenario. In light of this event, the nonimplemented education campaign against the non-emerging HIV-3 seems less incongruous: it prefigured this strange regime of biopolitical government, where the simulated mobilization against a fictive threat becomes a public health priority.

The public debates about avian flu gave Cameroonian journalists and

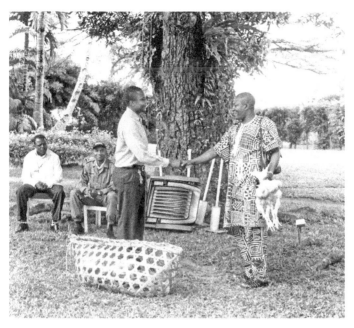

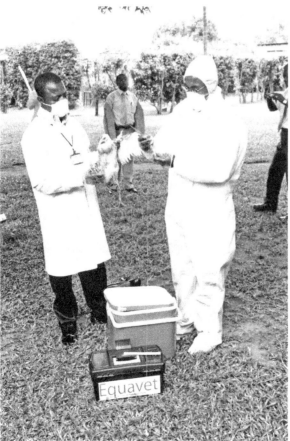

Figures 3.7 and 3.8. Simulating an avian flu outbreak at the Sawa Hotel, Douala (2008). Scanned photographs (author unknown) from the website http://www.cameractu.net, accessed on October 10, 2009.

scholars such as Joseph Owona Ntsama the opportunity to question, often with courage, the rather disproportionate response of the government and its international advisers[50]—two dead ducks, hundreds of ruined farmers, and billions of CFA francs spent. Popular reactions also systematized, in humorous ways, the critique of the emerging diseases rationale, which appeared about simian AIDS. The avian flu crisis inspired a well-known song from the Ivorian singer DJ Lewis. Named "Grippe Aviaire," the song is a *coupé-décalé* hit, which became a pan-African success in 2006. It was praised by government officials in the Ivory Coast as an attempt to "dedramatize" the problem of avian flu.[51] Its meaning, however, is more complex. In the video clip and during his live performances, DJ Lewis and his dancers transformed themselves into zombies (half naked and painted in white) dancing a "chicken dance." The shocking potential of the video contributed to the success of the song, as it played crudely with images of madness, disease, and death, as well as possession and exorcism: one of the repeated choruses of the song (coupé-décalé can be very repetitive) is "sors de ce corps!" ("move out of this body!"), as if a "chicken spirit" was asked to the leave the body of a sick dancer.[52]

Interpreting the song as an anecdotal example of an "African response" to the avian flu, as it has been done in the European press, is unfair. It is unfair because of its huge success and because of the rich African history of dances linked to epidemics—the 1958 Asian flu was named "cha cha cha" in Cameroon, after the Cuban dance that spread worldwide in the late fifties (Kuoh Moukouri 1963, 180), while AIDS inspired dozens of songs on the continent—and because it carries a precise and precious critique, the suggestion that the whole avian flu story is inherently insane, at least when it is seen from Africa. "On n'a qu'à être fou"—"Now, we just have to be mad": the second repeated chorus can also be understood as a more general proposition, that is, the reasonable way to react to the situation is to account for its insanity.

The Cameroonian reception of the song made this message more explicit. A group of humorists, led by stand-up artists Fingon Tralala and Tagne Condom, recorded their own (outrageous) video with DJ Lewis's music and lyrics.[53] Their work drew on the local taste for "play-backs"—many cabarets in Cameroon abandoned live music in 2003–5, assuming that play-back imitations were more modern than original performances. The video was controversial, but most amateurs argued that it was a successful attempt to prove more daring and shocking than the Ivorian DJ—that the imitation

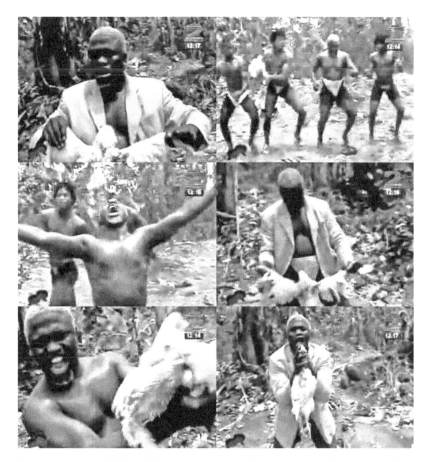

Figure 3.9. Fingon Tralala and Tagne Condom's parody of DJ Lewis's "Grippe Aviaire." Screengrabs from the video clip posted on YouTube, originally on the private TV channel Canal 2 (Douala), http://www.youtube.com/watch?v=9WiLsxbq8Vs&feature=related, accessed on June 1, 2009.

was definitely more interesting than the original. The Cameroonians won on the scale of scandal: the Tagne and Fingon video showed four madmen possessed by the "chicken disease," attained by epilepsy-like seizures, wearing women's underwear, playing with a live chicken, killing it, trying to eat it raw, and mimicking sexual relations with it.

Although its critical dimension is not explicit, this parody of a parody may refer to another insane theater play: the public performance of state and science power that followed the discovery of avian flu cases. DJ Lewis's and Fingon's comic gestures indicate that the old critique of medicine as farcical (Porter 2001, 24–25) can be reactivated in a context where preparedness plans for flu pandemics have transformed "exercises of simulations" into elaborated forms of inaction, which one may find, given the state of the local public health systems and the resources mobilized for such fictive actions, obscene and crazy.

This chapter has deliberately left aside most of the biomedical efforts done in Cameroon during the last two decades, which proceeded from more desirable modes of collaborations and health government (Gruénais 2001). By choosing an atypical story, my aim was not to make any great claim about "nihilism as the name of neoliberal biomedicine," but rather to propose a heuristic hypothesis to examine the place of hubris, simulation, and pretense in the politics and techniques of global health in Africa.

This study may help enrich our understanding of what neoliberal globalization did to science and medicine in Africa, and it may help us imagine critical ways to engage with this transformation.

First, the scientific effervescence that marked the hunt for Cameroonian HIVs complicates narratives on the "collapse of public health" and the retreat of the nation-state. Although the crumbling of public institutions formed the background of the hunt for Cameroonian viruses, such depiction would hinder the successful nature of the process, from the point of view of medical scientists themselves, and the reinforcement and valuation of their positions within the state apparatus (Hibou 2004) — that the most successful Cameroonian virus hunter was a colonel in the army makes it clear that the state did not "fail."

Second, the emerging diseases worldview, which framed most of the research related in this chapter, is often described as the age of security, surveillance, and global interconnectedness. The analysis developed above rather describes it as a regime of pretense and fictions, especially from a local African perspective where the material capacity of the state to intervene is constrained by its limited resources (to use a euphemism) and where the circulations that are supposed to perform the "global health era" have never been so restricted in recent history, above all by the European policies of "migration control" (to use another euphemism).

The fact that Nathan Wolfe, who likes to compare his work with "preventive" action against terrorism, has been a scientific consultant for the movie *I Am Legend* (a "viral apocalypse" film starring Will Smith) is not accidental:

spectacle, under this regime, is what matters. As scientists play at fighting imaginary public health threats, we should not forget that this way of pretending and dramatizing governmental interventions has a crucial function in the African context, which Jean and John Comaroff have well captured in their work on the simulation of car accidents by the South African police: that of a "simulacrum of governance, a rite staged to make actual and authoritative, at least in the eyes of an executive bureaucracy, the activity of those responsible for law and order. And by extension, to enact the very possibility of government" (Comaroff and Comaroff 2006, 289).

Notes

1 A detailed presentation of the project, with original publications as well as press coverage is available on the project website, http://globalviral.org/.

2 The expression appears under different versions in press releases, articles, and interviews. See, for example, Ratliff (2007).

3 Quoted from the portrait of Nathan Wolfe on the UCLA School of Public Health website. Accessed September 27, 2008. http://www.ph.ucla.edu/faculty _profiles.html.

4 The expression is equivalent for the French *viande de brousse*. It refers locally to the meat of wild game, from small rodents to bigger animals, and more specifically in the debates about viruses to the meat of monkeys and apes.

5 For a controversial example of a rationalization as necessary of nontreatment of Africa patients, see Marseille, Hofmann, and Kahn (2002).

6 For a radical critique of bioethical discourse as a form of nihilism, see Badiou and Hallward (2001).

7 On Céline's medical utopianism and nihilism, see Roussin (2005, chap. 2, 84–140). On colonial medicine and colonial epidemics, see Sartre (2007).

8 For a wide account of the politics of the AIDS fight in Cameroon, see Eboko (1996, 1999, 2002, 2005).

9 "Santé: Les options du gouvernement." *Cameroon Tribune*, no. 5688, September 27, 1994.

10 On the political and economic crisis, see also Collectif (1996), and especially Courade and Sindjoun (1996).

11 Interviews with the author, 2002, 2009.

12 Interview with the author, 2002.

13 For a general presentation, see Iliffe (2006, 65–79); and in the case of Cameroon, see Eboko (1999).

14 Interview with the author, 2008.

15 Memo from the FDA, Center for Biologic Evaluation and Research, "Interim Recommendations for Deferral of Donors at Increased Risk for HIV-1 Group O Infection," December 11, 1996.

16 An insider history of AIDS research at the Institute of Tropical Medicine (ITG) is available online. See the ITG website: "A Bridge between Two Worlds," http://www.itg.be/internet/geschiedenis/index.html. The story of the Projet Sida in Kinshasa, cosponsored by the ITM and the CDC, has been told several times, often in romanticized versions; for example, see Preston (1994).

17 The name HIV-3 appears in the patent number 88109200 (European Patent Office), deposited on June 9, 1988. On ANT-70, see Vanderborght, DeLeys, and Van Geel (1988); DeLeys et al. (1990).

18 For an overview of patents in the domain of AIDS diagnostic, see Reina (2003). For a more developed analysis of patents in the field of HIV in Cameroon, see Lachenal (2006).

19 Estimated from *Innogenetics Annual Report for the Year 2002* (58–59).

20 Peter Ndumbe had specialized in London as an immunologist and got his PhD from the London School of Tropical Medicine and Hygiene. He had come back to Yaoundé in 1985 with an appointment as a professor at the faculty of medicine. Though he was not directly involved in the fight against AIDS, he had several international commitments, being for example the local spokesperson of the WHO for vaccinations programs.

21 Unlike many other biomaterials (from cells to DNA) serums carrying the immunological trace of HIV infection are neither cultivable nor duplicable; they assume as such a quantitative economic value. The fact was well known: hospitals' "serums banks" (*sérothèques*) were frequently "hired" to serve as reference for the industry; small firms specialized in the trade of rare serums (namely, SeraCare Life Sciences and its subsidiary BBI Diagnostics); the saying goes that in the late 1980s, "in certain Parisian laboratories, a millilitre of HIV-2 serum would be sold for a fortune."

22 Interview with the author, 2002.

23 Interview with the author, 2002.

24 Total number of citations on April 26, 2007, via ISI-Web of Science, Research on "Cameroon" in all fields. Papers in earth sciences and plant sciences were excluded from the count.

25 For example, the meeting organized at the Royal Society in 2001 to discuss the origin of AIDS, in the presence of Ed Hooper, involved Leopold Zekeng and many other Cameroon-linked scientists (Zekeng 2001).

26 Beatrice Hahn is a former student of Robert Gallo and one of the world's leading specialists of HIV science.

27 Mark Schoofs won the Pulitzer Prize for his series of articles on AIDS in Africa. He extensively related the case of Cameroon in his paper on HIV basic science.

28 The use of the expression "HIV-3 or HIV-4" is a classical conclusion in oral presentations of the team at conferences (for example, Courgnaud, IAS 2003; Akogeng, ANRS 2005). The fact that it is likely to be unfounded may explain why it does not appear in publications.

29 Interviews with the author, 2002 and 2003.

30 The incident was reported in the *Post* (Limbe), no. 0071, June 1, 1998. It is evoked in Eboko (1999).

31 Leopold Zekeng and other Cameroonian researchers regularly denounced the "bushmeat" argument as racist. See, for example, Zekeng interviewed in Schoofs (1999).

32 Interview with the author, 2003.

33 On the depoliticizing effects of transnational discourses of ethics and rights, see Englund (2006).

34 I refer here to Boltanski and Chiappello's (1999) analysis of the ethos of neoliberal capitalism.

35 For a recent example, see Nathan Wolfe's profile in the *New Yorker*, December 20, 2010.

36 Interview with the author, 2003.

37 The misunderstanding has been mentionned in Eboko (1999).

38 On Chantal Biya's humanitarian project, see Eboko, "Chantal Biya: 'Fille du peuple' et égérie internationale."

39 Montagnier confirmed his position later in an interview with a local newspaper, "Le Sida ne vient pas du Cameroun," *Mutations*, July 3, 2006.

40 Interview with the author, 2002.

41 At the time of my latest inquiry in 2005.

42 For alternative views, see Drucker, Alcabes, and Marx (2001); Marx, Alcabes, and Drucker (2001); Schneider and Drucker (2006).

43 Personal communication, 2008.

44 Interviews with the author, 2003.

45 Ed Hooper, "'The Hollywooding of Science.' Beatrice Hahn's latest SIV Sequences from Cameroonian Chimps: An Alternative Interpretation," *AIDS Origins* (blog), June 16, 2006, updated August 5, 2006. Accessed September 16, 2007. http://www.aidsorigins.com/content/view/194/2/.

46 Interviews with the author, 2005.

47 See the projects website, http://www.globalviral.org.

48 For example, Altman et al. (2005). For a general overview, see Lakoff and Collier (2008).

49 For an example of official endorsement of nonintervention against bushmeat trade because of "economic and cultural dimensions," see the interview of Leopold Zekeng (then permanent secretary of the CNLS) in the daily *Cameroon Tribune*, November 1, 2004.

50 For a complete study of the response to avian flu in Cameroon, see Owona-Ntsama (2007).

51 See Habibou Bangré, "'La Côte d'Ivoire lance la danse de la grippe aviaire': Une initiative destinée à tordre le cou à la psychose," *Afrik.com*. http://www.afrik.com/article9834.html.

52 The video performance of DJ Lewis's song can be seen at http://www.youtube.com/watch?v=mJd1t-0Yvvc&feature=related. Accessed on June 1, 2009.

53 The video performance of Fingon Tralala and Tagne Condom can be seen at http://www.youtube.com/watch?v=9WiLsxbq8Vs&feature=related. Accessed on June 1, 2009.

References

Altman, S., B. L. Bassler, J. Beckwith, M. Belfort, H. C. Berg, B. Bloom, J. E. Brenchley et al. 2005. "An Open Letter to Elias Zerhouni." *Science* 307, no. 5714: 1409–10.

Anderson, Warwick. 2006. *Colonial Pathologies: American Tropical Medicine, Race and Hygiene in the Philippines.* Durham, NC: Duke University Press.

Apetrei, C., D. L. Robertson, and P. A. Marx. 2004. "The History of sivs and aids: Epidemiology, Phylogeny and Biology of Isolates from Naturally siv Infected Non-Human Primates (nhp) in Africa." *Frontiers in Bioscience* 9: 225–54.

Ayouba, A., P. Mauclere, P. M. Martin, P. Cunin, J. Mfoupouendoun, B. Njinku, S. Souquieres, and F. Simon. 2001. "hiv-1 Group O Infection in Cameroon, 1986 to 1998." *Emerging Infectious Diseases* 7, no. 3: 466–67.

Badiou, Alain, and Peter Hallward. 2001. *Ethics: An Essay on the Understanding of Evil.* New York: Verso.

Bayart, Jean-François. 2000. "Africa in the World: A History of Extraversion." *African Affairs* 99: 217–67.

Boltanski, Luc, and Eve Chiapello. 1999. *Le nouvel esprit du capitalisme.* Paris: Gallimard.

Charneau, P., A. M. Borman, C. Quillent, D. Guetard, S. Chamaret, J. Cohen, G. Remy, L. Montagnier, and F. Clavel. 1994. "Isolation and Envelope Sequence of a Highly Divergent hiv-1 Isolate: Definition of a New hiv-1 Group." *Virology* 205, no. 1: 247–53.

Collectif. 1996. "Le Cameroun dans l'entre-deux." *Politique africaine* 62: 3–14.

Comaroff, Jean, and John L. Comaroff. 2006. "Criminal Obsessions, After Foucault: Postcoloniality, Policing and the Metaphysics of Disorder." In *Law and Disorder in the Postcolony*, edited by J. Comaroff and J. L. Comaroff. Chicago: University of Chicago Press.

Courade, Georges. 2000. *Le désarroi camerounais: L'épreuve de l'économie-monde.* Paris: Karthala.

Courade, Georges, and Luc Sindjoun. 1996. "Introduction au thème: Le Cameroun dans l'entre-deux." *Politique africaine* 62: 3–14.

Deleuze, Gilles. 1962. *Nietzsche et la philosophie.* Paris: Presses universitaires de France.

DeLeys, R. J., B. Vanderborght, M. Vanden Haesevelde, L. Heyndrickx, A. van Geel, C. Wauters, R. Bernaerts, E. Saman, P. Nijs, B. Willems, H. Taelman, G. vander Groen, P. Piot, T. Tersmette, J. G. Huisman, and H. Van Heuverswyn. 1990. "Isolation and Partial Characterization of an Unusual Human Immunodeficieny Retrovirus from Two Persons of West-Central African Origin." *Journal of Virology* 64: 1207–16.

Dodier, Nicolas. 2003. *Leçons politiques de l'épidémie de sida, Cas de figure*. Paris: Editions de l'Ecole des hautes études en sciences sociales.

Dodier, Nicolas. 2005. "Transnational Medicine in Public Arenas: AIDS Treatments in the South." *Culture, Medicine, and Psychiatry* 19: 285–307.

Dondero, T., D. J. Hu, and J. R. George. 1994. "HIV-1 Variants: Yet Another Challenge to Public Health." *Lancet* 343, no. 8910: 1376.

Drucker, E., P. G. Alcabes, and P. A. Marx. 2001. "The Injection Century: Massive Unsterile Injections and the Emergence of Human Pathogens." *Lancet* 358, no. 9297: 1989–92.

Dry, Sarah, and Melissa Leach, eds. 2010. *Epidemics: Science, Governance and Social Justice*. London: Earthscan.

Eboko, Fred. 1996. "L'État camerounais et les cadets sociaux face à la pandémie du sida." *Politique africaine* 64: 135–45.

Eboko, Fred. 1999. "Logiques et contradictions internationales dans le champ du sida au Cameroun." *Autrepart* 12: 123–40.

Eboko, Fred. 2002. "Pouvoirs, Jeunesse et Sida au Cameroun." PhD diss., Sciences Politiques, Université Denis Diderot-Bordeaux II, Bordeaux.

Eboko, Fred. 2005. "Patterns of Mobilization: Political Culture in the Fight against AIDS." In *The African State and the AIDS Crisis*, edited by A. S. Patterson. Burlington: Ashgate.

Englund, Harri. 2006. *Prisoners of Freedom: Human Rights and the African Poor*. California Series in Public Anthropology, 14. Berkeley: University of California Press.

Farmer, Paul. 1999. *Infections and Inequalities: The Modern Plagues*. Berkeley: University of California Press.

Fassin, Didier. 2001. "Au coeur de la cité salubre: La santé publique entre les mots et les choses." In *Critique de la santé publique: Une approche anthropologique*, edited by J. P. Dozon and D. Fassin. Paris: Balland.

Fassin, Didier. 2007. *When Bodies Remember: Experiences and Politics of AIDS in South Africa*. California Series in Public Anthropology, 15. Berkeley: University of California Press.

Foucault, Michel. 2004. *Sécurité, territoire, population: Cours au collège de France, 1977–1978, Hautes études*. Paris: Seuil; Gallimard.

Gao, F., E. Bailes, D. L. Robertson, Y. Chen, C. M. Rodenburg, S. F. Michael, L. B. Cummins, L. O. Arthur, M. Peeters, G. M. Shaw, P. M. Sharp, and B. H. Hahn. 1999. "Origin of HIV-1 in the Chimpanzee Pan Troglodytes Troglodytes." *Nature* 397, no. 6718: 436–41.

Garrett, Laurie. 2000. *Betrayal of Trust: The Collapse of Global Public Health*. New York: Hyperion.

Goudsmit, Jaap. 1997. *Viral Sex: The Nature of AIDS*. Oxford: Oxford University Press.

Greene, Graham. 1961. *A Burnt-Out Case*. London: Heinemann.

Grmek, Mirko D. 1995. *Histoire du sida*. 2nd ed. Paris: Payot.

Gruénais, Marc-Éric, ed. 2001. "Un système de santé en mutation: Le cas du Cameroun." *Bulletin de l'APAD*, no. 21.

Gurtler, L. G., P. H. Hauser, J. Eberle, A. von Brunn, S. Knapp, L. Zekeng, J. M. Tsague, and L. Kaptue. 1994. "A New Subtype of Human Immunodeficiency Virus Type 1 (MVP-5180) from Cameroon." *Journal of Virology* 68, no. 3: 1581–85.

Hahn, B. H. 1999. "The Origin of HIV-1: A Puzzle Solved?" Keynote Lecture, Conference on Retroviruses and Opportunistic Infections, January 31, Chicago.

Hahn, B. H., G. M. Shaw, K. M. De Cock, and P. M. Sharp. 2000. "AIDS as a Zoonosis: Scientific and Public Health Implications." *Science* 287, no. 5453: 607–14.

Hibou, Béatrice. 1998. "Retrait ou rédéploiement de l'Etat?" *Critique Internationale* 1: 151–68.

Hibou, Béatrice. 2004. *Privatizing the State: The CERI Series in Comparative Politics and International Studies*. New York: Columbia University Press.

Hibou, Béatrice, ed. 1999. *La privatisation des Etats*. Paris: Karthala.

Hooper, Edward. 1999. *The River: A Journey to the Source of HIV and AIDS*. Boston: Little, Brown.

Hugeux, Vincent. 2007. *Les sorciers blancs: Enquête sur les faux amis français de l'Afrique*. Paris: Fayard.

Iliffe, John. 2006. *The African AIDS Epidemic: A History*. Oxford: James Currey.

Kalish, M. L., N. D. Wolfe, C. B. Ndongmo, J. McNicholl, K. E. Robbins, M. Aidoo, P. N. Fonjungo, G. Alemnji, C. Zeh, C. F. Djoko, E. Mpoudi-Ngole, D. S. Burke, and T. M. Folks. 2005. "Central African Hunters Exposed to Simian Immunodeficiency Virus." *Emergency Infectious Diseases* 11, no. 12: 1928–30.

King, Nicholas B. 2002. "Security, Disease, Commerce: Ideologies of Postcolonial Global Health." *Social Studies of Science* 32, no. 5: 763–89.

King, Nicholas B. 2004. "The Scale Politics of Emerging Diseases." *Osiris* 19: 62–76.

Kuoh Moukouri, Jacques. 1963. *Doigts noirs: "Je fus écrivain-interprètre sic au Cameroun."* Montreal: Editions à la page.

Lachenal, G. 2002. "Le Centre Pasteur du Cameroun. Trajectoire historique, stratégies et pratiques de la recherche biomédicale en coopération (1959–2002)." Mémoire de DEA en Epistémologie, Histoire des Sciences et des Techniques, Université Paris 7- Denis Diderot.

Lachenal, G. 2005. "Les réseaux post-coloniaux de l'iniquité: Pratiques et mises en scène de la recherche médicale au Cameroun." *Outremers* 93: 123–49.

Lachenal, G. 2006. "Scramble for Cameroon: Virus atypiques et convoitises scientifiques au Cameroun, 1985–2002." In *L'épidémie de sida en Afrique subsaharienne: Regards historiens*, edited by C. Becker and P. Denis. Louvain-la-Neuve: Academia Bruylant.

Lachenal, G. 2009. "Franco-African Familiarities: A History of the Pasteur Institute of Cameroon." In *Hospitals beyond the West*, edited by M. Harrison. New Delhi: Orient Longman.

Lachenal, G. 2010. "The Doctor Who Would Be King." *Lancet* 376, no. 9748: 1216–17.

Lachenal, G. 2010. "Le médecin qui voulut être roi: Médecine coloniale et utopie au Cameroun." *Annales HSS* 65, no. 1.

Lachenal, G. 2011. "The Intimate Rules of the French 'Coopération.'" In *Evidence, Ethos, and Experiment: The Anthropology and History of Medical Research in Africa*, edited by W. Geissler and S. Molyneux. Oxford: Berghahn.

Lakoff, Andrew, and Stephen J. Collier. 2008. *Biosecurity Interventions: Global Health and Security in Question*. New York: Columbia University Press.

Latour, Bruno. 2005. *Reassembling the Social: An Introduction to Actor-Network-Theory*. Oxford: Oxford University Press.

Le Carré, John. 2001. *The Constant Gardener*. New York: Scribner.

Loussert-Ajaka, I., T. D. Ly, M. L. Chaix, D. Ingrand, S. Saragosti, A. M. Courouce, F. Brun-Vezinet, and F. Simon. 1994. "HIV-1/HIV-2 Seronegativity in HIV-1 Subtype O Infected Patients." *Lancet* 343, no. 8910: 1393–94.

Marseille, E., P. B. Hofmann, and J. G. Kahn. 2002. "HIV Prevention before HAART in Sub-Saharan Africa." *Lancet* 359, no. 9320: 1851–56.

Marx, P. A., P. G. Alcabes, and E. Drucker. 2001. "Serial Human Passage of Simian Immunodeficiency Virus by Unsterile Injections and the Emergence of Epidemic Human Immunodeficiency Virus in Africa." *Philosophical Transactions of the Royal Society B Biological Sciences* 356, no. 1410: 911–20.

Marx, P. A., C. Apetrei, and E. Drucker. 2004. "AIDS as a Zoonosis? Confusion over the Origin of the Virus and the Origin of the Epidemics." *Journal of Medical Primatology* 33, nos. 5–6: 220–26.

Mbembe, Achille. 2001. *On the Postcolony*. Berkeley: University of California Press.

Monga, Célestin. 2009. *Nihilisme et négritude: Les arts de vivre en Afrique*. Paris: Presses Universitaires de France.

Muller-Trutwin, M. C., S. Corbet, S. Souquiere, P. Roques, P. Versmisse, A. Ayouba, S. Delarue, E. Nerrienet, J. Lewis, P. Martin, F. Simon, F. Barre-Sinoussi, and P. Mauclere. 2000. "SIVcpz from a Naturally Infected Cameroonian Chimpanzee: Biological and Genetic Comparison with HIV-1 N." *Journal of Medical Primatology* 29, nos. 3–4: 166–72.

Nguyen, Vinh-Kim. 2005. "Antiretroviral Globalism, Biopolitics and Therapeutic Citizenship." In *Global Assemblages: Technology, Politics, and Ethics as Anthropological Problems*, edited by A. Ong and S. J. Collier. Malden, MA: Blackwell.

Nguyen, Vinh-Kim. 2010. *The Republic of Therapy: Triage and Sovereignty in West Africa's Time of AIDS*. Durham, NC: Duke University Press.

Oppenheimer, Gerald M., and Ronald Bayer. 2007. *Shattered Dreams? An Oral History of the South African AIDS Epidemic*. Oxford: Oxford University Press.

Owona-Ntsama, Joseph. 2007. "La grippe aviaire au Cameroun: Une menace sanitaire et sécuritaire fondée?" *Enjeux* (Fondation Paul Ango Ela, Yaoundé) 31.

Peeters, M., V. Courgnaud, B. Abela, P. Auzel, X. Pourrut, F. Bibollet-Ruche, S. Loul, F. Liegeois, C. Butel, D. Koulagna, E. Mpoudi-Ngole, G. M. Shaw, B. H. Hahn, and E. Delaporte. 2002. "Risk to Human Health from a Plethora of Simian Immunodeficiency Viruses in Primate Bushmeat." *Emerging Infectious Diseases* 8, no. 5: 451–57.

Peterson, Dale 2003. *Eating Apes*. Berkeley: University of California Press.

Pollack, Andrew. 1994. "Variants of AIDS Virus Can Elude Blood Tests." *New York Times*, August 9, 1994.

Porter, Roy. 1997. *The Greatest Benefit to Mankind: A Medical History of Humanity from Antiquity to the Present*. London: HarperCollins.

Porter, Roy. 2001. *Bodies Politic: Disease, Death, and Doctors in Britain, 1650–1900*. Picturing History Series. Ithaca, NY: Cornell University Press.

Preston, Richard. 1994. *The Hot Zone*. New York: Random House.

Ratliff, Evan. 2007. "The Plague Fighters: Stopping the Next Pandemic Before It Begins." *Wired Magazine* 15, no. 5, April 24. Accessed September 27, 2008. http://www.wired.com/wired/archive/15.05/feat_firstblood.html.

Redfield, Peter. 2005. "Doctors, Borders, and Life in Crisis." *Cultural Anthropology* 20, no. 3: 328–61.

Reina, Domingo. 2003. *Etat des lieux dans le domaine du diagnostic du VIH: Les principaux acteurs, les brevets déposés, les licences et accords entre sociétés*. Rapport de recherche bibliographique, DESS RIDE.

Roques, P., D. L. Robertson, S. Souquiere, C. Apetrei, E. Nerrienet, F. Barre-Sinoussi, M. Muller-Trutwin, and F. Simon. 2004. "Phylogenetic Characteristics of Three New HIV-1 N Strains and Implications for the Origin of Group N." *AIDS* 18, no. 10: 1371–81.

Roussin, Philippe. 2005. *Misère de la littérature, terreur de l'histoire: Céline et la littérature contemporaine*. Paris: Gallimard.

Sartre, Jean-Paul. 2007. *Typhus* (unpublished scenario, c. 1944). Paris: Gallimard.

Schable, C., L. Zekeng, C. P. Pau, D. Hu, L. Kaptue, L. Gurtler, T. Dondero, J. M. Tsague, G. Schochetman, H. Jaffe et al. 1994. "Sensitivity of United States HIV Antibody Tests for Detection of HIV-1 Group O Infections." *Lancet* 344, no. 8933: 1333–34.

Schneider, W. H., and E. Drucker. 2006. "Blood Transfusions in the Early Years of AIDS in Sub-Saharan Africa." *American Journal of Public Health* 96, no. 6: 984–94.

Schoofs, M. 1999. "AIDS: The Agony of Africa. Part IV: The Virus, Past and Future." *Village Voice*, November 24–30.

Shah, Sonia. 2006. *The Body Hunters: Testing New Drugs on the World's Poorest Patients*. New York: New Press.

Simon, F., P. Mauclere, P. Roques, I. Loussert-Ajaka, M. C. Muller-Trutwin, S. Saragosti, M. C. Georges-Courbot, F. Barre-Sinoussi, and F. Brun-Vezinet. 1998. "Identification of a New Human Immunodeficiency Virus Type 1 Distinct from Group M and Group O." *Nature Medicine* 4, no. 9: 1032–37.

Stoler, Ann Laura, and Frederick Cooper. 1997. "Between Metropole and Colony: Rethinking a Research Agenda." In *Tensions of Empire: Colonial Cultures in a Bourgeois World*, edited by F. Cooper and A. L. Stoler. Berkeley: University of California Press.

Vanden Haesevelde, M., J. L. Decourt, R. J. DeLeys, B. Vanderborght, G. van der Groen, H. van Heuverswijn, and E. Saman. 1994. "Genomic Cloning and Complete Sequence Analysis of a Highly Divergent African Human Immunodeficiency Virus Isolate." *Journal of Virology* 68, no. 3: 1586–96.

Vanderborght, B., R. J. DeLeys, and A. van Geel. 1988. "Isolation and Identification of a Novel Human Immunodeficiency Virus from Two Cameroonians." Abstract no. 1552–1553. Paper read at International Conference on AIDS, Stockholm, June 12–16.

Wain-Hobson, S. 1998. "More Ado About HIV's Origins." *Nature Medicine* 4, no. 9: 1001–2.

Wolfe, N. D., P. Daszak, A. M. Kilpatrick, and D. S. Burke. 2005. "Bushmeat Hunting, Deforestation, and Prediction of Zoonoses Emergence." *Emerging Infectious Diseases* 11, no. 12:1822–27.

Wolfe, N. D., W. Heneine, J. K. Carr, A. D. Garcia, V. Shanmugam, U. Tamoufe, J. N. Torimiro, A. T. Prosser, M. Lebreton, E. Mpoudi-Ngole, F. E. McCutchan, D. L. Birx, T. M. Folks, D. S. Burke, and W. M. Switzer. 2005. "Emergence of Unique Primate T-Lymphotropic Viruses Among Central African Bushmeat Hunters." *Proceedings of the National Academy of Sciences USA* 102, no. 22: 7994–99.

Wolfe, N. D., T. A. Prosser, J. K. Carr, U. Tamoufe, E. Mpoudi-Ngole, J. N. Torimiro, M. LeBreton, F. E. McCutchan, D. L. Birx, and D. S. Burke. 2004. "Exposure to Nonhuman Primates in Rural Cameroon." *Emerging Infectious Diseases* 10, no. 12: 2094–99.

Wolfe, N. D., W. M. Switzer, J. K. Carr, V. B. Bhullar, V. Shanmugam, U. Tamoufe, A. T. Prosser, J. N. Torimiro, A. Wright, E. Mpoudi-Ngole, F. E. McCutchan, D. L. Birx, T. M. Folks, D. S. Burke, and W. Heneine. 2004. "Naturally Acquired Simian Retrovirus Infections in Central African Hunters." *Lancet* 363, no. 9413: 932–37.

Wynne, Brian. 1996. "Misunderstood Misunderstandings: Social Identities and Public Uptake of Science." In *Misunderstanding Science? The Public Reconstruction of Science and Technology*, edited by A. Irwin and B. Wynne. Cambridge: Cambridge University Press.

Yamaguchi, J., R. Coffey, A. Vallari, C. Ngansop, D. Mbanya, N. Ndembi, L. Kaptue, L. G. Gurtler, P. Bodelle, G. Schochetman, S. G. Devare, and C. A. Brennan. 2006. "Identification of HIV Type 1 Group N Infections in a Husband and Wife in Cameroon: Viral Genome Sequences Provide Evidence for Horizontal Transmission." *AIDS Research and Human Retroviruses* 22, no. 1: 83–92.

Yamaguchi, J., C. P. McArthur, A. Vallari, R. Coffey, P. Bodelle, M. Beyeme, G. Schochetman, S. G. Devare, and C. A. Brennan. 2006. "HIV-1 Group N: Evidence of Ongoing Transmission in Cameroon." *AIDS Res Hum Retroviruses* 22, no. 5: 453–57.

Zekeng, L. 2001. "Update on HIV/SIV Infections in Cameroon." *Philosophical Transactions of the Royal Society B Biological Sciences* 356, no. 1410: 799.

CHAPTER 4

What Future Remains?

Remembering an African Place of Science

P. Wenzel Geissler

Seeing a Place of Science in Africa

This chapter traces remnants of transformation, in forms of landscape and architecture and in divergent narratives of change—hope and promise, decay and disappointment—and their affective resonances and effects in the present, in a key place of African science some thirty years after its foundation. Rather than defining and critiquing the present in an unambiguous way, or explaining this present from past events, my main interest is in the diverse futures—past, present, and yet unimagined—held by the place, in monuments and buildings and its inhabitant's memories and objects.

Intertwined with diverse, sometimes contradictory traces of past futures—visible and meaningful for some, at certain times, and obscure to others—are two larger narratives of transformation. On the one hand, familiar stories of modernization and development, associated with mid-twentieth-century science and social science, which continue to be retold in the legitimizing texts of African science and in public claims to scientists. And on the other hand, interpretations of the present in terms of progressive loss, decay, and abandonment since the 1970s, sometimes shorthanded with reference to underlying economic processes as "neoliberalization," which have been fashionable among Africanists and critics of global health for a while and which also resonate with some of the local protagonists' viewpoints, at some moments, in certain situations.[1]

While in the first narrative, science equals progress and advancement, the second delineates—against the backdrop of science's potential to engender betterment and emancipation—the emergence of a new kind of governmentality, premised on economic and political "liberalization," and based on bioscientific knowledge, extending and transforming colonial and postcolonial "developmental state" biopolitics, radicalizing it toward "experimentality" (Nguyen, in this volume) or even "experimental domination" (see Rottenburg 2009).[2] While providing seemingly radically different outlooks onto the historical process, both narratives reiterate similar, postcolonial geographical distinctions of center and periphery, Africa and the West, and both share a similar temporality, the figure of a great transformation. My interest in time and place here is different; instead of pursuing a particular teleology, I want to explore the diversity of temporalities that is contained and simultaneously present in a given site, at one point in time.

WHAT FUTURES REMAIN

Transnational bioscientific interventions, funded by agencies outside Africa, implemented among African populations—exemplified by humanitarian emergency intervention, African anti-retroviral (ARV) programs and vaccine and drug trials (e.g., Redfield 2006; Nguyen 2009; Fassin and Pandolfi 2010)—lend themselves at first sight to critical interpretations in terms of *experimentalization* (see, for exemplary studies outside Africa, Rajan 2006; Petryna 2009). "Northern" control over scientific resources and outputs, the enclosure of scientific institutions, the sidelining of national academic and health care institutions, and the establishment of real-time transnational information flows resemble moreover the external control, outsourcing, and enclaving described for neoliberal African regimes of resource extraction, exploitation, and accumulation (see Ferguson 2006) or urban planning (e.g., Jürgens and Landman 2005; Murray 2010).

The institution explored below, the National Clinical Research Organisation (NCRO) of a sub-Saharan African country, shares certain traits—political-economic, organizational, topographic—of this description, and its history does coincide with the period of the "neoliberalization," which for the nation in question began with a momentous late 1970s governmental shift. Tied in with wider processes of privatization and drastic reductions of government funding, driven in part by external economic policies, the new government-founded NCRO, through a specific legal act that liberated bioscientific research from its previous place in government ministries and state universities, was encouraged to engage freely with academic bodies and other sponsors from outside the country.

Indeed, *collaboration*, as it came to be called, was not merely the institution's mandate—explicitly written into its statutes—but essential for its functioning, as government funding never allowed it to engage in sustainable, independent scientific endeavors. In the early 2000s, the NCRO's government-allocated budget was about £7 million a year, barely enough for core staff salaries and the basic maintenance of buildings, while its actual operating costs were six times this amount, the gap being filled by transnational partners and collaboration. The NCRO is thus a prototype of *parastatal* science, and its regional research center, my field site, which by contrast to other, neglected NCRO centers was blossoming with transnational funds, can seem its incarnation.

This constellation does not equal simply an order of "foreign domination."[3] As a leading NCRO scientist explained, countering such simplification, the NCRO bears full legal and scientific responsibility and ownership for its work. Global inequalities leave more subtle imprints and remain always contested. For example, the same scientist described that while new research projects indeed often are defined abroad and arrive at the center through the Global Health Agency (GHA) (subsequently approved by the NCRO), ultimately "if something happens" in the project, international PIs remember that the NCRO is the site's actual owner and turn to its director for help, who at that point is able to underscore his own role in the given project. But, he went on, his own and the NCRO's agency was curtailed, not just by who holds the purse strings, but also by the political leverage of the GHA, as major health donor, in the national capital. As such, collaboration is continuously contested and remade, an open-ended process (within obvious material limits) rather than a clear-cut hierarchical structure.

My aim here is not to reiterate the vision of an epochal shift or to provide a critique of the present structures (nor to counter such narratives of rupture with evidence of continuity). I want to suspend the desire to unequivocally describe the present and instead try to render visible some of its layers and inherent contradictions. To do so I shall focus on the (asymmetrical) coexistence of different pasts in the present, conflicting narratives of transformation and persistence in one place, positioning our own analytical timelines among other stories. Such ethnographic reading of this place of science in Africa, attending to material forms, movements, and stories, shifts our attention from the contrast of past and present (purifying the present as a specific "regime") to the compression of multiple temporalities within lived-in space, open to continuous interpretation and contestation by multiple actors. As such, the past constitutes a reservoir for the future rather than a mere counterfoil to the present.

This chapter is about science in time. Examining one major site of African scientific production, engaging the lay of the land, commemorative events, and narratives about past and future, I trace relationships between past and present and between diverse pasts in the present. First, I describe the place, the research center, exploring its geography, architecture, and circulations around one social event: the thirtieth anniversary celebrations of the collaboration between the NCRO and its main partner, the GHA. This reveals certain forms of memory and representation and also registers absences, amnesia, and invisibilities. Subsequently, I will extend my gaze beyond first impressions, and beyond the moment of institutional memorialization, and attend to other traces and remains, less prominent movements and circulations, and other evocations of memory. This reexamination of the present landscape will lead us, finally, to the memories and expectations of those who for generations have lived around the research station.

Rather than showing that "the place of science has changed" (which it certainly has), I show that the place—as material object and collective—contains ongoing engagements between pasts, presents, and futures. This is not just the (important) point that different actors (African doctors, visiting expatriate scientists, European anthropologists, local staff, research participants) hold different "perspectives" on one material world and history, shaped by position, identity, and interest. The place itself contains different pasts that engage and collide in concrete practices and specific events and that extend, through the present, into diverse possible futures.

A Social Situation in Global Health Science

THE NCRO

Some kilometers outside the major provincial city where the NCRO station is situated, one turns off the battered tarmac road onto a smooth side road—streetlights, pavements, sign-posted speed bumps. After one kilometer one passes a first gate, and after another short drive along a security wall one reaches the second gate, flanked by cameras, operated by an international security company. The guards check one's pass or confirm with one's host inside before opening the double gates. Outside the wall is what seems like dry wastelands, similar to the surrounding bushland partially used for small-scale agriculture; at some distance one makes out thatched village homes. A small Researchers Cafe offers soft drinks—its ramshackle construction from recycled timber and iron sheets rising from black cotton soil provides a stark contrast to what one glimpses through the gate: lush, well-trimmed lawns, straight alleys of palms and shade trees, demarcated parking and pavements, and shiny buildings with newly tiled roofs: this is the NCRO Centre for Global Health.

Depending on the speaker's affiliation and the conversational context, the place is variously referred to as the NCRO, the NCRO/GHA, the GHA/NCRO, or the GHA field station.[4] This multitude of names may be indicative of different ways of seeing the place and remembering its past, although the variation and slippage is also due to inattentiveness and habit. Aware of the contested politics of naming, after discussions with the NCRO, the GHA management standardized the terminology to the NCRO/GHA field station—replacing the GHA stickers on new cars with an NCRO/GHA label, and correcting the language of research proposals and e-mails—although lapses into GHA/NCRO or GHA remain common in everyday talk.

Local staff and participants consider themselves proudly linked to the GHA—a resource-rich organization and a source of global scientific knowledge and policy (see, e.g., Fairhead et al. 2006). The GHA is by far the largest of the center's collaborators, paying the salaries of over a thousand African staff. Involving hundreds of thousands of research participants in surveillance and clinical trials (with attendant financial and medical benefits), and managing, in addition to research, HIV care and treatment in large areas, it is a highly visible and much admired regional source of medical care and knowledge.[5]

The field station is the central node through which staff, samples, and results of scientific investigations circulate: most staff live in town and travel back and forth either by private cars or, for the majority, with GHA shuttle buses; international scientists are regular visitors. In the opposite direction, field staff and data collectors travel from the field station out "to the field"—that is, the GHA funded "health and demographic surveillance system" covering several neatly mapped rural districts with over 200,000 inhabitants that have been surveyed for a decade, and upon which most clinical trials are conducted—to access rural study populations and collect specimens and other data that are transported back to the laboratories to be processed and analyzed.[6] Data, in turn, can be transmitted from the station to other research centers and the distant coordination points of multisite clinical trials. The field station is, thus, a well-connected conduit of people, materials, and data linking peripheral villages to global centers of scientific investigation, an intersection in rapid global circulations. At the same time, this enclave of world-class scientific possibilities is physically separated from the surrounding countryside—and the circulation of people, specimens, and data between this realm of science and surrounding public health and care institutions is at times more challenging than information flows and travel to international centers.[7]

Inside the NCRO/GHA compound, one passes a turn toward single-story 1980s bungalow structures with the national flag in front of them. Overshadowed by the more imposing buildings behind them, a visitor would be forgiven to overlook these, although this is the actual center of the center, the offices of NCRO scientists and the director of the Global Health Centre. However, the main landmark and the first destination an uninitiated visitor would direct herself to is the new, multistory building, with antisun windows, air-conditioning, uniformed guards, security checks, and magnetic access badges, which houses the offices of the research programs funded by the GHA collaborative agreement. Next to it are the collaboration's extensive laboratories, housing, and state-of-the-art equipment, such as DNA sequencers, serviced and maintained by international laboratory suppliers. On the neat lawns between them, spacious pavilions and the clean staff canteen offer a pleasant meeting space, and on the parking lot stand the 4×4s of lead scientists and some of the station's white Land Cruisers, many of which at the time of our ethnographic fieldwork still bore red diplomatic number plates.

In such comfortable conditions, expatriate and African scientists produce and analyze data and manage trials, overseen by the GHA heads of disease-specific divisions and the scientific director of the GHA field station and his administrator, who at the time of fieldwork were still expatriates.[8] Although the station director at the time of our research, genuinely committed to the ideal of collaborative partnership, had removed his own national flag from the office entrance, the premises are recognizably different in style and atmosphere from others in the nearby city. The young staff's dress, comportment, and communication styles leave little doubt that one is within a leading international organization. As staff occasionally remark, one feels "out of Africa," which is why African staff jokingly refer to the field station by the name of the distant GHA headquarters. To scientists, the field station presents an island of possibility and validity, security and hygiene, a place not only out of Africa but also ahead in time, beyond the prevailing temporality of the surrounding lands, which in terms of science and public health fall further and further behind global standards.

To an anthropologist of postcolonial science, the field station's spatial order and resources, and the material inequalities between those inside and people living around, between science workers and trial participants, and between international and local research staff—may give the impression of a scientific enclave shaped by foreign scientists and funding. The combination of seeming local disconnect and global high-speed connectivity—transferring resources and data, bypassing local entanglements—is reminiscent of critical anthropological analyses of "neoliberal" topography and its "modularity."[9] One discerns the outlines of an "offshore" science production, with connotations of domination and exploitation.[10]

Such interpretation does reflect some important features of the station's institutional and architectural order. Many people inhabiting the site, including anthropologists, scientists and technicians, expatriates and locals, observe inequalities and exclusions—and experience tension between them and their own personal morality, as well as the inherent egalitarianism of public health work. Few of them would agree with a unifying interpretation of their endeavor as "neoliberal science" or worse, "neocolonial science" (Boshoff 2009) or "scientific imperialism" (Wilmshurst 1997), but many—Africans and expatriates alike—experience occasional discomfort with current arrangements, which may be articulated in private conversations or ironic comments, through detachment or absences, or confronted through cultivation of friendships, egalitarian leisure activities, charity work, and other social engagements that aim to transcend inequality and boundaries.[11]

I therefore suggest that the narrative of African science's regress into *experimentality* (or whatever other pejorative epithet one may chose) is not a conclusive diagnosis, but one story among many that emerge from this territory's layered morphology. A narrative that gives preeminence to certain forms and objects—the largest, most obvious ones—and overlooks or deems irrelevant more subtle features.

Spatial configurations and size—power, wealth—are certainly important; they render visible or invisible, constrain circulation and movement, prevent or enable action, exercise force. But the visibility of structures and remains, of pasts and futures, is also affected by characteristics of the beholder—position and associations, historical experience, intentionality—and different people weave different stories out of the available, more or less recognizable materials, connecting past and present toward different futures. This is not simply about setting the record straight—"bringing to the fore" alternative renderings of place and history, for the sake of it, irrespective of their relative visibility, force, and effect. Tracing multiple historical trajectories from past to future cannot erase inequality, but attention to their intersections, tensions, and potential alliances may restore unpredictability to a seemingly monolithic and static present. In the next section, I will begin to pursue the intertwined stories embedded in this place of science around the celebration of the thirtieth anniversary of the NCRO/GHA collaboration, which does reiterate some obvious features—inequalities, maybe "dominance"—observed above, but also reveals alternative teleologies, contradictions, silences, and absences.

Happy Anniversary

CELEBRATING 30 YEARS OF NCRO/GHA

The official celebrations of thirty years of collaboration between the GHA and NCRO, the country's largest research infrastructure, lasted several days, moving from the capital city out to the field by way of the field station, where the main event was held.

This was a "smart" occasion. Participants were influential and wealthy people, including an ambassador and members of Parliament, senior scientists, leading NGO representatives, and some civil servants. Dress ranged from the dark suits of local officials and embassy guests and the uniforms of security personnel to the emphatically informal, often Africanized, attire of younger expatriate scientists, to the carefully tailored wax-cloth dresses, in recent West African fashion, of female research staff. It was matched by the quality, cleanliness, and uniformity of the white awnings erected on the center's well-kept lawns, plastic chairs, table decorations, and flower bouquets, hired from an event management business run by an expatriate wife. Preprinted badges, conference packs with glossy brochures on the collaborations activities, uniformly wrapped presents, handed out by cheerful junior female staff, added a flavor of corporate hospitality and emphasized resources; PowerPoint presentations screened on multiple screens gave the occasion a scientific, "international" outlook.

It is not easy to pinpoint the material and aesthetic qualities that brand this event as distinctive. And yet, having taken part in a range of similar events by the GHA/NCRO collaboration, they have commonalities. None of the material objects at display—awnings, decorations, technology—is unique, but as a whole, things appear as cast from one mold, neat and efficient. Key participants and prominent speakers belong to the expatriate community whose self-confidence and leisurely dress give it a distinguished yet informal feel. Many of the materials are expensive and not easy to get locally. And small aesthetic decisions—the decorations and entertainment at the anniversary, the decision of what might constitute fun, or, at other occasions, the kinds of games played, the role of sports, competitions, and physical team building exercises—create a setting "out of Africa." Their peculiar materiality, order, and cleanness conveys, against the background of a provincial African town, a sense of stability and strength—the ability to control space in a setting where such control is otherwise rarely attained. Such control is something of a luxury and as such also a pleasant experience for all participants.

Yet it is not simply a matter of size, cost, or exclusivity. "Time management" is in these events not limited to the proceedings, which progress without the otherwise common technical hitches and delays. The up-to-date smoothness and cleanness of materials and surfaces themselves exercises control over time by insisting on the primacy of the present; lacking historical reference, erasing traces and leaving none, avoiding material frictions and seemingly untouchable by decay.[12]

Local Pasts in Global Present

The celebration's imposition of a certain temporality not only defines a static present but also creates its own versions of a given past. As a highlight of the celebrations, the directors of the GHA field station and NCRO center honored their "elders": previous GHA field station directors and senior scientists, who had come from overseas; senior NCRO scientists who had worked alongside shifting generations of overseas visitors for up to thirty years, and leaders of important research programs; and also some elderly local technical staff, including an octogenarian laboratory technician who had been recruited as a malaria microscopist twenty years ago, after retirement from decades of government service. The award consisted of a custom-made traditional stool—associated with elder-hood and kinship—embroidered with NCRO/GHA logos in colorful beads. After receiving the stools, wrapped in bright gift paper, the elders squatted upon them and presented some pertinent memories. These circled around the poor material state of things when they began working on the site, and the vast improvements since.

The idiom of elder-hood, the stools and the other memorial gift—an African waistcloth, printed with the anniversary logo and the slogan: "NCRO/ GHA research and public health collaboration: Celebrating 30 years"—as well as performances by traditional musicians and dancing schoolchildren reflect a conscious effort to take up "local" forms in the transnational celebration and reference a particular localized past associated with "the community."[13] The posters the GHA made for the memorial celebrations praise accordingly "the community . . . our most important partners without whom any form of research would not be possible," under a photograph of a traditional dance group with painted faces and elaborate traditional headgear; another one shows the mentioned congregation of GHA/NCRO elders and the wrapped stools with the caption: "The African stool is a sign of leadership and respect. Previous and current directors as well as the long serving staff received African stools."

While some of these aesthetic decisions and representations can seem idiosyncratic, it is important not to overlook that they also reflect a genuine desire, on account of the organizers, to "bring in the community" and to break through the separations that uncomfortably mark the overall situation. The complementary aesthetics of presentist high-tech material perfection and the imagined past of "traditional culture," contrasting "local" or "community" (also "grass-roots," "ground-level") elements with transnational science, which is characteristic for GHA events, is at least partly owed to the progressive and egalitarian morality of many public health scientists, and in particular the leadership of the GHA at the time of our fieldwork. The performance of being part and parcel of place and community references collaborative values of respect and recognition and seeks legitimacy from localized togetherness. Yet this collage achieves not simply a move toward the local pole of a local-global continuum but also the opposite: a confirmation of the celebration as "international"—as local parlance has it—or maybe "expatriate."[14] Resourceful enough to incorporate seemingly incongruous but carefully selected elements among its decorum, while leaving out others; demarcating radical otherness between modern science and a particular rendering of traditional culture. This otherness implies social distance, and it suggests a historical trajectory in which science, and the establishment of the research station, constitutes a rupture away from a very different past—a narrative of creation that I shall presently return to.

Juxtaposing present, universal science and local traditions represented as curios and ancestor worship, something in between is less visible. What would the occasion look like had it been organized by Ministry of Health employees or the staff of a nearby dispensary or school—local agents, too, but not quite as much as grass skirts and drums? As a senior observer commented, "savvy events," skillfully staged and funded by international research budgets, are trademarks of the NCRO/GHA collaboration. Certain characteristics of ordinary local public events are not visible in this NCRO/ GHA occasion. And it is their invisibility that is the point: it is not whether those more typical local celebrations, with their more improvised furnishings and equipment, long speeches, conspicuous displays of respect and hierarchy, extensive meals and fluid timings, are preferable or more authentically "local"; they are, obviously, equally hybrids of sedimented postcolonial traditions, nongovernmental inspiration, and government habits, and given ample resources, the ministerial staff very likely would have preferred the GHA's styles. The point is that the sedimented routines, time-hallowed symbols, and well-worn materials characteristic of the local administrative, medical, and academic elite are not there on this occasion, making the event to some extent alocal and atemporal. These absences are noticed by some but not others.

Another absence from this event is the anniversary of the NCRO itself, which was not celebrated, partly because of political unrest during its anniversary year and because of transitions in the leadership of the NCRO itself, after its long-serving founding director had been dismissed after misappropriating the GHA's research funds as well as, as later emerged, his own staff's pension funds. The limited role of the NCRO was underlined by the fact that permanent, senior NCRO scientists (that is, those paid by the national government rather than GHA funds) and local health system representatives were less visible at the celebrations. As one of the co-organizers explained, the celebration "was on a Saturday and we really had to convince some guests to come." Experiencing the celebration as "a bit of a GHA thing," some of them, though of course invited, only made brief appearances. Such absences are visible to those who have been in the place for a long time and know who else could be present. They are invisible or irrelevant for others, including foreign visitors who lack these memories.

Absence from an event like the anniversary can be due to more pressing local or political commitments or the choice of an inconvenient weekend day. But it may also express critique in a local idiom. Such critique by silence or invisibility is open to multiple readings: a transnational visitor, ignorant of local institutions, might not observe it at all; for a resident expatriate scientist, the absence, if noticed, may confirm the impression of "weak state structures" or can be explained away with a particular absentee's personal idiosyncrasies; an African scientist colleague might read the absence of a senior colleague as an act of defiance, but she or he might equally understand it as acceptance of defeat and accordingly judge it as a sign of strength or of weakness, wisdom or stubbornness.[15]

The absences reinforce the impression of the collaborative celebration being a GHA thing; as one senior NCRO scientist privately expressed a propos the anniversary: "I keep wondering: what *is* the NCRO?" His statement led our conversation back to an earlier speech by the then overall NCRO director to staff, GHA colleagues, and distinguished foreign visitors, which was vividly remembered among NCRO/GHA staff, even after the director had been discredited. The director generally considered himself as the NCRO's "founding father" and missed few opportunities to narrate the story of the NCRO's creation as a nationalist postcolonial project. In his speech he drew upon African patrilineal idiom—"a house has only one door and one kitchen"—to underline that that there was only one institution, the NCRO, to which people belonged. Visitors to his house should not assume the role of the host, and the home's children, that is, staff, should remember which father they belonged to, in the end a remark that took on an ironic tone after the director's misappropriation of staff pensions had become known. Recalling this event in a conversation with the author, the NCRO director reiterated proudly: "I said this to them last time I went there, even in the presence of their ambassador," and went on stressing that there was "one, only one" institution, the NCRO, and that the foreign collaborating institutions "do not exist," adding that "the research center is the NCRO only. The GHA has no title deeds. It is all property of the NCRO!"

These memorable statements resonated with the inclination of other older NCRO scientists and might have momentarily enhanced the director's legitimacy and authority with some staff, before his downfall. Local scientists' insistence on the profoundly national character of their institution was frequently reiterated, for example, by an NCRO scientist who contested my rendering of the NCRO as a *mere* para-statal collaborator in an earlier draft of this chapter. He rightly stressed that the NCRO was a truly *national* agency—though of course ruefully underfunded at present and thus, in the long meantime, entirely reliant upon foreign funding. Rather than accepting a representation in terms of dependency, he drew attention to the contradictions this meant for his position, being "answerable to the MoH" as well as responsible to foreign funders. This double bind, and the nationalist undercurrent, are important, not only as a key feature of twenty-first-century African politics (open to populist misuse), but also because it marks the presence of another potential future, seeded in the founding moment of the NCRO, when young scientists shed the (post)colonial yoke and took the helm of African science (as the disgraced ex-director recalled)—and this is all but forgotten.

Yet such evocations of other futures easily go unnoticed by expatriate colleagues or they are, as in the case of the ex-director, dismissed as "mere talk," counterfactual posing in the face of forceful political-economic realities (and of personal culpability): proclaiming ontological or legal doubts about the GHA's existence will not make it go away. And more crucially, who would want it to go away? Least of all those recalcitrant orators, who enjoy the good working conditions at the field station and whose careers and scientific opportunities have co-evolved with the GHA collaboration. Thus, rather than voicing actual opposition to collaborative research, the nationalist narrative opens, between fiction and reality, a space for one's imagination of alternative futures, and as such it finds resonance and is remembered and retold by the center's inhabitants. It ties the present transnationalized situation back to the NCRO's origins in nationalist science and modernizing African biomedicine—origins that still have effects despite contemporary neoliberalized fictions of the NCRO as profit-generating biotech producer-to-be. Rather than simply countering manifest reality with a fiction, this narrative seeks to counter the dominant story of the GHA's making of the NCRO, relating the present to a different past and possibly to a different future.

MEMORIALIZING THE PRESENT
Untouched by these deeper historical memories, the public historical narratives during the anniversary focused on the GHA/NCRO collaboration and began accordingly from the GHA's arrival in the country. An official GHA website remembered: "30 years ago, a doctor from the GHA arrived in [the capital city] to start a research station with the NCRO. That time, which for him was one of the best in his life, started the GHA/NCRO field research station, what has now become one of the largest investments in the history of medical research [in the country]."

This short story on the collaboration's beginnings could be understood to imply—enhanced by the anniversary iconography—that the GHA came to an empty space. Yet before the lonely medical officer's arrival, the local scientific community had been anything but a void. Indeed the country was one of the leading science nations in Africa during the decades after independence, and the NCRO recruited many of its first staff from a respected group of regional research institutes, which had led African science for decades. The first director of the research center—prior to the beginning of the collaboration—had previously been the first African director of one of these well-renowned research institutes, from where he had come back to his native area when the regional collaboration dissolved in the late 1970s. Together with his staff, he had, prior to the GHA's arrival, laid the foundation of what became the NCRO's Global Health Centre.

The NCRO website places less emphasis on these shared regional roots and seeks its own origins instead in the capabilities and needs of the postcolonial nation-state: the NCRO was here founded out of the drive of a new generation of African protagonists—led by young, often U.S.-trained specialists in new scientific fields such as immunology—in a particular innovative nationalist moment when a new government took over. In this narrative many different international organizations collaborated (the GHA hardly features) in the creation of a *national* medical science, but the leadership lay in the hands of a new generation of postcolonial scientist-entrepreneurs.

During the official anniversary celebrations of the collaboration, this nationalist narrative was not prominent. Addresses by the minister of health and the directors of the NCRO and GHA, published in a major advertising feature in a national newspaper, emphasize instead transnational resource transfers. The minister stresses the gift-like nature of collaboration, expressing thanks for: "technical support and capacity building," "infrastructure as well as manpower," "donations of state of the art equipment and renovations," adding up to an "invaluable contribution to the health of [local people] and indeed, the world." The NCRO director praises the GHA's contribution to producing research capacity and laboratory facilities, while also mentioning—by contrast to other contributors—the fact that the NCRO had already been in existence when the collaboration started. The GHA country director—with long personal experience of research in the region—recalls how the GHA "began a partnership with the organization newly mandated to carry out public health research . . . [the] NCRO, . . . starting in a small office at the . . . district hospital, [and since then] the partnership has grown extensively." He underlines that the collaboration falls "within GHA's international focus, which is to protect the health of all people," to which end the "GHA employs more than 14,000 employees . . . in [the country], the NCRO/GHA collaboration has about 1,200 dedicated staff compared with an initial two in 1979." While emphasizing partnership and expressing thanks to the ministry "for enabling the GHA to build a strong partnership with the NCRO," the text includes what actually are NCRO staff among the global GHA workforce and describes the emergence of the NCRO as intertwined with the GHA's contribution; the highly trained and experienced NCRO staff already present when the collaboration started, and who had laid the foundations for the collaboration's malaria research when they moved from the postcolonial malaria research station to its present location, do not feature.

In his keynote speech at the anniversary celebration itself, the GHA country director similarly began by focusing on the GHA's contribution. One of his slides, "30 years—Then and Now," contrasts the access road in the 1980s and today, mud versus tarmac, and (West African) drums and a network diagram over Internet "Connectivity by GHA," underlining progress in communications and transport (a theme reiterated also in many official anniversary posters, which documented achievements by way of contrasting old and new: "NCRO/GHA has come a long way in terms of infrastructure"). This message is amplified by the next slide that presents a young student Obama in front of an African hut and then President Obama at the handover ceremony, under which is written: "The journey is long and we have come from far . . . yes we can."

However, what at first seems like an unabashed praise of northern achievements is quickly qualified by this leading public health man's modernist, meliorist, and egalitarian commitments when—during the subsequent slides—President Obama is quoted promising to use government to "restore science to its rightful place" and address "the needs of the poor," moving on to John Snow's, or scientific knowledge's, famous victory over cholera in London, emblematic of progressive public health science. The GHA features here—common among the progressive and highly dedicated GHA staff—as public governmental project, reminding us that the GHA itself is a state entity with a strong public ethos and its staff are government officers with an outspoken ethos of serving the public through science.

The speech by this highly respected international scientist dedicated to life and work in Africa contains diverse renderings of history and possible futures and defies easy categorization. The audiovisual "monument" to the anniversary, a ten-minute video produced by the GHA communications team, conveys, at first sight, a simpler message. The opening scene shows a man's back on the side of the driveway to the station. After putting on traditional headgear, he squats on the ground and commences playing a lyre, singing a praise song to the NCRO/GHA and specifically to the first overseas scientist of the collaboration who had arrived in 1979, accompanied by images of gardens, lawns, and the large GHA building.[16] The song fades over to a telephone interview with the same scientist, who recalls the foundational moment: "I was the one who started the station, I was the first person there." He goes on explaining how they started research with few resources, "nothing," borrowed from the Ministry of Health. His voice speaks over the images of rundown government hospital premises and laboratories. Yet the old doctor praises his host country as a "beautiful country—our time there was one of the best in our lives." The video meanwhile underscores radical infrastructural progress through superimposed before—and after—photos.

After a short interval with the singer, a GHA station director from the early 1990s describes how he, on a minute budget, "struggled with bats in the laboratory" and lived and worked with little communication with the headquarters, against a background showing hypermodern laboratory technology and the celebration of the laboratory's ISO accreditation. Two African scientists working with different GHA programs then briefly remember that they had found the compound "overgrown," with "just one administration building, and a very bad road, no tarmac, purely mud." A former lead scientist recalls how there had been no water supply in the early 1990s, and as the NCRO water tower was broken, the GHA had drilled its own borehole, "so for the first time there was running water in the toilets." He goes on to say that the canteen then had only had a wooden table, and the chickens for lunch had still roamed under the tables at breakfast.

The skillfully edited video focuses the site's story on the trajectory from one man's initiative to a large-scale endeavor. Similar to practical arrangements and commemorative discourses at the anniversary, it assigns a dominant role to the overseas partner. Yet the inevitably truncated quotes do not exhaust the speakers' experience, which can point us to different pasts and other ways of remembering. For example, the video's apparent "first scientist" draws in his CV upon the time's characteristically modest idiom of "participation" to underline that local "people . . . maintained control of the program throughout," and that he himself had been "mentored by . . . the senior project leader" (an African doctor), and in a subsequent conversation he placed strong emphasis on the firm rooting of science in Africa—and indeed his and other GHA scientists' long ties to Africa—and the fact that he was part of a strong team of brilliant local scientists who "shaped the agenda" and who then all were equal staff members of a NCRO center, rather than a GHA station.

Likewise, the video interviewee's graphic descriptions of distance from headquarters, practical tinkering and improvisation, and scientific commensality, although emphasizing rough conditions and by implication the long way traversed, also reveal excitement. The time in Africa had been one of contingency and pleasure precisely because things were less well defined and controlled then. Thus, the previous director, who had overseen the main building work, described not only—to a background of historical images of construction work, fading into recent images of shiny roads—"mud everywhere and big equipment," but concluded that "it was by far the best job I ever had. It is surely fun to think about." In similar words, many other GHA veterans enjoyed remembering what many described as a "great time."

The last witness was the long-term African NCRO center director. He, too, appreciated what had been achieved and what "keeps us together here as a family." Although the *family* terminology suggests togetherness, he also implied that his perspective might be different from that of the expatriate witnesses who only saw sections of the overall process, while he has seen it all. In the same vein as his expatriate colleagues, he too appreciated, in a later conversation, the "early days" of improvisation, before the establishment of a massive, rolling bilateral funding program, when "there was a different working model" and fluid structures, and when he, for example, together with his overseas PhD supervisor had creatively made ends meet by jointly applying for various smaller grants.

This underlying praise of openness, of ongoing future making, underwritten by fond memories of improvised work and small surprises and shared by scientists of different origins, is an important, if less visible, take-home message from the anniversary video. Upon first viewing the film—rounded off by a series of staff members saying "Happy anniversary NCRO/GHA"—seems to present a linear narrative of creation ex nihilo, driven by the resources of the foreign partner; a narrative of "bare fields rendered fertile" that recalls older mission narratives (or corporate historiography's "rags to riches"). Yet what its protagonist's recollections evoke is much less bold pride in achievement, teleological satisfaction, than a shared yearning for an original sense of possibility.

MULTIPLE NARRATIONS, MOMENTARY POSITIONINGS

The tensions between the protagonists' progressive commitment to public health—with its egalitarian, social justice undertones and a palpable desire to cooperate and do "the right thing"—and the anniversary celebration's materiality reveals divergent and contradictory intentionalities and interpretations within the present situation. Different actors experience and interpret the anniversary celebrations setting differently, and one actor may account for it differently at different times: while the linear, congratulatory version seemingly dominated official representations, many people held more differentiated views in private, especially people who worked in the site for a longer time, or independently of the GHA, held different versions of history—if not necessarily *a* different history as such. The anniversary celebration (and by extension the collaboration) can thus be read as a consensual performance; a collective ritual that works and takes effect—if for the moment—irrespective of participants' "belief" in its narration or full commitment to its practices.

The anniversary resembled in this regard other public events by the GHA/ NCRO—targeted either at the collaboration's internal public, such as team building, or at a wider public, as in dissemination and mobilization. Although usually working smoothly and to most participants' satisfaction (if of very diverse expectations), these events, too, were commonly accompanied by a running commentary by participants (across diverse institutions and origins) concerning perceived incongruities, ethical tensions, or aesthetic oddities. Awareness of occasional absurdity and futility is certainly also found among expatriate scientists, one of whom summarized her experience of the anniversary as "a waste of time and money" (which did not prevent her from enjoying the party). Such observations do not necessarily oppose the celebration or what it stands for; rather than nascent ruptures, they form part of the connective tissue. Voiced in private, ironic, or self-conscious remarks, they sometimes express a sense of detachment (notably when physical team-building exercises are involved) that runs counter to the optimistic, inclusive thrust of the activities, speeches, and displays, but this skepticism also makes inclusive participation possible.

This coexistence of contradictory elements within and between descriptions of the present (and underlying different historical narratives) qualifies the overly simple dichotomous interpretation of northern versus African institutions and reveals a potential of contestation and change inherent to the present condition.

Mutually engaged memories are also contained and engendered by buildings, ruins, traces, and other objects, as people engage with the landscape and things they live and work with (see Tousignant 2013). In the remainder of this chapter, I will explore the foundations—architectural and geographical—upon which the present field station is erected and which are palpable to some (but not all, nor at all times) of those inhabiting the present. From this, I hope, we will gain a better sense of the lasting contradictions—and thus also of the possibilities—of the edifice.

Foundations of the NCRO: Traces of Futures

BLUEPRINT AND LANDSCAPE

When the anniversary visitors approached the field station, most would have perceived the second gate as the actual entrance, because of its materiality and the rigid protocol, and because only the space behind it displays the distinctive aesthetic features described above. The space between the gates looks much like the surrounding countryside. Yet it is the first gate, manned by elderly NCRO staff rather than private security, which opens into the territory of the NCRO center, while the second gate gives access to an enclosure covering less than a third of the NCRO site. Today's field station was thus carved out, in the early 2000s, from the original forty acres acquired by the NCRO around 1980.

Between the gates one passes a modernist water tower and multistory housing block; well-worn concrete structures, which few foreign visitors would have given much thought to. Only long-term NCRO staff, such as the center director and his age-mates among the permanent staff (who share a marked sense of their own historicity), know the significance of these spatial arrangements and structures. In a drawer of his desk, the director keeps the original 1980s blueprint, by a local architect, for the NCRO center.

The drawing is striking in its vision: an entire scientific-cum-civic community, complete with laboratories, workshops, and administration, as well as staff housing for different ranks, from subordinate to senior scientists, flats for visiting scientists, and communal facilities: clinic, kindergarten and school, tennis courts and pool. This self-contained science city was projected at a time when the country's actual cities and municipal services were declining under a new government that, advised by foreign institutions, demolished or shrunk governmental structures—from commodity boards to health care, from universities to transport and public works. The blueprint reformulates, under changed political-economic conditions, an older dream of the polis, a civic space guided by rational government and scientific advance. It proposes a contraction of the erstwhile dream of national development and expanding modernity—but does not abrogate it.

This vision of a science city, a few miles outside the actual municipal entity, is different from older postcolonial landscapes of science. The leading site of national medical-scientific research—and government public health—between the 1940s and the 1970s had been a division of the national Ministry of Health, whose fifty stations reporting to a headquarters in the capital city had covered the country, radiating outward in order to transform the nation. Its local research station was located at the city center, adjacent to other administrative and health institutions with whom it worked. When northern government institutions started to work in the city from the late 1970s, they initially utilized these by then underused government staff and laboratories in the city and subsequently took technicians and scientists along with them to the NCRO center outside town. These now elderly staff hold memories of a different way of conducting scientific inquiries and public health work, more firmly integrated into the texture of city and nation.

Similar experiences were brought along by those who joined the NCRO/GHA after commencing their laboratory and scientific careers within the aforementioned regional research institutes, a network of disease-specific scientific institutions located in different sites across the wider region, which produced world-leading science and advised postcolonial national governments. Like the ministry's research division, these were integrated with the state apparatus and informed national governments. When regional collaboration collapsed, the first African director of the oldest of these famous research institutes came with his staff to the NCRO research center's present location to build up national malaria research. His plans for the NCRO center, including suggestions for new buildings and extensive staff housing for a large malaria center (see Hutchinson, forthcoming), were never built. Yet they lived on in the field station blueprint, which moved the center out of town and contracted these flights of fancy into a seemingly more achievable scale.

These two layers of unrealized blueprints for an African place of science had in turn an architectural precursor in the aforementioned regional research institute, where the first African director, immediately after his institute had been "Africanized" in the 1970s, had commissioned plans for an impressive multistory modernist laboratory block. To make room for this vision he demolished—to the chagrin of his European predecessors—the existing functioning laboratory built in colonial times. Today a short flight of stairs leads to a level patch of grass where the grand laboratory should have been erected: a void that variously references colonial infrastructures and postcolonial hopes—as well as serving as a conveniently canopy-free lawn for meteorological measurements.

Underneath the present NCRO/GHA center depicted in the opening of the chapter is thus a deep genealogy of unrealized projects for postcolonial African scientific futures; while not ruins in a conventional material sense, these ruined visions—underscored by stories about the ruined lives of some of the protagonists, which are told among older African scientists—form part of the research center's landscape. To those who remember them, like the NCRO center director and his elderly secretary—who began with the regional research institutes and retired one year before the anniversary—they reference buried hopes and aspirations, failure and disappointment. To the many young staff born in the 1980s, let alone to many short-term expatriate staff, they are invisible.

Remembered (by some) in the transnational research center at the time of its anniversary, the project of 1970s national governmental science exemplified by the national ministry's research arm or the regional research institutes has an exotic feel, as if a radical break had happened since. But this departure was not obvious in the early 1980s, when new forms took shape within older plans and landscapes. The blueprint's field station did not propose a radical break with the idea of scientific government and citizenship, representative of the mid-twentieth-century developmental nation-state. On the contrary, the NCRO's foundational rhetoric was emphatically nationalist, proposing a step up in decolonization, away from British colonial funding toward more diverse and especially North American collaboration, replacing colonial remnants with new institutions. Little suggested the return of transnational inequalities. Instead of proposing something radically new, the blueprint merely adapted an older vision of national science-as-government. It leaves the city behind, proposes a center in and by itself, but it preserves the dream of civic unity, a polis that integrates life and science.

PARTIAL REALIZATION

The building of this hypermodern fiction, extending the lease of scientific modernity by exaggerating traits of the modern imagination,[17] was stopped during "phase 1" of the envisioned three-stage building process. When I first came to the center in 1993, one administration and laboratory bungalow, a few staff houses, and the water tower had been built on the forty-acre site. When the GHA, around the year 2000, resumed building to accommodate its expanding program, it was based on a new architectural outline, drawn by an international architectural firm and covering only a section of the site.

The older blueprint's island city was reduced, a smaller enclosure super-imposed and surrounded by a protective wall. Only laboratory and administrative sections were included; housing, welfare, leisure, education, procreation, and transport did not feature here as parts of the science site. The few staff houses originally realized remained outside the perimeter wall and have not been further developed—apart from vegetable cultivation coordinated by NCRO staff. Today—and apparently after a period when nobody wanted to live in these isolated houses—the flats, owned by the NCRO, are in demand on account of their stable water and electricity supplies and their security, in contrast to similarly priced housing in the city. They are mainly inhabited by senior NCRO scientists who avoid the city's choked traffic and skyrocketing rents. Other staff commute from their rented accommodation in town, relying on private cars or the GHA shuttle bus. Short of either, it is a long walk from the nearest main road's minibus services. Periurban circulations with the National Railways—the center site had originally been chosen next to a railway station—have ceased to work after decades of neglect and privatization.

FURTHER INSCRIPTIONS: MOVING ACROSS THE PLAN

Today's research station's apparent centerpiece is the GHA administration building and laboratory (both with provisions for doubling their size). The GHA plan left untouched the single-story NCRO administration bungalow and laboratory, apart from redoing walls, windows, and roofing, achieving a consistent overall impression.

The idea of the GHA building as the center of the center—not merely a project within it—is reflected in its size and the fact that the GHA planners imagined the NCRO's administrative structure to be incorporated into the building: in the senior management wing we find, in the architects drawings, two large offices, reflecting the partners' collaborative symmetry, complete with identical desks and seating groups, for respectively the director of the GHA and the director of the NCRO.

Adjacent to these offices one finds senior staff and administration for the entire field station. The building also contains spaces for researchers, including individual offices for the GHA section chiefs of malaria, HIV, and the other larger GHA funded programs. The inclusion of the NCRO center director and his administration into the GHA designs resonates with the historical narrative discussed above. For some of the permanently employed NCRO staff, the incorporation of the NCRO into the GHA plan, as equal partner, appears less generous than gregarious—too much of a collaborative embrace. For them the NCRO center remains to be found in the small, older buildings separate from what they refer to as the GHA building—or more to the point: they are engaged in a struggle to maintain a vision according to which the GHA building is, in the NCRO center director's words related above, "only a project among others" of the NCRO and in which the NCRO is, in accordance with the legal situation, the sole owner of the site.

This alternative gaze onto the historically formed landscape took material form when the then NCRO center director decided not to move into the office designated for him by the GHA architects but to remain, with his elderly secretary and a handful of permanent NCRO staff, in the pleasant older bungalow accommodation. He explained his decision with the fact that he was "not GHA," that the proposed equivalence between the directors did not reflect the legal situation or the NCRO's vision. He perceived his proposed position in the GHA plan as a misinterpretation of collaborative relations and chose to inscribe his opposite view, adding: "I prefer to be on my own." As a result, the equivalent office of the GHA field station director was not used by the NCRO director but for the GHA employed, expatriate deputy field station director, administering collaborative program funds. Thus, the senior management section of the new building was in 2009 inhabited by those who oversee GHA funding and activities, reflecting political-economic realities maybe more appropriately than the architects' symmetrical vision of collaborative partnership.

A practical choice by the NCRO center director provides here a lasting commentary on competing historical narratives about the origins and purpose of the NCRO center and inscribes an alternative interpretation into the landscape—waiting to be transposed into an alternative future.[18] I hasten to stress that this gesture, though resonating with critical remarks and telling absences noted above, does not express opposition to the collaborative arrangement; the director himself is a pillar of the collaboration and has developed his scientific career within it—and for all scientists related to it, its resourceful laboratories and effective management provide vital conditions for scientific creativity and innovation and professional satisfaction. But alternative futures can remain latent in spatial distributions and circulations, potentially to be reanimated when the opportunity arises.

The blueprint, the remnants and ruins of its vision, and the circulation and placement of people in the resulting landscape reveal diverging memories and historical narratives—and diverging intentionalities and futures— are tangible alongside the more prominent shapes of the contemporary order and their myths of origin. They remain present in the seemingly over-determined social situation of the anniversary celebration, not only in participants' inscrutable consciousness but also in buildings and landscape. But who actually notices and engages with these traces, and who doesn't? For a young foreign visitor, the archaeology of past projects is at first invisible. A long-term African scientist, on the other hand, might know everything outlined above, and more, about the history and original visions attached to the place, but in the given situation, his eyes might be focused on the necessities at hand: maintaining collaborative relations, sustaining funding for staff, getting access to laboratory equipment, and learning, jointly with others, how to make better science.

The ethnographic tracing of such other histories is only a first step in responding to dominant strands of commemoration; from here begins the task of discerning what people *do* with memories of past projects, and how they practically engage contradictory histories, pursue divergent futures, and associate with others positioning themselves on different historical narratives. How does a senior African scientist, long familiar with the place and since recently employed by the GHA, make his way, every day, between the 1980s senior staff housing on a field outside the center, into the scientific enclave? And how does his expatriate colleague, driven by her origins in progressive health politics and committed to ideals of justice and equality, travel from her 1940s bungalow in the former colonial administrative district? How do international visitors (including the ethnographers), in search of collaborative field sites, enter and move across the center, which locations do they engage, and to what ends? Which temporalities are evoked by addressing the site as, respectively, the NCRO or the GHA? And what difference does it make who speaks and where? And how does telling and juxtaposing stories—as in this chapter—evoking the affective resonance of traces, contribute to ongoing struggles?

Memories of the Land Returning

Around the time of the official anniversary celebrations, partly triggered by the publicity attendant to it, communities living in villages around the center or involved in long-term research asked yet another time what benefits research, after thirty years, had brought to the place and its people. Such encounters between villagers and scientists, in Community Advisory Board meetings and community consultations at the field station or at local *barazas* in the field, preparing new research projects, turned around concrete material outcomes: employment, health care provision, and infrastructure development, including education and sanitation.

These historically rooted local claims resonated somehow with African scientists' commentary on political and economic inequality, encountered above. Yet, rather than justice, the issue here was responsibility within hierarchical relations of accepted inequality. While scientists aspired to an equal place in universal scientific space, and for sovereign national science, villagers did not challenge unequal distributions of power, resources, and knowledge or evoke global and national frames, but they sought to access the scientists' local resources, evoking shared responsibilities for human well-being that arise from conjoined lives upon one piece of land. After three decades of cohabitation, the argument ran, some local development— the concrete localized effect of science (and its production process)—some benefits toward the original owners of the land were due. *Development* (in the local vernacular also *growth*)—a prominent term in local praise for the NCRO and GHA, as well as in critical demands—has here implications of sharing substance, recognizing local relations in resonance with local kinship idioms of belonging and becoming.

Such claims are based on a different strand of memory from the institutional remembrance examined above. They are raised by those who, since they decades ago signed a piece of land over to the NCRO, witnessed or bodily participated in the NCRO/GHA's research and enjoyed benefits and nurtured hopes attached to scientific field trials of new treatments and vaccines, and who felt that the larger promise of scientific development had not been fulfilled—for them, in their place.

Development references here also local histories of progress. The NCRO center is part of a periurban area, where since independence hopes for development and modernization ran high. A prominent national politician hails from here—a modernist, pro-Western trade union leader trained in the United States and murdered by political opponents, who remains for many the embodiment of disappointed political hopes for modern, improved lives. Moreover, the area is the location not only of the scientific center but also the recently expanded international airport, itself embroiled in over five decades of legal controversy with local landowning clans over compensation and benefits and subject to recurrent speculative hopes, and an enormous but dysfunctional industrial plant, built around the same time as the NCRO center and owned by one of the country's leading industrial and political families, involving corruption scandals leading back to the mentioned politician's murder. The question as to what local benefits the appropriation of fertile lands for such quintessentially modern enterprises accrues is thus ripe in the area.

The NCRO/GHA site, with its securitized concentration of resources, technology, and expertise, and its connection to circulations beyond local control, raises similar questions as a huge factory that never produced but made its owners rich(er) or an expanding airport most people only ever see through its fence and land speculation along its boundaries. Sometimes this is expressed in rumors about nefarious practices, be it the popular lore about political murder, rumors about the Chinese contractors expanding the airport, or indeed about scientists stealing local people's blood, but much more commonly these questions are put forth in concrete practical requests: for water supplies, food aid, employment opportunity, school buildings, and a local hospital, which are directed at the NCRO/GHA collaboration rather than the NCRO as such.

The institutions' response to such demands, raised repeatedly over decades, must, despite everyone's best intentions, remain limited. Human resource procedures and scientific meritocracy do not allow preferential employment of neighbors, and at the time of field research, funding levels were stabilizing or declining in response to the financial crisis and hiring stagnated. Requests for infrastructure projects or permanent health care provision could not easily be accommodated because of cyclical project funding and because the NCRO and GHA are research bodies, not aid organizations.[19] Sometimes the questions did not even reach their addressees: in public discussions, community representatives supporting the NCRO/GHA's argumentation thus sometimes criticized or silenced allegedly "selfish" compatriots' excessive demands, presumably because they were considered inappropriate and potentially harmful to working relations with the NCRO/GHA.

The fact that the institutions could not adequately respond to these demands does not mean that the individual actors—African and expatriate scientists as much as local field staff—did not wish to respond and assist. An earlier GHA director had thus given neighboring homes the right to use water from the center's borehole via a tap near the gate and to utilize the center's electricity and telephone exchange for further connection; the center's staff clinic was opened to patients from neighboring villages; in various meetings, the NCRO/GHA promised, if possible, to utilize (and thereby partially support) local clinics for future research; individual scientists did commonly try, on an ad hoc basis and limited by regulations, to use some research funds for improvements of health care standards. On a more personal level, field staff often felt compelled to assist individuals with small personal donations, and some senior scientific staff engaged in considerable charitable projects as funders and fund-raisers. After the end of my fieldwork, a more systematic "corporate responsibility program" began to take shape, which included suggestions to pool staff contributions for ad hoc charitable responses and an initiative to pass on waste paper and decommissioned furniture for income generation to villagers living around the center.

Another, more sustained response to persistent and occasionally accentuated local requests was the field station's expanding community engagement program.[20] Considering communication, rather than just material exchanges, as a panacea to strained relations, its tools were information focused: public meetings, dissemination events, a newsletter, and a magazine. One important strategy was to hold events in schools around the field station, which would contribute to knowledge about research and general health education and improve relations between community and researchers.

One larger school event included an essay and painting competition, where pupils were given opportunities to articulate ideas about medical research and the GHA. The prizes for the best essays and drawings were gifts, donated by the staff of the field station.[21] The celebrations involved performances of poems and songs, school milk donations, and health lessons to the children by disease-specific researchers. The shining white awnings, Land Cruisers, plastic furniture, loudspeakers, and the elegantly dressed female NCRO/GHA staff, presenting neatly wrapped prizes, side by side with decayed rural primary school buildings without electricity or water and children in worn uniforms on coarse wooden benches confronted the timeless, near-perfect materiality of the anniversary celebrations, described above, with the surrounding landscape. The well-intended gesture toward engagement certainly provided an enjoyable and instructive occasion for the local children and their teachers, both because of the new medical knowledge and because of the material displays and the physical contact with NCRO/GHA staff and resources it involved. The wider historical hopes for material development will remain lingering inside and outside the research center's fence, engaging particular interests with the overlapping temporalities of nation, place, and habitation in the memories and aspirations of scientists as well as local schoolchildren.

As for the latter, the competition images depicting the field station in its place give us some idea of the memories that the present will leave behind in future generations. Many of the drawings depict hopes for the future fulfilled by the NCRO/GHA: health care, enlightenment, and improved lives. Others focus on the present sufferings of families and children, implying the need for the NCRO/GHA's assistance to make present ailments past. Others again focus on the shiny surfaces of the present field station—the Land Cruisers with embassy number plates, the uniforms and cars of the expensive security company, the beautiful houses rented out to international NCRO/GHA staff, and their fences. One picture is split in the middle by a fence and gate, with colorful and neat buildings and cars inside the research station, and mud houses, graves, and a family without shoes outside the massive gate. Attention to these alternative narratives of science, history, and place—told outside the center and out of the limelight of the anniversary celebrations—gives us some idea of the memories and hopes that are embedded and continuously reinscribed and revised by those who live, work, and engage with each other upon this place of science in Africa. This is not a matter of contrasting narrations by those inside and outside, researchers and community, foreigners and Africans. On the contrary, the interest of this ethnographic-archaeological inquiry lies in the intertwining, within one place and in the lives and stories of its inhabitants, of diverging and contradictory attempts to connect past, present, and future.

Looking at a place of science in a moment when it looks at itself and represents itself to the public has opened our view to different ways of seeing and being in one place at one time. These are not just positions shaped by different stakes and interests, different perspectives onto the same material reality. Rather, the historically shaped landscape and the narratives occasioned by it—different for different storytellers—co-constitute a present on its way between past and future. Attention to the place and its stories renders the present as process rather than as the outcome of global transformative causalities operating shifts between states. Such "processual ethnography" of an African present suspended between diverging pasts and multiple futures (Moore 1987), which reads diagnostic events as localized intersections of historical processes, reveals the present as a site of struggles, past and present, and the terrain of future possibility. It dissolves visions of the present as stable "regime"—defined by contrast to a past historical state—revealing instead diversity and opportunity. Instead of telling one history, it provides starting points for new stories.

The succession of failed projects for an African science—the 1970s grand laboratory in the regional research institute's station or the 1980s NCRO blueprint—are invisible ruins in the landscape and the memories of the protagonists above. These ruins do not simply reference nostalgia, but neither do they emanate mere resentment (Stoler 2008, 207). To those who can see them, their resonances shape present visions of the future, guide attempts to change the order of scientific space, and avoid the pitfalls of change. This chapter on an African science site's past and futures is offered to those working on the site not as testimony to failure nor as nostalgic time travel but as a contribution to ongoing contests about the shape of the future and an extension of many a pleasant conversation.

Notes

This chapter draws on materials generated as part of Wellcome Trust GR077430 and ESRC-ORA RES0360-25-0032.

1 Neoliberalization's temporal-cum-spatial implications have been described in broad strokes by Harvey (e.g., 2006; see also 1990; May and Thrift 2001); for more specific accounts, see, e.g., Ong (2006); Sassen (2006); for Africa, see, e.g., Ferguson (2005); Comaroff (2007); see also Rottenburg (2009).

2 Rottenburg (2009) proposes that Africa has become progressively marginal in political and economic terms and yet evermore central to global forms of experimentation and knowledge production.

3 For a discussion on "legitimate domination" and global health, see, e.g., McFalls (2010).

4 The NCRO was founded by government act in the late 1970s as one of several para-statal scientific institutions. The GHA is a main collaborator, conducting research on malaria, HIV, and emergent diseases. The NCRO and GHA have, since the late 1970s, jointly built the field station, which expanded during the 1990s to become one of the leading medical research sites in Africa, with an annual budget around US$30 million (2009)—excluding projects funded by other sources and expatriate staff salaries and allowances. It engages over 1,000 national staff on renewable short-term NCRO contracts (paid for by the GHA), some NCRO staff scientists on permanent, pensionable contracts paid by national government funds, a handful of expatriate scientists, and thousands of participants involved in surveillance and clinical trials.

5 While all staff members funded by the GHA collaboration formerly are NCRO employees, the perception among staff and outsiders is that the collaborative work between the NCRO and GHA is set apart from the smaller non-GHA activities on the site—which is why it is variously referred to as the NCRO/GHA or the GHA—and the staff members in question (most staff working on the site) are different from ordinary NCRO employees (also referred to as NCRO-NCRO) in that they are not permanently employed but usually on rolling one-year contracts and describe themselves commonly as "being with the GHA" (just like volunteers and trial participants do).

6 Data generated by rapid testing or interviews in a rural home or field laboratory can be transferred through local wireless networks and satellite connections in real time for analysis at the research center or in the distant centers of multisite clinical trials.

7 Contact, through meetings and direct information exchange with local public health authorities, although universally deemed desirable, is not always easy; due to the limited capacity and cost of the ISO accredited laboratories, these cannot simply extend their services to surrounding health care facilities, and due to the processes of careful institutional data validation and academic publishing, findings must be circulated widely before being fed back into national health policy (although preliminary results are presented at regular seminars at the field station).

8 During the time of fieldwork, some major changes concerning the role of African scientists were set in motion: in accordance with some major funders' regulations, many projects began to employ local principal investigators (PIs) on project-funded contracts, while previously PIs had usually been expatriates and research coordinators had been locals. Moreover, several heads of disease-specific sections were during subsequent years replaced with African scientists. At the time of publication, this shift includes also the station director, who for the first time is not an expatriate. Expatriates serve thus increasingly as mere advisors; while continuities and change always remain intertwined in such efforts to establish new patterns, their significance lies in the intentionalities they indicate and in the horizons of possibility they open.

9 For example Ferguson's (e.g., 2006) description of African resource extraction enclaves run by multinational companies and global "capital hopping" associated with foreign direct investment (see also Appel 2012 on "modularization"); Ong's (2006) analysis of Asian export production zones and "variegated sovereignty"; or Caldeira's (2000) seminal studies of urban segregation (see also Murray 2010).

10 This evokes the work of Petryna (2009; see also Rajan 2006) on the recent off-shoring of (for-profit) clinical research by the pharmaceutical industry. An important difference between the literature on pharmaceutical outsourcing and biocapital and the present case—indeed most African bioscience—is that most African research is not for profit but funded by and accountable to national governments and public charities.

11 Indeed, these features are so obvious that the critical anthropologist's task cannot be limited to exposing—as in the old Enlightenment vision of revelatory and iconoclastic critique—the "truth" of the place. Rather, it raises the question of how inequalities and exclusions can be "public secrets" open to view and yet seemingly unchangeable and irrelevant to the working of public health science and how this reading coexists, articulates, and conflicts with other descriptions and historical narrations inscribed in the place.

12 The atemporality of materials that (seem to) reject traces and resist decay, and their use in architecture and domestic life in an African village setting, is also discussed in Geissler and Prince (2010).

13 The particular vision of the "local" embodied by these artifacts points toward the role of community, widespread in transnational collaborations, as the deserving recipient of support and collaboration, with which progressive global forces link up directly, rather than through national government.

14 The concept of the *expatriate* and processes of *expatriation* deserve further unpacking as a key to contemporary forms of dwelling and political ethics; as, e.g., Redfield (2012) shows, the peculiar commitment to no-place, while residing and acting upon specific places, makes not only for particular patterns of consumption and work but also for characteristic moral conundrums.

15 When I asked GHA colleagues why the NCRO had not played a more central role in a particular event, or why a particular senior scientist or official had not attended, answers had a resigned tone, although they certainly recognized the desirability of a more "balanced" collaboration: "Had it been up to them [the NCRO], this [celebration] would not have happened"; "You know that he never attends these things"; "We keep inviting them, but you know."

16 The traditional song's lyrics were directed at the grandchildren of a fictive "white man, son from abroad, who is a gentle man wearing spectacles"—presumably a reference to the scientist and medical doctor who started malaria work on behalf of the GHA in the 1970s—who is the hero figure praised by the song. The singer refers to being called by a relative "from abroad, who calls me when I'm inside the interior bush" and being told of the arrival of the said white man, evoking images of backwardness and progress as well as transnational connections.

17 The architectural blueprint of the field station resembles the legal foundations of the NCRO itself: a law from the late 1970s facilitated the creation of new, so-called para-statal, research institutes, which at least in the vision of their founders aimed to replace much of the research activity that earlier had been carried out by government institutions. This document is strikingly Janus faced—calling for reinvigorated post-postcolonial, nationalist government science, while at the same time establishing the foundations of science as transnational and, to some extent, private business. The earlier sections of the act emphasize the duty to advise government and guide the nation through science; the latter sections do not mention the nation but describe instead the future research institutes as corporate bodies, holding private property rights in their assets as well as their future scientific findings and attracting, generating, and administering income, separate from government budgets.

18 This move kept options open. At the time of this chapter's publication, after another change of the station's directorship, the former NCRO center director has been appointed to replace his expatriate predecessor as director of the GHA/NCRO collaboration. He now inhabits the office formerly designated as belonging to the director of the GHA. While these were momentous changes, outcomes of contestation, they do not resolve built-in tensions but constitute another move on a historically layered board.

19 This explanation was not always understood well, partly because of the official slogan of the NCRO/GHA collaboration, "for research and public health," and the public acclaim for the collaboration to have benefited the health of local people (see discussion of anniversary advert above), and partly because the NCRO and GHA have long been involved in HIV treatment and care in the area, which makes this sort of institutional "therapeutic misconception" at least understandable.

20 In her recent doctoral thesis, Chantler (2012) traces how "community engagement" in global health research has come about since the 1980s in response to the growing gap between science and its national public, and how it evolved out of "participatory" approaches in the 1980s to become a professional domain preoccupied with "communicating" science to study participants and their communities in order to facilitate research.

21 This insistence on "real" gifts was meant to emphasize personal relations between those inside and outside the station. Moreover, the station had no designated budget for this, and using research budgets could have appeared as unethical "undue inducement."

References

Adams, Vincanne. 2002. "Randomized Controlled Crime: Postcolonial Sciences in Alternative Medicine Research." *Social Studies of Science* 32, nos. 5–6: 659–90.

Anderson, Warwick. 2009. "From Subjugated Knowledge to Conjugated Subjects: Science and Globalisation, or Postcolonial Studies of Science?" *Postcolonial Studies* 12, no. 4: 389–400.

Appel, Hannah. 2012. "Offshore Work: Oil, Modularity, and the How of Capitalism in Equatorial Guinea." *American Ethnologist* 39, no. 4: 692–709.

Boshoff, Nelius. 2009. "Neo-Colonialism and Research Collaboration in Central Africa." *Scientometrics* 81, no. 2: 413–34.

Comaroff, Jean. 2007. "Beyond Bare Life: AIDS, (Bio)Politics, and the Neoliberal Order." *Public Culture* 19, no. 1: 197–219.

Dahdouh-Guebas, Farid, et al. 2003. "Neo-Colonial Science by the Most Industrialised upon the Least Developed Countries in Peer-Reviewed Publishing." *Scientometrics* 56, no. 3: 329–43.

Fairhead, J., M. Leach, and M. Small. 2006. "Where Techno-Science Meets Poverty: Medical Research and the Economy of Blood in the Gambia, West Africa." *Social Science and Medicine* 63, no. 4: 1109–20.

Fassin, Didier, and Mariella Pandolfi. 2010. *Contemporary States of Emergency: The Politics of Military and Humanitarian Interventions*. New York: Zone Books.

Ferguson, James. 2006. *Global Shadows: Africa in the Neoliberal World Order*. Durham, NC: Duke University Press.

Harvey, David. 2006. *A Brief History of Neoliberalism*. Oxford: Oxford University Press.

Hutchinson, Lauren. Forthcoming. "Independence and Malaria Research in Kenya, 1977–1985." PhD diss., University of London.

Jürgens, U., and Karina Landman. 2005. "Gated Communities in South Africa." In *Private Cities: Global and Local Perspectives*, edited by G. Glasze, C. Webster, and K. Frantz. London: Routledge.

Lave, Rebecca, Philip Mirowski, and Samuel Randalls. 2010. "Introduction: STS and Neoliberal Science." *Social Studies of Science* 40, no. 5: 659–75.

May, Jon, and Nigel Thrift. 2001. "Introduction." In *TimeSpace: Geographies of Temporality*, edited by J. May and N. Thrift, 1–46. London: Routledge.

Moore, Sally Falk. 1987. "Explaining the Present: Theoretical Dilemmas in Processual Ethnography." *American Ethnologist* 14, no. 4: 727–36.

Murray, Martin J. 2010. *City of Extremes: The Spatial Politics of Johannesburg*. Durham, NC: Duke University Press.

Nguyen, V. K. 2009. "Government-by-Exception: Enrollment and Experimentality in Mass HIV Treatment Programmes in Africa." *Social Theory and Health* 7: 196–217.

Petryna, Adriana. 2009. *When Experiments Travel: Clinical Trials and the Global Search for Human Subjects*. Princeton, NJ: Princeton University Press.

Rajan, Kaushik Sunder. 2006. *Biocapital: The Constitution of Postgenomic Life*. Durham, NC: Duke University Press.

Redfield, Peter. 2006. "A Less Modest Witness." *American Ethnologist* 33, no. 1: 3–26.

Sassen, Saskia. 2006. *Territory, Authority, Rights: From Medieval to Global Assemblages*. Princeton, NJ: Princeton University Press.

Tousignant, Noemi. 2013. "Broken Tempos: Of Means and Memory in a Senegalese University Laboratory." *Social Studies of Science* 43:729–53.

Verran, Helen. 2002. "A Postcolonial Moment in Science Studies." *Social Studies of Science* 32, nos. 5–6: 729–62.

Wilmshurst, Peter. 1997. "Scientific Imperialism." *BMJ* 314, no. 7084: 840.

CHAPTER 5

International Health and the

Proliferation of "Partnerships":

(Un)Intended Boost for State

Institutions in Tanzania?

Rene Gerrets

This chapter focuses on the rapid proliferation of transnational public-private partnerships (PPPs) in international health during the past decade, a multifaceted phenomenon that is deeply intertwined with the enormous contemporary expansion of infectious disease research and control efforts across the Global South (Ravishankar et al. 2009). A rarity in international health until the late 1990s, *partnerships* expanded in number and influence during the past decade, transforming prevailing thinking and practices in this domain and attracting historically unprecedented levels of attention and resources to fight diseases mainly afflicting the world's poor (Buse and Walt 2000a, 2000b).[1] Combining the strengths of institutions from the public and for-profit sectors as well as civil society, so goes the reasoning, partnerships can mobilize the extensive skills and resources needed to address complex, border-transgressing health problems such as malaria or AIDS, which cannot be tackled by organizations working in isolation (Barrett et al. 1998). Collectively, these entities are considered markedly effective in terms of achieving their intended goals, despite disappointing results or outright failure of some partnerships (Peters and Phillips 2004). Evidence to support such claims comes from various sources. For example, hundreds of millions are currently receiving vaccines, drugs, and technologies that erstwhile were either nonexistent or unavailable to people who need them most (Caines et al. 2004; Serdobova and Kieny 2006). Likewise, seemingly intractable public health problems that used to disable millions, such as guinea worm or river blindness, are nearing elimination (Barry 2007; Traore et al. 2009). Finally, interventions funded by the Global Fund to Fight AIDS, Tuberculosis, and Malaria (GFATM)—the largest partnership established to date—are estimated to have prevented millions of deaths (Komatsu et al. 2010).

Directly and indirectly affecting the lives, livelihoods, and well-being of hundreds of millions of people across the world, these partnerships are key features of a nascent system of global health governance (Aginam 2005; Gostin 2005). Network-based, this emerging global health architecture is arising alongside and intersecting with the existing nation-state–centered multilateral system (Kickbusch 2005), which, according to many critics, is poorly equipped to address infectious disease–related problems in a globalizing world marked by steadily intensifying movements of people, germs, objects, and ideas (Cooper et al. 2007; Fidler 2004). Professionals and scholars alike have taken an interest in partnerships as emergent modes of global governance, generating a burgeoning literature that focuses primarily on the ramifications of this phenomenon on the international plane (Bartsch 2006; Gostin and Mok 2009; Kickbusch et al. 2007; Ruger 2007). By comparison, very little has been written about the impact of partnerships on, or their shaping by, low-income country settings, even though their activities are concentrated in these kinds of places (Crane 2011; Corbin 2006; Hein et al. 2007).

This oversight is peculiar for two interrelated reasons. First, while (public-private) partnerships are well-established *neoliberal tools for shrinking* the public sector (especially in wealthy countries), in low-income countries (LICs) these entities are *assuming core functions* that public sector agencies either are unable or unwilling to conduct. A useful illustration is Avahan, the Gates Foundation–sponsored HIV control partnership involving 300 million inhabitants of six Indian states (Chandrasekaran et al. 2008). Moreover, partnerships have also assumed enormous responsibilities on the transnational plane and nowadays often feature prominently in activities that used to be dominated by multilateral agencies (e.g., the Global Alliance for Vaccines and Immunization, which emerged out of and eclipsed the floundering WHO-led Childhood Vaccine Initiative [Muraskin 2002]). Second, the spectacular growth of partnerships is fueled by enormous amounts of (donor) money. Partnerships often involve funding streams that far exceed those available to public sector institutions in LICs. For example, in 2009 the GFATM awarded US$680 million to expanding malaria treatment and prevention in Tanzania, a sum three times the annual operating budget of the entire Ministry of Health.

With partnerships still growing in number and in financial clout, and public sector institutions (such as ministries of health) infrequently playing a dominant role in them, it might be tempting to presume that the proliferation of these entities probably weakens nation-states further, especially those already highly dependent on foreign aid (Abrahamsen 2004; Miraftab 2004). The following case study cautions against such reasoning. Based on nearly two years of ethnographic fieldwork among CONTACT, a transnational malaria research and control partnership operating mainly in Tanzania, it shows how several Tanzanian partners, through their participation in CONTACT, bolstered state influence in health governance at the district and the national level. These effects were mostly unplanned and arose through complex and often markedly indeterminate and idiosyncratic processes.

To trace and unpack these governance effects of CONTACT, this chapter highlights a feature that many partnerships share but that is scarcely considered in the literature: their limited *makeability*. Like countless other interventions, partnerships such as CONTACT are conceived in terms of persuasive sets of goals, inputs, outputs, and desired impacts. However, transforming such a plan into a functioning organization is easier said than done. As will be shown below, it is in the slippery space that separates ideas from practice that actors mobilized the partnership to further their agendas, with variable degrees of success. These agendas were neither uniform nor readily predictable. While some used this slippery space to pursue material and economic gains for themselves or relatives, others used it to advance their organization or to pursue broader social, political, and civic interests. In addition to exposing the processes by which actors and institutions "crafted" CONTACT out of its constituent parts, exploration of this slippery space also sheds light on the para-statal space that the partnership settled into, shaped, and was influenced by. In the Tanzanian case explored here, this para-statal space was at times quite distant from the state but on other occasions barely distinguishable from it.

To contextualize the data and argument presented in this chapter, it begins with a brief historical sketch of malaria research and health services in Tanzania. Then the focus shifts to the notion of partnership and the scientific aims of CONTACT. Drawing on theoretical insights by Mosse and Rottenburg, I explore why CONTACT lacked a detailed plan of action. In the two subsequent ethnographic sections, I chart the dynamic processes through which the partnership was assembled and turned into a running whole, examining how this trajectory was profoundly shaped by interactions with contexts characterized by enormous flux and unpredictability. Throughout these processes, actors' and institutions' variable, often indeterminate interactions with the partnership enabled some to pursue agendas that helped strengthen various Tanzanian state institutions, illustrating how these could thrive in the para-statal space that, at first glance, appeared more conducive to the interests and priorities of non-state actors.

A Historical Glimpse at Malaria Research
and Health Services in Tanzania

Throughout Tanzanian history, malaria was the leading public health problem across the country except in disease-free high-altitude regions (Iliffe 1979). Attempts to reduce sickness and death caused by the scourge commenced under German colonial rule, several years after Ronald Ross determined in 1898 that anopheline mosquitoes transmitted the parasitic disease (Ollwig 1903; Ross 1898). Initially, these efforts focused on groups deemed relevant to the colonial economy, such as whites, urban residents, and some African laborers. Following the First World War, when the British took over the reins, renaming the colony Tanganyika, the authorities began expanding the tiny allopathic rural health system, exposing a slowly growing proportion of the general population to malaria control measures (Beck 1977; Clyde 1967). These efforts took off in earnest after independence in 1961, when the government led by Julius Nyerere embarked on building an extensive rural health care system that became the envy of many African nations (Jonsson 1986; Turshen 1989).

Nyerere's socialist vision for Tanzania rested on maximizing government control over economic and social life, so, correspondingly, he banned all commercial involvement in the health sector during the 1970s. Church missions continued to play an important role in health services provision in some parts of the country (Beidelman 1982), but the health sector was increasingly dominated by public sector institutions, notably the Ministry of Health, its subsidiaries (e.g., the National Malaria Control Programme, NMCP), and various para-statal organizations (e.g., the National Institute for Medical Research, NIMR).[2] By the 1980s, economic demise and withdrawal of donor support spelled the end of Tanzania's socialist experiment. Facing bankruptcy, the government requested assistance from the International Monetary Fund (IMF), which, in exchange, demanded implementation of a Structural Adjustment Program (SAP) aimed at cutting government spending on the health sector and other "social services" (Turshen 1999). Following this decision, donors resumed offering Tanzania financial assistance. This was insufficient to prop up the health system, which remained a state monopoly and was hollowed out by years of chronic underinvestment, becoming largely dysfunctional in much of the country (Jonsson 1986). From 1993, after the Tanzanian government tacitly permitted private sector involvement in the health sector, this situation changed very quickly. Two years later, nearly 40 percent of all health facilities were classified as private sector operations (Tripp 1997). However, while private enterprise flourished in the health sector, public sector institutions languished, caught between the cash-strapped Tanzanian government and donors unwilling to support these notoriously ineffective organizations.

Collaboration and Partnership in International (Health) Development

Better times for (Tanzanian) public sector institutions arrived with the shift from economic to political conditionality in development thinking that gradually took hold during the 1990s. In this new paradigm, attention shifted away from imposing economic reforms (e.g., SAPs) to fostering "good governance," "capacity building," "participation," and "local ownership" (Edwards and Hulme 1995; Moore 1997). Coinciding with the rise of the good governance agenda, criticism was mounting in international health circles that neoliberal reforms promoting involvement of the private sector and civil society in the health sector had done little to alleviate the health problems that primarily affect the poorest people on the planet, in particular the so-called neglected (tropical) diseases (Moran et al. 2001). In this context, a growing number of players in the health arena acknowledged that many health problems in poor countries were so complex and tenacious that these could not possibly be resolved by institutions working in isolation—only collective efforts of multiple "stakeholders" could muster enough skills and resources to make a dent in these problems. However, the field of international health had become enormously fragmented, contentious, and competitive during the 1980s and 1990s. Actors routinely called for greater collaboration and coordination, yet few led the way to make this happen (Walt and Buse 2000). This fragmented and contentious landscape proved fertile ground for the spread of *partnership*, a term that became widely used during (and that symbolizes) the shift from economic to political conditionality. This notion is central to the consensus belief that took hold during the late 1990s: the currently dominant idea that partnership is an "unavoidable necessity" for combating complex health problems in poor countries (Buse and Walt 1997; Richter 2004).

This changing ideological context, wherein competition gradually gave way to collaboration as a dominant urge, set the stage for the rise of PPPs (Gerrets 2010). A novelty in international health until the late 1990s, these entities began to flourish at the turn of the twenty-first century, their proliferation fueled by skyrocketing donor funding for infectious disease research and control efforts (Ravishankar et al. 2009; Shiffman 2006). Even though the lion's share of these funds went to the fight against HIV/AIDS, many other diseases also received greater attention and funding. Annual disbursements for malaria, for instance, soared from US$35 million to US$652 million between 2000 and 2007, an eighteen-fold increase (Ravishankar et al. 2009; Roll Back Malaria 2009). This funding boom and the concomitant proliferation of partnerships offered unprecedented opportunities to Tanzanian public sector institutions such as the NMCP and NIMR, whose activities, severely eroded by decades of neglect and cutbacks, became critically dependent on foreign funding (Gaillard 2003).

The rise of partnership ideology helped generate a more favorable—or less hostile—environment for public sector institutions. This change of wind, however, does not predetermine which branches of government might benefit, let alone in which ways. Moreover, collaboration—an indispensable building block in any partnership—means a range of different things to people and institutions. While some collaborate to pursue mutually agreed-upon and beneficial objectives, others are inclined to dominate collaborators and impose their views, whereas others still make commitments they cannot meet or sponge off their partners. In other words, collaborating is anything but homogeneous, self-evident, automatic, or easy, in partnerships as in other types of organizations. Rather, collaborating is a skill that actors need to develop and cultivate. As with other acquired skills, some actors become highly competent, while others fail outright (Goffman 1967). Given the finesse and continuous work needed to keep a collaboration on track, it is not surprising that some partnerships collapse during the planning stages due to insurmountable differences (e.g., interpersonal, sociocultural, economic, disciplinary, institutional) between actors (Huxham and Vangen 2005; Lasker et al. 2001; Reich 2002). Moreover, there is little reason to assume that these issues vanish once a partnership is up and running. Turning partnerships from plans into well-functioning wholes, no matter how well conceived in terms of inputs and outputs, requires substantial effort and ongoing fine-tuning of partners' contributions, activities, and relationships (Fowler 2000; Lister 2000).

Moreover, partnerships such as CONTACT must not only successfully navigate complex social landscapes in order to thrive but also overcome hurdles emanating from the physical landscape in which they operate. Problems such as power or water outages, communication and infrastructure breakdowns can disrupt even the best-prepared endeavors, demanding considerable flexibility and ingenuity from actors intent on achieving their goals. As the following section shows, some CONTACT partners were more adept than others in juggling these multifaceted challenges, just as they displayed diverse skills in mobilizing the partnership for individual or organizational agendas.

Assembling and Running CONTACT in Tanzania

CONTACT was conceived in 2001 by experts from two institutions that spearheaded the partnership, the Tanzania-based Ifakara Health Research and Development Centre (IHRDC — a preeminent center of research on the African continent, independently run though affiliated with NIMR) and the U.S.-based Centers for Disease Control (CDC — the largest public health institution in the world, a branch of the U.S. government). Together with several other key partners such as the NMCP and the District Medical Officer (DMO) of Rufiji District, these core experts co-developed the primary objectives of CONTACT. The overarching goal of CONTACT was straightforward: to determine the efficacy of artesunate combination therapy (ACT),[3] a potent new antimalarial drug, under "real world" conditions in a rural African setting. ACT was already being used extensively in Southeast Asia, however, at around US$6 per dose,[4] it was considered too costly for widespread use in sub-Saharan Africa. Yet spreading antimicrobial resistance was rapidly rendering affordable alternatives obsolete, so pressure was mounting on the Global Fund to finance the switchover to ACTs in order to stave off soaring morbidity and mortality rates (Snow et al. 1999; Trape et al. 1998). In anticipation of this change, CONTACT set out to assess the effectiveness of ACT in a "typical" rural African district marked by a weak health system, chronic shortages of staff, resources, and supplies, and poor communications. Multidisciplinary in design, CONTACT examined the clinical, biomedical, and biological aspects of ACT as well as its sociocultural, economic, policy, and health systems implications. Since Tanzania was planning to switch to ACTs in the coming years, the partnership expected to generate invaluable operational information for the Ministry of Health, which faced considerable difficulties in 2001 when replacing chloroquine with sulfadoxine-pyrimethamine (SP) (Eriksen et al. 2005; Mubyazi and Gonzalez-Block 2005).

Like most externally funded collaborative health interventions, CON-TACT experts formulated the objectives of the partnership in a research proposal that was sent to potential donors to solicit funding and to regulatory agencies in Tanzania and the United States for (ethical) approval. Led by two counterparts, Michael, an American epidemiologist from the CDC, and Abdul, a Tanzanian epidemiologist from the IHRDC, this effort involved several dozen experts who co-developed different elements of the undertaking. In 2003 Michael sent me a copy of the grant proposal that he had submitted to USAID (the U.S. government agency providing economic and humanitarian assistance) so that I could familiarize myself with the objectives of the endeavor. Measuring well over 140 pages, the CONTACT proposal described in abundant detail each partner's contributions to the endeavor. To my surprise, the blueprint offered scant details as to when, where, or how these activities would take place. Moreover, the document barely addressed the organizational dimensions of this complex undertaking that was going to last more than five years. So how were CONTACT experts going to put together this transnational partnership, which involved actors and organizations from five continents and activities radiating out globally from three Tanzanian locations? How were they going to keep the partnership running for several years?

The absence in the grant proposal of a clear organizational plan for implementing CONTACT was neither an oversight nor an error. Exploring a similar disjuncture between plans and their implementation in international development organizations, the anthropologist David Mosse (2004, 640) argues that protocols and policies guiding interventions are a poor guide for "understanding the practices, events and effects of development actors, which are shaped by the relationships and interests and cultures of specific organizational settings." A key reason for this disjuncture, so argues Mosse (2004, 640), is that the things that make for "good policy"—policy which legitimizes and mobilizes political support—in reality make it rather unimplementable within its chosen institutions and regions. Akin to these development planners, the brains behind CONTACT developed a "good" proposal with persuasive scientific and political objectives—their plan was fully funded and approved by relevant authorities (Mosse 2004). In sharp contrast, the designers of CONTACT *wanted* to implement the objectives spelled out in the plan and do so *without* a detailed plan of action. As the following two ethnographic sections illustrate, this vagueness can be attributed to what Rottenburg (2005) calls a "metacode"—a tacit view of social reality, especially issues that (should) remain unsaid, invoked by actors when attempting to overcome difficulties and challenges through concerted action. Among CONTACT actors, this metacode pivoted on a deeply shared faith in, and a reliance on, organizational flexibility and ambiguity. This faith helped them surmount unexpected challenges that likely would have derailed more tightly planned undertakings and rendered CONTACT "makeable" notwithstanding the absence of even a rudimentary organizational plan.

Partnership from Plan to Practice: Getting and
Keeping CONTACT on Track

Reflecting its partnership framework, CONTACT included various Tanzanian partners from different branches of government (e.g., the Ministry of Health, NMCP, and the Council Health Management Teams [CHMTs] responsible for health matters at the district level). It also involved several nongovernmental organizations (e.g., the Tanzanian Essential Health Interventions Project or TEHIP, which managed the Rufiji demographic surveillance system that provided CONTACT with vital statistics). Beyond Tanzania, CONTACT involved partners from institutions such as the Australian National University, the Swiss Tropical Institute (STI) and the London School of Hygiene and Tropical Medicine (LSHTM). The French pharmaceutical company Sanofi—supplier of artesunate, the key ingredient of ACT—was the sole private sector organization involved in CONTACT. On closer scrutiny, however, boundaries between public and private sector partners are quite unclear and permeable, for organizations such as the IHRDC can be considered PPPs themselves.

The involvement of these partners was not uniform and often varied notably across the life span of CONTACT. The planning phase, for example, mainly involved experts from the CDC, the IHRDC, and the LSHTM who developed the research agenda in cooperation with representatives from the Ministry of Health and the NMCP. By contrast, partners such as the TEHIP and the Rufiji CHMT were mainly involved during the implementation stage. Expected to last around four to five years, CONTACT's evaluation of ACT was anchored in three principal sites in Tanzania. The main offices were located at IHRDC headquarters in Dar-es-Salaam, and most field activities occurred in two rural districts, Rufiji and Kilombero/Ulanga.[5] Rufiji District served as the experimental site, where some 200,000 residents would be treated with ACT for uncomplicated malaria. Kilombero and Ulanga Districts were the control site, where around 300,000 inhabitants received SP, the standard first treatment for uncomplicated malaria across Tanzania from 2001 to 2006.

The experts behind CONTACT—all seasoned researchers with long-term experience in African settings—asked various Tanzania government officials to get involved during the planning stage. Doing so, they reasoned, would facilitate the design and implementation of CONTACT, for example, by making it easier to factor in current and future government activities, especially those that might influence, hamper, or jeopardize the undertaking. This approach usually worked well, except when branches of government deviated from their own plans and commitments. Since communication about such changes often left much to be desired, CONTACT experts regularly had to adapt their plans on the spot. Examination of CONTACT experts' ad hoc responses to—oftentimes only partially understandable—extraneous events renders visible their reliance on and faith in organizational flexibility and vagueness. The following ethnographic vignette illustrates CONTACT experts' reliance on this metacode when navigating a drug supply crisis that could have damaged the trial.

Faith in Flexibility and Vagueness among CONTACT
Actors in Kilombero/Ulanga

Two years before planning for CONTACT started in earnest, in 1999, the Ministry of Health announced that SP would replace chloroquine as the first-line treatment for malaria in Tanzania. However, the ministry did not specify a date for this transition and repeatedly pushed forward the implementation of this decision, eventually settling on August 1, 2001, as the deadline. Since CONTACT was primarily interested in examining ACT, experts had no choice but to modify their plans and shelve activities that could only be conducted after the government would begin distributing SP, such as studies exploring community perceptions of the drug. Importantly, these adaptations were not necessarily considered setbacks. Michael regularly noted, with some irony, that these delays enabled CONTACT to collect superb baseline data about the pre-switchover situation. The three annual data sets, two more than originally planned, were an unexpected boon for longitudinal analysis that, in hindsight at least, was worth the additional costs and stress.

Obviously, the Ministry of Health representatives were well aware that these delays and other unforeseen changes could have negative consequences for CONTACT. Highlighting their stake in the success of the partnership, they repeatedly offered assurances that the introduction of SP would proceed as smoothly as possible in the trial sites of Rufiji and the Kilombero/Ulanga Districts. However, these assurances meant little in practice, for drug distribution was not in the hands of the Ministry of Health but the responsibility of the Medical Stores Department (MSD). An independent arm of the Ministry of Health established in 1993,[6] this para-statal has supplied government health facilities subsequently, a task it has not done very satisfactorily judging by the almost taken-for-granted regularity of medicine outages across the country (Mubyazi et al. 2006). Fitting this pattern, the MSD delivered the first batches of SP several months after the formal switchover date to a fraction of the health facilities in Kilombero/Ulanga. A half year later, by mid-2002, it had managed to supply most health facilities in the area with SP. During this period, a large number of facilities had no choice but to continue using chloroquine despite the formal ban on this drug. Yet with chloroquine rapidly losing efficacy due to mounting antimicrobial resistance, a steadily growing proportion of practitioners and patients started buying SP through commercial outlets. Thus usage of SP increased steadily in Kilombero/Ulanga despite the MSD's failure to deliver the drug, and eventually CONTACT could commence with research activities that had been scheduled for the preceding year(s). These activities proceeded well for about nine months until trouble from an unexpected corner reduced the availability of antimalarials in Kilombero/Ulanga yet again.

The 2003 troubles were triggered by a novel CONTACT partner, the Tanzanian Food and Drugs Authority (TFDA), established earlier that year as the semiautonomous body of the Ministry of Health responsible for regulating pharmaceuticals and enforcing pertinent laws. For TFDA officials, the chaotic antimalarial market constituted an opportunity to assert their freshly minted authority. Tanzanian pharmaceutical law distinguished between over-the-counter drugs, which may be sold by "Part I pharmacies" or *maduka la dawa baridi*, "cold drug stores," and prescription drugs, available only through "Part II pharmacies." However, the TFDA's predecessor, the Pharmacy Board, upheld this law inconsistently so that for years prescription drugs and over-the-counter medicines were available through myriad licensed and unlicensed providers (e.g., general shops, iterant drug peddlers; see Geest and Whyte 1988; Geest et al. 1996). Chloroquine, the most widely used drug in Tanzania, epitomized this ambiguity: formerly classified as a Part I drug, it was obtainable through general stores and other types of outlets that formally were not permitted to sell the drug (Goodman et al. 2004). Keen on enforcing pharmaceutical laws more strictly, the TFDA did not break entirely with the law-bending habits of its predecessor and made an exception for SP. Due to rare but potentially life-threatening side effects, SP was formerly classified as a Part II pharmaceutical. However, Part II pharmacies were few and far between in rural areas, so to ensure that Tanzanians living in rural areas had sufficient access to SP, the TFDA declared that it would condone sales of the drug by maduka la dawa. Moreover, as if to underscore its ambition to improve compliance with (its interpretation of) national pharmaceutical laws, the TFDA announced that it would immediately prosecute general stores and other unlicensed providers selling SP (Goodman et al. 2004; Hetzel 2007; Kachur et al. 2006).

However, as happens in organizations everywhere, the implementation of the TFDA guidelines was not uniform and was profoundly shaped by players and priorities at the district level. The TFDA representative for Kilombero and Ulanga Districts, Mr. Magombe, interpreted these guidelines more strictly and directed his staff to look for and to fine any unlicensed providers that stored and sold SP. Within weeks, the availability of SP and several other antimalarials dropped sharply due to these measures. Since all nineteen maduka la dawa baridi in Kilombero/Ulanga were located in several big villages, SP availability plummeted in smaller villages and rural areas, where 319 general shops were no longer permitted to sell SP, antibiotics, and other prescription drugs (Hetzel 2007). The far-reaching ramifications of this severe drop in antimalarial availability became painfully apparent during the farming season, when villagers moved en masse to their *mashamba* (farmsteads) just as hunger and transmission of malaria and other infectious diseases peaked. Since TFDA staff also targeted itinerant peddlers, mashamba residents lost easy access to SP and would have to travel to villages with maduka la dawa baridi to obtain the drug. However, due to flooding, poor roads, and long distances, such journeys could take a day or more and inevitably elicited high costs, monetary (e.g., transportation expenses or consultation fees)[7] as well as nonmonetary (e.g., lost time tending the crop) (Kamat 2006). Except for obvious emergencies, most farmers were reluctant to risk such high—and potentially catastrophic—losses (Jowett and Miller 2005; Somi et al. 2007). Instead, many resorted to more easily accessible therapeutic options such as amodiaquine (the second-line antimalarial, an over-the-counter drug widely available through general stores) or herbal preparations (often of questionable efficacy). In Kilombero/Ulanga, the implementation of TFDA policy thus inadvertently promoted what biomedical experts call "irrational" or "inappropriate" treatment behavior (Trostle 1988). Moreover, it likely brought more sicknesses, deaths, and suffering to rural residents of Kilombero/Ulanga, though reliable data to back up this claim are lacking (Hetzel 2007).[8]

CONTACT experts could ill afford to ignore these events in Kilombero/ Ulanga. As the control site, changes in this location could influence the study and, in extreme cases, disrupt or damage it. For instance, if SP use among Kilombero/Ulanga residents were to drop too sharply or if amodiaquine use were to rise enormously, then this site would at some point no longer be considered an appropriate control for the experimental district Rufiji. In turn, this could diminish the validity of research findings. Fortunately, the size of the population under study (around 75,000 people) ensured that statistically reliable claims could be made even if antimalarial use were to fluctuate by a factor of ten. Furthermore, since CONTACT aimed to study ACT under "real world conditions," problems such as SP supply disruptions actually constituted valuable data. Since the partnership had sufficient financial reserves, delays did not pose a risk to the endeavor as staff could be assigned to other tasks (such as collection of baseline data sets that were not in the original work plan). Finally, CONTACT experts were also disinclined to intervene in Kilombero/Ulanga—for example, by supplying SP to government health facilities during stock outs—because this might raise hackles among MSD and TFDA staff, something they wanted to avoid at all costs.

In Rufiji CONTACT experts' hands-off approach—and underlying faith in organizational flexibility and fluidity—would face greater challenges than in Kilombero/Ulanga for two key reasons. First and quite obviously, as the intervention site, Rufiji was of pivotal importance to the CONTACT experiment. Hence, a problem in Rufiji could potentially cause greater damage than in Kilombero/Ulanga. Second, partners' interpersonal dynamics and relations had even greater influence on the unfolding of CONTACT in Rufiji than in Kilombero/Ulanga. The following section examines these dynamics by taking a closer look at the CONTACT artesunate supply system. Exploration of how this system was set up, kept running, and (almost) collapsed illustrates how partners' faith in organizational flexibility and ambiguity, the metacode guiding their activities (Rottenburg 2005), rendered CONTACT makeable in the face of enormous, largely unforeseeable hurdles.

Partnership, Flexibility, and the Maintenance of Artesunate Distribution in Rufiji

The principle objective of CONTACT—evaluating the efficacy of ACT under real world conditions over a period of several years—hinged on a (sufficiently) reliable artesunate distribution chain. Yet as was the case with other organizational aspects of CONTACT, the grant proposal offered few clues about the procurement, transportation, and distribution of artesunate. One day, after months in the field (and slightly worried that my question might be interpreted as brazen), I asked Michael why the artesunate distribution received such limited attention in the grant. Chuckling, Michael said that although the planners obviously considered the distribution system a vital component of CONTACT, they merely had a rough idea about the form it would take. Rather, they expected to work out its details during the implementation phase, in close collaboration with partners from the MSD and the Rufiji CHMT, by drawing on individual and collective experiences and knowledge and after assessing possibilities and limitations.

The first component of the distribution chain, procurement of artesunate, was relatively straightforward to set up. When Abdul and Michael began searching for potential suppliers in 2002, global demand for artesunate far exceeded production (Mutabingwa 2005). Complicating matters further, only some manufacturers were willing to make a several-year commitment to three monthly shipments of high-quality artesunate at the WHO-negotiated at-cost rate (nearly $2 per treatment dose). The French pharmaceutical giant Sanofi was the company of choice. However, since CONTACT intended to distribute artesunate for free in Rufiji,[9] Sanofi insisted on measures to prevent the drug from "leaking" into the commercial sector where artesunate sold for about $5 to $6 per dose (2004 prices). Sanofi did not want leaked artesunate from Rufiji to ruin this market, so as part of the contract CONTACT agreed to do its utmost to prevent leakage.

Ensuing discussions about designing effective artesunate delivery systems were profoundly shaped by issues surrounding leakage prevention. CONTACT experts took up these issues with key Tanzanian partners (e.g., the Ministry of Health, the NMCP, the MSD, the Rufiji CHMT) during the preparatory phase of the endeavor, well before the first batch of the drug arrived. It quickly became clear that accommodating Sanofi's demands regarding leakage prevention meant abandoning the original plan to work through the existing MSD distribution system. Even if significant improvements were made, the MSD could not possibly meet Sanofi's requirements regarding the monitoring of supplies, consumption, and storage of artesunate. Faced with this hurdle, CONTACT scientists had to embark on a task they had not envisioned doing—creating, from the ground up, a distribution system for artesunate that met Sanofi's criteria.

The task of building this distribution and monitoring system de novo was eased by the fine cooperation between CONTACT experts and Dr. Omari, the DMO and head of the CHMT in Rufiji District. A crucial partner, Dr. Omari went out of his way to facilitate the implementation of CONTACT. As in other rural areas across Tanzania, the government health system in Rufiji was beset by multiple persistent problems such as staff shortages, crumbling facilities, recurrent shortages of supplies and equipment, and poor transport and communication. For Dr. Omari, collaboration with CONTACT provided invaluable opportunities for achieving his major goal: improving health services in Rufiji District. Native to the area, Dr. Omari worked tirelessly, often against overwhelming odds, to achieve this goal, acquiring a reputation as a DMO who fought hard for "his" district. Together with Dr. Mkimbuga, the district pharmacist responsible for medicines, supplies, and equipment in the sixty facilities composing the government health system in Rufiji, Dr. Omari helped Michael, Abdul, and Joseph (the CONTACT staff members hired to oversee artesunate distribution) to develop an artesunate delivery mechanism. After weighing their options, they decided on a two-tier, hybrid system: CONTACT would take care of transporting artesunate from Sanofi in France to the CHMT storage facilities in Rufiji (in the towns of Kibiti and Utete). In Rufiji CHMT would be responsible for distributing the drug to all health facilities, and CONTACT's sole task would be monitoring drug use, both licit consumption and "leakage."

It soon became clear that this hybrid setup did not function as well as planned. Due to staff, transport, and communication problems, the CHMT task—distribution within Rufiji—was less dependable than CONTACT wished for and, more importantly, than Sanofi required. Impelled by these realities on the ground, CHMT and CONTACT reconsidered the originally conceived division of labor and devised a new, more fluid artesunate distribution system. As in the preceding arrangement, CONTACT remained responsible for transporting artesunate to Rufiji warehouses, at which point CHMT gained formal ownership over these stocks. However, unlike in the preceding arrangement, CHMT was no longer solely responsible for distributing the drug within Rufiji. Instead, CONTACT would henceforth take care of supplying the forty-eight health facilities on the mainland, whereas CHMT would provision the remaining twelve facilities in the Rufiji River delta, remote sites that can only be reached by boat or canoe. This adaptation of the original plan is unsurprising given that CONTACT resources and mobility were far superior to those of the CHMT and health facility staff. CONTACT staff not only received handsome per diems for distributing artesunate, as opposed to CHMT staff for whom it was an unpaid activity that was added to their regular workload. In addition, CONTACT staff conducted restocking trips in an air-conditioned luxury Land Cruiser, a far more efficient (and prestigious) means of transport than the mopeds, bicycles, or buses used by CHMT and health facility staff to redistribute artesunate across Rufiji.

The privilege of CONTACT staff, apparent in numerous ways, easily could have fueled envy among CHMT members and health facility staff wanting their share of the pickings, with negative consequences for artesunate distribution and other partnership activities. However, CONTACT actors regularly offered valued benefits (e.g., trainings with relatively high per-diems) and provided nonmaterial assistance, creating goodwill that helped curtail resentment. For example, Joseph, the CONTACT implementation manager, routinely offered rides to nurses and clinical officers working in remote health facilities. He also transported MSD supplies to these sites, more than once preventing or ending a drug outage. Such deeds were appreciated by the DMO and CHMT team members, whose tasks he alleviated by taking over a time-consuming responsibility, as well as by dispensary staff, who often resented sending sick community members back home for lack of treatment. One sign of the deepening mutual appreciation between CONTACT and the Rufiji CHMT was the growing regularity with which Dr. Omari began presenting CONTACT study findings. For instance, in 2005 Abdul and Michael swung by his office in Utete to share their latest data showing that the percentage of patients seeking care for malaria and other febrile illnesses at government health facilities increased sharply, from 32 percent in 2002 to 48 percent following the introduction of ACT in 2003. Visibly excited by these findings, Dr. Omari said that he would like to use these data to pressure the Ministry of Health to send him more nurses and clinicians, a perennial obstacle in his efforts to improve the health system in Rufiji. He also proposed to report these data at the upcoming annual meeting of Tanzanian DMOs. Similarly thrilled, Abdul and Michael sent Dr. Omari a specially prepared PowerPoint presentation that the DMO used for his visits to the Ministry of Health and the national DMO meeting.

The informal comanagement by CONTACT and CHMT of the Rufiji-wide artesunate distribution system functioned smoothly for nearly three years. While other rural districts of Tanzania had to contend with recurrent shortages and outages, health facilities in Rufiji provided uninterrupted access to antimalarials. Noticing this difference, inhabitants of adjacent districts began flocking in growing numbers to Rufiji health facilities, especially when antimalarials ran out in surrounding areas. Then, in 2005, havoc struck. Precipitated by miscommunication between the MSD and Ministry of Health, SP shortages and stock outs began rippling across Tanzania, eventually affecting much of the country.

As regularly happens with large-scale problems, the 2005 nationwide SP stock out could be traced to a small error, in this case a miscalculation that occurred several years earlier. In 2001 the MSD purchased a huge lot of SP based on erroneous calculations of projected consumption.[10] Sufficient to treat all Tanzanians for a decade, this batch had an expiration date of four years. Since the Ministry of Health was planning to switch over to the next first-line antimalarial artemeter-lumefantrine (ALu) before the expiration date, the MSD decided against replenishing expiring SP stocks. A sensible decision, it became problematic when the Ministry of Health delayed the switchover to ALu, leaving the MSD insufficient time to procure a new load of SP to replace aging stocks. Not permitted (or ordered) to distribute expiring drugs, the MSD omitted SP in standard three-month medicine kits from mid-2005 onward. Predictably, government health facilities across Tanzania reported running out of SP supplies soon thereafter. In Rufiji similar problems could have occurred but this was prevented by the swift action of the CHMT, which promptly redistributed remaining stocks across health facilities. Since SP supplies were abundant in Rufiji, uninterrupted provision could be guaranteed across the district, at least until the next MSD shipment was due three months later. When the next kit to arrive also lacked SP, despite promises to the contrary, the CHMT and CONTACT knew that they had a crisis on their hands.

Upon hearing that the MSD kit yet again contained no SP, Dr. Omari immediately phoned Michael to discuss how they could address the impending SP outage. By law, Dr. Omari had to purchase SP through the MSD, unlike CONTACT. Keen to avoid any interruption of SP provision, Michael promptly instructed staff to purchase a three-month supply for treating the 200,000 residents of Rufiji. At about US$0.10 per dose, SP was nearly twenty times cheaper than artesunate, so the price tag was not a big hurdle. However, it was the end of the budget year and CONTACT had insufficient money to purchase the drug. Unwilling to wait another three weeks until the CONTACT account would be replenished, Abdul raised the problem with the director of the IHRDC, who promptly authorized an emergency loan. It took Joseph several days to scrounge together a three-month stock of SP from various suppliers, after which he departed by Land Cruiser for Rufiji to restock the forty-eight health facilities on the mainland, a task that took four long days to complete. Meanwhile, his assistant Bakari and CHMT colleagues resupplied the remaining twelve facilities in the delta by boat. Through their collaborative effort, CONTACT and the CHMT successfully avoided a disruption of SP provisions in Rufiji while the drug ran out in districts across Tanzania. Dr. Omari received praise for averting an SP outage just as CONTACT experts were pleased that their assessment of ACT proceeded without interruptions. The next mishap, which erupted in 2006, would pose a greater threat to the distribution system.

This mishap also started with a seemingly minor glitch. For reasons that never became fully clear, the electronic payment made by Saidi, the CONTACT administrator, to Sanofi in late 2005 did not land into the right account. Awaiting this payment (of around US$60,000), Sanofi temporarily halted shipments to CONTACT, a routine procedure that it did not notify Saidi about. By the time Saidi figured out what had gone wrong and had managed to trace and resend the missing payment, several months had passed and messages began trickling in at CONTACT headquarters that a growing number of Rufiji health facilities was running low on artesunate. Alarmed by this news, Abdul and Michael immediately started searching for alternate sources of artesunate. However, unlike SP, artesunate was costly and scarce. Finding enough artesunate to treat a district of 200,000 inhabitants for several weeks was a daunting task—as in 2002, global demand for the drug still outstripped supply. After searching frenetically for two weeks, the co-directors identified a source in Zanzibar that was willing to loan them 50,000 doses of artesunate. This solution brought a sense of relief that, however, proved to be short-lived. When opening the shipment at the customs office in Dar-es-Salaam harbor—Zanzibar and Tanzania are separate states within the same nation—Joseph's assistant Anna counted 8,000 instead of the promised 50,000 doses of artesunate. Although this amount barely sufficed for two weeks of consumption in Rufiji, Joseph hurriedly devised an artesunate redistribution plan so as to ensure that all health facilities could offer ACT for another couple of weeks. Just after this redistribution was concluded, word arrived that Sanofi had received the back payment and sent off an artesunate shipment. In a joint operation, CONTACT and CHMT members distributed the new three-month supply of artesunate, narrowly averting a disruption of ACT provision across Rufiji District.

Several months later, in spring 2006, a similar mishap would end less fortunately, resulting in the only major disruption of artesunate distribution in Rufiji. Once again, it was triggered by seemingly minor and distant events, in this case the period of political uncertainty that followed the election of Kikwete as president of Tanzania in December 2005. Shortly thereafter, the customs office postponed all transactions "due to the elections," an allusion to the anticorruption campaign that President Kikwete announced after his election. Like other imported products, Sanofi's March 2006 delivery was sequestered at the customs office in the harbor of Dar-es-Salaam. Efforts to sway officials to release the drugs were fruitless. Fueling anxieties further, CONTACT received two disconcerting notifications. First, Sanofi informed the directors that the company would comply with new WHO guidelines aimed at thwarting microbial resistance and discontinue sales of artesunate monotherapy. Sanofi would only produce preformulated ACTs, effectively cutting off artesunate supplies to CONTACT. Second, the Tanzanian Ministry of Health announced that the switchover from SP to ALu was delayed (yet again), from May to November 2006. This presented a major problem, for CONTACT was scheduled to wind down field activities and did not have US$90,000 to purchase six more months of artesunate to continue treating Rufiji residents until ALu would become available.

Reflecting this unprecedented convergence of bad news, Dr. Omari, Michael, and Abdul jointly approached the head of the NMCP, Dr. Semali, to discuss the impending malaria treatment crisis in Rufiji. For scientific, public health, moral, and ethical reasons they agreed it was unacceptable to deprive inhabitants of Rufiji of ACT just before the rest of the nation was about to shift to ALu. Since the Ministry of Health had already secured large stocks of the drug, Dr. Semali proposed a creative solution: Rufiji would be permitted to transition "quietly" to the new antimalarial one or two months before its official launch in a neighboring district. Combined with careful redistribution of remaining stocks, this solution meant that CONTACT would need to find "merely" US$55,000 to purchase 30,000 to 35,000 extra doses of artesunate. Joining forces, Abdul, Michael, Dr. Omari, the director of IHRDC Dr. Semali, and other partners pleaded with their contacts at Sanofi, WHO, USAID, the CDC, and the Global Fund to help out. Their efforts were successful: the partners not only secured additional funding but also a commitment from Sanofi to ship one final six-month supply of artesunate. The crisis seemed averted.

The artesunate shipment arrived in Tanzania as scheduled, but due to "elections" the Tanzanian customs office could not release the medicines, which sat for weeks in its warehouse, decaying in the tropical humidity. CONTACT staff left no stone unturned to try to release the shipment, but all efforts failed. One Rufiji health facility after another ran out of artesunate. Instead, staff switched to SP or amodiaquine monotherapy, less effective treatments that required higher dosages. After several weeks facilities started running out of these antimalarials as well. The one "real world" situation that CONTACT tried to prevent at all cost, a district-wide breakdown of ACT provision, progressed inexorably mid-2006. Lasting around six weeks, it ended as it had begun: citing delays caused by the elections, the customs office released Sanofi's shipment of artesunate. The following day, CONTACT and CHMT began restocking Rufiji health facilities with artesunate and SP. The hybrid artesunate distribution system operated without any further interruptions until late 2006, when ALu replaced ACT as scheduled.

Concluding Comments

During the past decade, skyrocketing donor funding has spurred the proliferation of partnerships aimed at tackling a range of infectious diseases in low-income countries. Collectively, these partnerships are attracting sizeable resources, expertise, and skills that often dwarf those available to ministries of health and other public sector institutions, rendering them critical players in infectious disease research and control efforts at the national and the international level. While partnerships are regularly praised for their effectiveness in terms of achieving health goals (Komatsu et al. 2010; Kumaresan et al. 2004), they are also criticized for various "unhealthy habits" such as opaque governance and accountability structures, questionable representation, wasteful duplication of activities, sapping public sector institutions, and the favoring of single-disease approaches (Buse and Harmer 2007). Moreover, public sector institutions and actors from southern countries infrequently play leading roles in partnerships—the Global Fund, wherein southern NGOs exert substantial influence, is an often-cited exception (Bartsch 2007). Finally, the funding/partnership boom has made many southern countries even more dependent on external financing for health interventions (Kirigia and Diarra-Nama 2008; Piva and Dodd 2009).

Given these problematic ramifications, it is unsurprising that some critics deride partnerships as Trojan horses for advancing northern priorities and neoliberal private sector agendas (Miraftab 2004), the contemporary face of "scientific colonialism" (Binka 2005), and "scientific imperialism" (Tucker and Makgoba 2008). Such characterizations, while no doubt applicable to certain partnerships and, in some regards, to the enterprise of international health as a whole, sit uncomfortably with this ethnographic case study of the CONTACT partnership. Although northern funding, institutions, actors, and priorities featured centrally in CONTACT from start to finish, Tanzanian actors and institutions profoundly shaped the partnership at all stages by supporting, ignoring, exploiting, hindering, or jeopardizing its various aims, and by drawing it into varied, at times conflicting, agendas. For actors such as Dr. Omari, the DMO of Rufiji, CONTACT constituted a valuable resource in his ongoing struggles with the Ministry of Health about upgrading health services in his district, illustrating how the partnership possibly served as a Trojan horse, though—contrary to Miraftab's claim (2004)—primarily involving local agendas, issues, and priorities.

That CONTACT was enmeshed in and became a resource for all kinds of local issues and concerns is hardly surprising; similar processes have been described for all sorts of development interventions across the world (Arce and Long 2000; Cooper and Packard 1997; Gupta 1998). However, analysis of the ways in which the partnership was appropriated into the Tanzanian context adds relevant insights to the central theme of this book—the para-statal space. In some regards, Tanzania differs markedly from many other LICs, states typically described as weak, distant, or ineffective (Bierschenk and Olivier de Sardan 1997; Reno 1997). Although among the twenty poorest countries of the world, Tanzania government institutions are strong, stable, and prominent, a legacy dating back to the Nyerere era and strongly related to the de facto continuity of one-party rule since independence (Snyder 2008; Tripp 1997). As described at the outset of this chapter, the 1980s financial crisis and 1990s structural reforms hollowed out Tanzanian government institutions, which, nonetheless, retained considerable political and social clout. The Tanzanian government used this influence with remarkable success to garner high levels of foreign financial assistance for its expenditures, especially in the health sector and the sciences, which are highly dependent on foreign funding (Brautigam and Knack 2004).

It is against this backdrop that the prominence of various Tanzanian public sector actors and institutions in this ethnographic account of CONTACT becomes legible. Both the partnership's makeability and its planners' faith in organizational flexibility and ambiguity opened up new opportunities for representatives of public sector institutions to assert their claims and pursue their interests, fostering a para-statal space that enables the Tanzanian state to reassert authority that was corroded during the preceding era of neoliberal reforms. Deviating from patterns observed in many other LICs, this appropriation of partnership in Tanzania points to the variable forms that para-statal spaces take across different contexts.

Notes

1   In this chapter, mirroring common practice, the term *partnership* is used in two ways: as shorthand for a class of hybrid organizations—public-private partnerships (PPPs)—and to denote collaborative relationships between organizational and/or individual actors. Ideally, partnerships are a subset of relationships—those characterized by equity, mutuality, and joint decision making (Brinkerhoff 2002). For various reasons, this ideal is not easy to attain in practice, not least because social life is riddled with all kinds of inequalities.

2   Founded in 1979, the Tanzanian National Institute for Medical Research is a para-statal organization under the aegis of the Ministry of Health. It was created by an act of Parliament (No. 23) to run all research institutions in Tanzania, which had been managed by the East African Medical Research Council (EAMRC) until the East African Community collapsed in 1977. Established toward the end of the colonial era in 1961, the EAMRC succeeded the Bureau of Research in Medicine of colonial East Africa, the organization that coordinated and stimulated science and medicine in British-ruled Kenya, Tanganyika, and Uganda (Beck 1977).

3   Strictly speaking, ACTs are a class of drugs that combine artesunate with another antimalarial, in this case SP (short for sulphadoxine-pyrimethamine), the first-line treatment for uncomplicated malaria from 2001 to 2006. SP replaced chloroquine, the mainstay of malaria treatment for decades. Should the first-line antimalarial fail to cure the patient, then treatment ought to be switched to the second-line drug (from 2001 to 2006, amodiaquine (AQ) was the second-line antimalarial on mainland Tanzania).

4   In 2005 artesunate monotherapy, the principal component of ACT, was available

in pharmacies in Dar-es-Salaam and several other large cities at around US$6 per dose. The price of fixed dose ACTs such as Coartem was even higher, around US$8 per dose.

5 Kilombero and Ulanga are neighboring districts separated by the Kilombero River, located about 450 kilometers southwest of Dar-es-Salaam, the principal city of Tanzania. The IHRDC runs a demographic surveillance system (DSS) that is situated on both sides of the Kilombero River, in Kilombero and Ulanga Districts. This DSS—a defined geographical area wherein all births, deaths, and migrations are continuously monitored—serves as the backdrop for many studies in the area, hence Kilombero and Ulanga are often considered as a unit, Kilombero/Ulanga.

6 The Tanzanian parliament created the MSD in 1993. Through the Medical Stores Department Act of 1993, Parliament transformed the medical supplies division of the Ministry of Health into a para-statal organization. Financially self-sustaining and operating on a commercial basis, the MSD is formally an autonomous department of the Ministry of Health. Since the Ministry of Health plays a key role in financing and purchasing certain drugs (e.g., ARVs and, since 2006, antimalarial combination therapies paid for by the Global Fund), the MSD is less independent than its statute suggests. See the website for the MSD, especially its "About Us" section, accessed March 17, 2011, http://www.msd.or.tz/index.php/aboutus.

7 Unlike Rufiji, where government health services remain free of charge (though imposition of informal fees by health workers is quite common), cost sharing has been introduced in Kilombero and Ulanga Districts, so patients are expected to pay a fee for services and many medicines. By contrast, when patients visit maduka la dawa, they are only charged for drugs while shop attendants typically "diagnose" ailments for free, thus saving time and money.

8 In Tanzania as in many other sub-Saharan countries, reliable morbidity and mortality statistics are scant. The Kilombero/Ulanga DSS described earlier generates such data. However, the farmlands are outside the DSS, so accurate mortality and morbidity data for these areas are not available.

9 Although cost sharing had been introduced in many Tanzanian districts, in Rufiji government health facilities still provided medicines and services at no cost to residents. CONTACT followed this arrangement and did not charge for artesunate.

10 The calculation error was essentially about converting a therapeutic dose of chloroquine into a therapeutic dose of SP. For example, a therapeutic dose for an adult involved multiple tablets of chloroquine but merely one SP pill. The MSD overlooked this difference in the calculations of anticipated consumption, and several times more SP was purchased than needed. Since SP was a cheap drug, this mistake did not have serious financial consequences and was not considered a major issue until it turned into a national sellout.

References

Abrahamsen, Rita. 2004. "The Power of Partnerships in Global Governance." *Third World Quarterly* 25, no. 8: 1453–67.

Aginam, Obijiofor. 2005. *Global Health Governance: International Law and Public Health in a Divided World*. Toronto: University of Toronto Press.

Arce, Alberto, and Norman Long. 2000. *Anthropology, Development and Modernities: Exploring Discourses, Counter-Tendencies and Violence*. New York: Routledge.

Barrett, Ronald, et al. 1998. "Emerging and Re-Emerging Infectious Diseases: The Third Epidemiological Transition." *Annual Review of Anthropology* 27: 247–71.

Barry, M. 2007. "The Tail End of Guinea Worm: Global Eradication without a Drug or a Vaccine." *New England Journal of Medicine* 356, no. 25: 2561–64.

Bartsch, Sonja. 2006. "The South in Global Health Governance: Perspectives on Global Public-Private Partnerships." Conference Paper. International Studies Association.

Bartsch, S. 2007. "The Global Fund to Fight AIDS, Tuberculosis, and Malaria." In *Global Health Governance and the Fight against HIV/AIDS*, edited by W. Hein, S. Bartsch, and L. Kohlmorgen, 146–71. New York: Palgrave Macmillan.

Beck, A. 1977. "Medicine and Society in Tanganyika, 1890–1930: A Historical Inquiry." *Transactions of the American Philosophical Society* 67, no. 3: 5–59.

Beidelman, T. O. 1982. *Colonial Evangelism: A Socio-Historical Study of an East African Mission at the Grassroots*. Bloomington: Indiana University Press.

Bierschenk, Thomas, and Jean-Pierre Olivier de Sardan. 1997. "Local Powers and a Distant State in Rural Central African Republic." *Journal of Modern African Studies* 35: 441–68.

Binka, F. 2005. "Editorial: North-South Research Collaborations: A Move Towards a True Partnership?" *Tropical Medicine and International Health* 10, no. 3: 207–9.

Brautigam, D. A., and S. Knack. 2004. "Foreign Aid, Institutions, and Governance in Sub-Saharan Africa." *Economic Development and Cultural Change* 52, no. 2: 255–85.

Brinkerhoff, J. M. 2002. *Partnership for International Development: Rhetoric or Results?* Boulder, CO: Lynne Rienner Publishers.

Buse, K., and A. M. Harmer. 2007. "Seven Habits of Highly Effective Global Public-Private Health Partnerships: Practice and Potential." *Social Science and Medicine* 64, no. 2: 259–71.

Buse, K., and G. Walt. 1997. "An Unruly Melange? Coordinating External Resources to the Health Sector: A Review." *Social Science and Medicine* 45, no. 3: 449–63.

Buse, K., and G. Walt. 2000a. "Global Public-Private Partnerships: Part I—A New Development in Health?" *Bulletin of the World Health Organization* 78, no. 4: 549–61.

Buse, K., and G. Walt. 2000b. "Global Public-Private Partnerships: Part II—What Are the Health Issues for Global Governance?" *Bulletin of the World Health Organization* 78, no. 5: 699–709.

Caines, Karen, et al. 2004. *Assessing the Impact of Global Health Partnerships: Synthesis of Findings from the 2004 DFID Studies.* DFID Health Resource Centre.

Chandrasekaran, P., et al. 2008. "Evaluation Design for Large-Scale HIV Prevention Programmes: The Case of Avahan, the India AIDS Initiative." *AIDS* 22, no. 5: S1–15.

Clyde, David F. 1967. *Malaria in Tanzania.* Oxford: Oxford University Press.

Cooper, Andrew Fenton, John J. Kirton, and Ted Schrecker. 2007. *Governing Global Health: Challenge, Response, Innovation.* Burlington, VT: Ashgate.

Cooper, Frederick, and Randall M. Packard. 1997. *International Development and the Social Sciences: Essays on the History and Politics of Knowledge.* Berkeley: University of California Press.

Corbin, J. H. 2006. *Interactive Processes in Global Partnership: A Case Study of the Global Partnership of the Global Programme for Health Promotion Effectiveness.* IUHPE. Research Report Series, Bergen, Norway, Research Centre for Health Promotion.

Crane, J. 2011. "Scrambling for Africa? Universities and Global Health." *Lancet* 377, no. 9775: 1388–90.

Edwards, Michael, and David Hulme. 1995. "Too Close for Comfort? The Impact of Official Aid on Nongovernmental Organizations." *World Development* 24, no. 6: 961–73.

Eriksen, J., et al. 2005. "Adoption of the New Antimalarial Drug Policy in Tanzania: A Cross-Sectional Study in the Community." *Tropical Medicine and International Health* 10, no. 10: 1038–46.

Fidler, D. P. 2004. "Germs, Governance, and Global Public Health in the Wake of SARS." *Journal of Clinical Investigation* 113, no. 6: 799–804.

Fowler, Alan F. 2000. "Beyond Partnership: Getting Real About NGO Relationships in the Aid System." In *Questioning Partnership: The Reality of Aid and NGO Relations*, edited by A. Fowler. *IDS Bulletin* 31, no. 3: 1–13.

Gaillard, Jacques. 2003. "Tanzania: A Case of 'Dependent Science.'" *Science Technology and Society* 8, no. 2: 317–43

Geest, S. van der, S. R. Whyte, and A. Hardon. 1996. "The Anthropology of Pharmaceuticals: A Biographical Approach." *Annual Review of Anthropology* 25: 153–78.

Geest, Sjaak van der, and Susan Reynolds Whyte. 1988. *The Context of Medicines in Developing Countries: Studies in Pharmaceutical Anthropology.* Boston: Kluwer Academic.

Gerrets, Rene. 2010. "Globalizing International Health: The Cultural Politics of Partnership in Tanzanian Malaria Control." PhD diss., New York University.

Goffman, Erving. 1967. "On Facework: An Analysis of Ritual Elements in Social Interaction." In *Interaction Ritual: Essays on Face-to-Face Behavior.* New York: Anchor Books.

Goodman, C., et al. 2004. "Retail Supply of Malaria-Related Drugs in Rural Tanzania: Risks and Opportunities." *Tropical Medicine and International Health* 9, no. 6: 655–63.

Gostin, L. O. 2005. "World Health Law: Toward a New Conception of Global Health Governance for the 21st Century." *Yale Journal of Health Policy, Law and Ethics* 5, no. 1: 413–24.

Gostin, L. O., and E. A. Mok. 2009. "Grand Challenges in Global Health Governance." *British Medical Bulletin* 90: 7–18.

Gupta, Akhil. 1998. *Postcolonial Developments: Agriculture in the Making of Modern India*. Durham, NC: Duke University Press.

Hein, Wolfgang, Sonja Bartsch, and Lars Kohlmorgen. 2007. "Introduction: Globalization, HIV/AIDS and the Rise of Global Health Governance." In *Global Health Governance and the Fight against HIV/AIDS*, edited by W. Hein, S. Bartsch, and L. Kohlmorgen, 1–17. Basingstoke, UK: Palgrave Macmillan.

Hetzel, M. W. 2007. "Access to Prompt and Effective Malaria Treatment in the Kilombero Valley, Tanzania." PhD diss., University of Basel.

Huxham, Chris, and Siv Vangen. 2005. *Managing to Collaborate: The Theory and Practice of Collaborative Advantage*. New York: Routledge.

Iliffe, John. 1979. *A Modern History of Tanganyika*. New York: Cambridge University Press.

Jonsson, U. 1986. "Ideological Framework and Health Development in Tanzania, 1961–2000." *Social Science and Medicine* 22, no. 7: 745–53.

Jowett, M., and N. J. Miller. 2005. "The Financial Burden of Malaria in Tanzania: Implications for Future Government Policy." *International Journal of Health Planning and Management* 20, no. 1: 67–84.

Kachur, S. P., et al. 2006. "Putting the Genie Back in the Bottle? Availability and Presentation of Oral Artemisinin Compounds at Retail Pharmacies in Urban Dar-Es-Salaam." *Malaria Journal* 5: 25.

Kamat, V. R. 2006. "'I Thought It Was Only Ordinary Fever!' Cultural Knowledge and the Micropolitics of Therapy Seeking for Childhood Febrile Illness in Tanzania." *Social Science and Medicine* 62, no. 12: 2945–59.

Kickbusch, I. 2005. "Action on Global Health: Addressing Global Health Governance Challenges." *Public Health* 119, no. 11: 969–73.

Kickbusch, I., G. Silberschmidt, and P. Buss. 2007. "Global Health Diplomacy: The Need for New Perspectives, Strategic Approaches and Skills in Global Health." *Bulletin of the World Health Organization* 85, no. 3: 230–32.

Kirigia, J. M., and A. J. Diarra-Nama. 2008. "Can Countries of the WHO African Region Wean Themselves Off Donor Funding for Health?" *Bulletin of the World Health Organization* 86, no. 11: 889–92.

Komatsu, R., et al. 2010. "Lives Saved by Global Fund–Supported HIV/AIDS, Tuberculosis and Malaria Programs: Estimation Approach and Results between 2003 and End-2007." *BMC Infectious Diseases* 10: 109.

Kumaresan, J., et al. 2004. "The Global TB Drug Facility: Innovative Global Procurement." *International Journal of Tuberculosis and Lung Diseases* 8, no. 1: 130–38.

Lasker, Roz D., E. S. Weiss, and R. S. Miller. 2001. "Partnership Synergy: A Practical Framework for Studying and Strengthening the Collaborative Advantage." *Milbank Quarterly* 79, no. 2: 179–205.

Lister, Sarah. 2000. "Power in Partnership? An Analysis of an NGO's Relationships with Its Partners." *Journal of International Development* 12, no. 2: 227–39.

Miraftab, Frank. 2004. "Public-Private Partnerships? The Trojan Horse of Neoliberal Development?" *Journal of Planning Education and Research* 24, no. 1: 89–101.

Moore, Donald B. 1997. "Issuing a New Ruling Class: 'Good Governance' and the African Capacity Building Foundation." In *The Post-Colonial Condition: Contemporary Politics in Africa*, edited by D. Ahluwalia and P. Nursey-Bray, 177–88. New York: Nova Science.

Moran, M. K., C. M. Hewison, and R. D. Gillies. 2001. "Medical Research into 'Neglected Diseases.'" *Medical Journal of Australia* 175, nos. 11–12: 667–69.

Mosse, David. 2004. "Is Good Policy Unimplementable? Reflections on the Ethnography of Aid Policy and Practice." *Development and Change* 35, no. 4: 639–71.

Mubyazi, G. M., and M. A. Gonzalez-Block. 2005. "Research Influence on Antimalarial Drug Policy Change in Tanzania: Case Study of Replacing Chloroquine with Sulfadoxine-Pyrimethamine as the First-Line Drug." *Malaria Journal* 4: 51.

Mubyazi, G., et al. 2006. "User Charges in Public Health Facilities in Tanzania: Effect on Revenues, Quality of Services and People's Health-Seeking Behaviour for Malaria Illnesses in Korogwe District." *Health Services Management Research* 19, no. 1: 23–35.

Muraskin, W. 2002. "The Last Years of the CVI and the Birth of the GAVI." In *Public-Private Partnerships for Public Health*, edited by M. R. Reich, 115–68. Cambridge, MA: Harvard Center for Population and Development Studies.

Mutabingwa, T. K. 2005. "Artemisinin-Based Combination Therapies (ACTs): Best Hope for Malaria Treatment but Inaccessible to the Needy!" *Acta Tropica* 95, no. 3: 305–15.

Ollwig, H. 1903. "Die Bekaempfung der Malaria." *Zeitschrift für Hygiene und Infektionskrankheiten* 43: 133–55.

Peters, D. H., and T. Phillips. 2004. "Mectizan Donation Program: Evaluation of a Public-Private Partnership." *Tropical Medicine and International Health* 9, no. 4: A4–15.

Piva, P., and R. Dodd. 2009. "Where Did All the Aid Go? An In-Depth Analysis of Increased Health Aid Flows over the Past 10 Years." *Bulletin of the World Health Organization* 87, no. 12: 930–39.

Ravishankar, N., et al. 2009. "Financing of Global Health: Tracking Development Assistance for Health from 1990 to 2007." *Lancet* 373, no. 9681: 2113–24.

Reich, Michael. 2002. *Public-Private Partnerships for Public Health*. Cambridge, MA: Harvard Center for Population and Development Studies.

Reno, William. 1997. "African Weak States and Commercial Alliances." *African Affairs* 96, no. 383: 165–86.

Richter, Judith. 2004. "Public-Private Partnerships for Health: A Trend with No Alternatives?" *Development* 47, no. 2: 43–48.

Roll Back Malaria. 2009. *The World Malaria Report—2009*. World Health Organization.

Ross, Robert. 1898. "The Role of the Mosquito in the Evolution of the Malarial Parasite." *Lancet* 152, no. 3912: 488–90.

Rottenburg, Richard. 2005. "Code-Switching, or Why a Metacode Is Good to Have." In *Global Ideas: How Ideas, Objects and Practices Travel in the Global Economy*, edited by B. Czarniawska and G. Sevon, 259–74. Malmö and Copenhagen: Liber and Copenhagen Business School Press.

Ruger, J. P. 2007. "Global Health Governance and the World Bank." *Lancet* 370, no. 9597: 1471–74.

Serdobova, I., and M. P. Kieny. 2006. "Assembling a Global Vaccine Development Pipeline for Infectious Diseases in the Developing World." *American Journal of Public Health* 96, no. 9: 1554–59.

Shiffman, J. 2006. "Donor Funding Priorities for Communicable Disease Control in the Developing World." *Health Policy and Planning* 21, no. 6: 411–20.

Snow, R. W., et al. 1999. "Estimating Mortality, Morbidity and Disability Due to Malaria Among Africa's Non-Pregnant Population." *Bulletin of the World Health Organization* 77, no. 8: 624–40.

Snyder, Katherine A. 2008. "Building Democracy from Below: A Case from Rural Tanzania." *Journal of Modern African Studies* 46, no. 2: 287–304.

Somi, M. F., et al. 2007. "Economic Burden of Malaria in Rural Tanzania: Variations by Socioeconomic Status and Season." *Tropical Medicine and International Health* 12, no. 10: 1139–47.

Traore, S., et al. 2009. "The Elimination of the Onchocerciasis Vector from the Island of Bioko as a Result of Larviciding by the WHO African Programme for Onchocerciasis Control." *Acta Tropica* 111, no. 3: 211–18.

Trape, J. F., et al. 1998. "Impact of Chloroquine Resistance on Malaria Mortality." *Comptes Rendus de l'Académie des Sciences III* 321, no. 8: 689–97.

Tripp, Aili Mari. 1997. *Changing the Rules: The Politics of Liberalization and the Urban Informal Economy in Tanzania*. Berkeley: University of California Press.

Trostle, James. 1988. "Medical Compliance as an Ideology." *Social Science and Medicine* 27, no. 12: 1299–1308.

Tucker, T. J., and M. W. Makgoba. 2008. "Public-Private Partnerships and Scientific Imperialism." *Science* 320, no. 5879: 1016–17.

Turshen, Meredeth. 1989. *The Politics of Public Health*. New Brunswick, NJ: Rutgers University Press.

Turshen, Meredeth. 1999. "Disinvesting in Health." In *Privatizing Health Services in Africa*, 114–33. New Brunswick, NJ: Rutgers University Press.

Walt, G., and K. Buse. 2000. "Partnership and Fragmentation in International Health: Threat or Opportunity?" *Tropical Medicine and International Health* 5, no. 7: 467–71.

CHAPTER 6

Working and Surviving: Government
Employees on ART in Uganda

Susan Reynolds Whyte

African states are employers—even in these times of neoliberalism or post-
neoliberalism. In Uganda hundreds of thousands of people are on the government payroll and their situations cast another light on recent discussions
of the African state. In contributing to these discussions, this collection proposes the notion of the *para-state* as a way of exploring the range of forms
into which African states have diversified. They are para-states in the sense
that they are more or less like their earlier postindependent selves. Dependent on a complex variety of external funding, unable to provide the level
of services expected today, they seem in many ways to operate according to
new rationales, as Geissler suggests in the introduction to this collection.
Many state functions are carried out in such intimate collaboration with
"development partners" that it is not always clear what is national and what
is foreign, what is governmental and what is nongovernmental. Other services that could have been government responsibilities are offered by NGOs
or charities or international research projects or commercial interests.

Yet the idea of the state remains vital in Uganda. It is not just the memory of the state or what is left over of the state—although these figure too,
especially for older people. The state is the arena for national politics. It
is what people struggled to make functional again after the suffering and
abuses of "the regimes" of Amin and his immediate successors. It is what the
National Resistance Movement (NRM) created anew with decentralization
and the tiered system of local councils down to village level. At its core is
the military, a whole army of government employees (Tripp 2010). It basks
in the reflected gleam of foreign-funded development projects, which in
many ways lend it credibility. With all its faults, the state touches the lives
of every citizen through its teachers, health workers, district officials, and

police. They carry out their jobs with more or less corruption and commitment, cynicism and idealism, with greater or fewer resources from outside the government. But for many people, themselves included, the bottom line is that they have salaried jobs.

This is by no means usual. The last national census reported that wage and salaried employees constituted only 16 percent of the workforce. Self-employed workers—those in the informal economy, petty business, and small-scale trading—accounted for 43 percent. Unpaid family workers made up 41 percent of the workforce, comprising those occupied with subsistence agriculture and domestic chores.[1] With inflation, big families, and increasing needs for cash, with high population growth and ever-greater numbers of hopeful young people completing their education and desperately searching for work, it is hard to overemphasize the desire for work.

The nature and social value of work, especially the qualities of regular employment, were brought into sharp relief with the advent of antiretroviral therapy (ART), and it is this optic I adopt for examining bioscience in Uganda's present (para-)state.[2] Before ART was widely available for free, it was those with good jobs who had access to it. Later, when many more people got a "second chance" through ART, regaining life meant getting back to work. Being on ART cast their occupations in a new light. This chapter focuses on the qualities of government employment as experienced by people trying to get on with the lives that ART made possible. Those qualities can be understood by contrast with the work situations of the majority of Ugandans on ART, whose livelihoods are a "gamble." They are also illuminated by comparison with the work opportunities emerging from the very bioscientific interventions providing the lifesaving treatment.

Taking the perspective of government employees re-centers recent discussions of the shifting character of the state in the face of increasing private enterprise and foreign-funded interventions (Ferguson 2006; Ong 2006; Comaroff and Comaroff 2000; Tsing 2004). Whereas government facilities present a façade that allows citizens to imagine the state—and complain about its lack of resources and services (Masqulier 2001)—the view from behind the façade provides different angles. We can examine the ways in which positioning within a national political economy affects appropriation of transnational biopolitical initiatives. To put it pointedly: our informants are alive today because of those interventions, but they are alive while others have died because they are government employees. There is no doubt that life science research and treatment programs, heavily funded from the

Global North, have changed the nature of health care in Uganda. But in order to paint a picture with greater nuance, we must recognize the persisting significance of national government, as do those whose livelihood depends upon it. While the arguments of Nguyen (this volume, 2009, 2010) emphasize the therapeutic domination of international donors and NGOs upon whom entire populations now depend (Nguyen 2009), a closer look reveals that those who enjoy the benefits of "therapeutic domination" are but segments of the population. Nguyen saw this when ART first became available in West Africa: those who adopted the "confessional technology" of the first NGOs survived because they achieved access to the ARVs (Nguyen 2010). In the Ugandan context, the most important key to ART in the early days was an income.

Listening to the accounts of government employees re-centers our conceptual apparatus in another way too. From their viewpoint, survival is not "mere survival" or "somatic individuality" (Rose 2001). While continued biological existence may be the main objective of some health professionals, policy makers, and donors, the concern of our Ugandan informants was also the social survival that made individual life possible. Family support carried people through periods of severe illness and weakness; connections to treatment programs and encouragement to stay on medication came through other people. When they had regained strength, people went back to work, and the nature of their work conditions was key to *survival*, in the sense that it has in Ugandan English—that is, getting by in difficult circumstances, managing somehow, creatively making it through with the help of others. This chapter is thus an attempt to understand the para-state from the inside perspective of those who work for a national government, depend on foreign life science interventions, and survive in the broadest sense within a given historical and social context.

Civil Service since the "Original Uganda"

Since independence in 1962, the fortunes of civil servants have shifted radically. In the 1960s, teachers, health workers, and other government officers were relatively comfortable, compared to farmers and traders. They enjoyed a decent standard of living, staff housing, and reasonable, reliable wages. In 1969 salaries were so regular that our schoolteacher neighbor used to remark that she loved February because she got her pay after only twenty-eight days. In retrospect, it is a time imagined as foundational. "You knew the original Uganda," remarked an acquaintance upon hearing that we first lived in Uganda from 1969 to 1971. Not that he was nostalgic for a past he had lost. Most Ugandans do not remember the time before Amin's coup in 1971, and even if they do, the tumultuous history thereafter has overshadowed the immediate postindependence period of the 1960s (Rice 2009). Nevertheless, the legacy of civil service, inherited from the colonial period and reinforced in the first decade after independence, persists in some important ways.

The pattern of Milton Obote's "original Uganda," which actually extended into the first years of Amin's regime, was the centralization of political and administrative power, a tendency common in many African states immediately after independence. Under Obote, firms were nationalized and para-statals (in the old sense—not to be confused with the para-state, as distinguished in Geissler's introduction) were increased (Nabuguzi 1995, 193–94). The para-statals of that period took the form of boards for marketing (lint, coffee, produce, and dairy) and provision of public services (electricity, insurance, transport, telecommunications, banking). The postcolonial state was seen as representing popular aspirations, a view that donors also shared, in that foreign aid was transferred to the state in order to strengthen public sector–led development (Hyden 1995, 41). It was the civil service that had the mandate to realize the visions of independence. Government employees were respected for their education and specialized training and for their incomes. Wage earners were a "labor aristocracy" compared to farmers; the minimum wage rose fivefold between the late 1950s and the late 1960s, while cotton and coffee prices, upon which the majority depended for cash income, declined (Jamal 1991, 84; Grillo 1973, 9–10).

Amin's expulsion of 50,000 Asians in 1972 at first seemed a further step toward strengthening the state, in that it brought their property and businesses into the hands of government. But these resources were distributed as patronage and mismanaged; shortages became the order of the day. The para-statal marketing boards collapsed and were replaced by another kind of *para-*, or parallel, informal economy. The *magendo* black market flourished. Civil servant salaries were insufficient, delayed, or not paid at all, while hyperinflation made the salaries almost meaningless anyhow (M. Whyte 1990, 131–32, 143–45). People kept their government jobs but simultaneously engaged in all kinds of "survival strategies" to eke out a livelihood. The Public Service Salaries Review Commission (1980–82) wrote of a "retainer fee syndrome," whereby token salaries functioned as means of retaining civil servants in their positions, rather than providing a living wage (Obbo 1991,

101). The "retainees" were unable to devote full time to their government jobs, but many were happy to be retained because of benefits like housing and transport.[3] Their civil service jobs positioned them and gave them legitimacy. Those with access to public resources were able to turn them into income generating endeavors in myriad creative ways (Obbo 1991).

When Yoweri Museveni assumed power in 1986, his NRM government began to implement structural adjustment policies. Some of the existing para-statals (still in the old sense), such as the National Insurance Company and the Uganda Electricity Board, were privatized and the old para-statal marketing boards were never revived. Efforts were made to cut back on the civil service; this meant retrenchment (dismissal) for some and the loss of housing privileges for others (though occupants of urban staff residences benefited from the opportunity to buy their houses on favorable terms). Between 1993 and 1996, a demobilization program aimed to cut the army by 30 percent (Twaddle and Hansen 1998, 4–5). Whether due to the effects of structural adjustment or simply the improved efficiency and stability after fifteen years of misrule, working conditions and salaries were slowly regularized. By the turn of the millennium civil servants were being paid more or less on time.[4] Compared to the 1960s, civil servants were worse off, but compared to the 1970s and 1980s, their conditions were much improved. Nevertheless, patterns of *para-work* as salary supplementation continued: health workers ran small clinics and drug shops, teachers offered extra tutoring for a fee, policemen took on shifts as private watchmen.[5]

The NRM government attracted large amounts of donor funding, but the nature as well as the scale of funding had shifted since the immediate postcolonial period. There was a move from para-statals to para-statism, which took several forms yielding a complicated and often unclear picture of what is state and what is not. One pattern was that donor-funded agencies took over institutions and functions established under state auspices. For example, the Joint Clinical Research Centre (JCRC), a leader in treatment and research for HIV that began as a joint initiative of the Ministries of Health and Defense and Makerere, the premier national university, now calls itself an NGO and is supported by foreign research funds and the President's Emergency Program for AIDS Relief (PEPFAR). The Uganda Virus Research Institute, once a government agency (and earlier an institution of the three East African countries), is now also a research station of the British Medical Research Council. Another tendency was that donors established new separate development and service activities, such as supplying food to internally displaced people in northern Uganda, a task that the government might have taken on given that the army had forced them into camps. Perhaps most common of all was the weaving of donor programs into existing government institutions, for example, providing resources for training the police and building new classrooms for government schools.

Whereas the old para-statals were monopolistic boards and agencies primarily controlled by the state using public and private funds, or authorities that regulated private companies, the new generation of agencies are statutory organizations (established by legal statute) designated as "semiautonomous bodies" or "semiautonomous institutions." They are often reincarnations of former government units that receive core funding from government and are able to enter into "partnerships" with NGOs, businesses, or multi- and bilateral donors in order to carry out their functions.[6] For example, the Uganda Wildlife Authority (formerly the Game Department and Uganda National Parks), which administers the national parks and wildlife reserves, has partners, including Tullow Oil (the major player in oil exploration), USAID, several tourism associations, and the International Gorilla Conservation Programme.

Employees of donor-supported NGOs and nongovernment projects were generally better paid than civil servants, although their contracts were time limited. However, civil servants also benefited from external funding through resources for extra activities, equipment, and training that were funneled into government structures. An example close to hand is the Enhancement of Research Capacity program that supported Makerere University staff and the research collaboration upon which this chapter is based.[7]

Work in the Time of AIDS

Work first captured the attention of AIDS researchers and policy makers because of its link to transmission. Soldiering, long-distance truck driving, cross-border trading, fishing, and labor migration have all been seen as high-risk for men. Women who served these men in bars or engaged in trading were also categorized as doing work that put themselves and others at risk (Iliffe 2006, 25; Barnett and Blaikie 1992, 68–85). The epidemic was early on associated with the "fat cats," the *mafuta mingi*, prosperous mobile traders (Kinsman 2008, 58–9). During the magendo era of the late 1980s, that category included some civil servants involved in business, with money to spend on sexual partners. (Indeed, the first person I knew who admitted he had

AIDS was a local magistrate posted in a border town, who returned to the village to die.) An oft-repeated story about Museveni's early strong stand on HIV is that Cuban doctors alerted him to the high prevalence of the virus in the army soon after he came to power (Kinsman 2008, 69; Putzel 2004, 23). Thus, government employees were affected by the epidemic from the beginning, but so were people in other kinds of occupations. As the disease spread, it became clear that HIV was for everyone. In Uganda the focus on risk groups was quickly tempered by recognition that HIV was "our sickness," not just "theirs" (Epstein 2007, 161).

When ART became available, its cost was prohibitive for all but the wealthy. As the South African judge Edwin Cameron said to an international AIDS conference in 2000: "I can take these tablets, because on the salary I earn as a judge, I am able to afford their cost. . . . In this I exist as a living embodiment of the iniquity of drug availability and access in Africa. . . . Amidst the poverty of Africa, I stand before you because I am able to purchase health and vigour. I am here because I can afford to pay for life itself" (quoted in Barnett and Whiteside 2002, 183). With the advent of generics, prices began to fall around 2001. People with regular reasonable incomes were able to buy the medicines, although this entailed great sacrifices and they often had to skip doses when they were short on cash (Whyte et al. 2004; Byakika-Tusiime et al. 2005; Kabugo et al. 2005). Those were years when a good job, or a family member with a good job, literally meant the difference between life and death.

Starting in mid-2004 with resources from the Global Fund and taking hold in 2005 when PEPFAR came in, ART became widely available for free. There was a dramatic uptake within a few years. In 2003 the Uganda AIDS Commission reckoned that 10,000 people were receiving antiretroviral medicines. WHO estimated Ugandans receiving ART at 44,000 in 2004, increasing to 115,000 in 2007. This corresponded to a rise in coverage of those in need of treatment from 12 percent to 33 percent (WHO 2008 factsheet). From early on, Uganda welcomed support from donors in the fight against AIDS (Parkhurst 2005), and financially the country is heavily dependent on external support for AIDS activities. For the period from 2008 to 2009 it was estimated that the Ugandan government contributed 7 percent to the AIDS response, while multilateral donors covered 4 percent, and bilaterals 89 percent. The United States alone contributed over 80 percent of the funds for HIV/AIDS prevention and treatment (UNGASS 2010, 55–56).

The donor funds supported a plethora of programs both within and without the government health system. New units were constructed at or near existing hospitals. The U.S.-supported AIDS Information Centres, which provided most HIV testing for many years, were mainly located within government hospital compounds. The AIDS Support Organisation (TASO) frequently built facilities just at the edge of hospital grounds. While the NGO Joint Clinical Research Centre has its own complex near Kampala, it supports HIV treatment at a long list of government health centers under its TREAT program. It is thus difficult to disentangle national from external management of HIV and AIDS. As one client of an ART program fervently declared: "I really thank this government—I don't know—whoever brought these drugs."

In late 2005 a team of four Danish and four Ugandan anthropologists undertook a study of living with ART.[8] It became a kind of ethnography of contemporary Uganda through the lens of the first generation of people to benefit from widespread free ART. They shared historical circumstances. They had seen their relatives and friends die; some had been close to death themselves. They experienced a second chance—the prospect of taking up their lives again, albeit with the strictures and opportunities of being clients in treatment programs (S. Whyte et al. 2013). But the conditions of their lives and work were as varied as Ugandan society itself.

We first undertook life history interviews of forty-eight people receiving ART. They were from seven different treatment programs: three in Kampala and four in eastern Uganda. Of these forty-eight, we identified twenty-three who were willing to let us continue visiting them seven more times over the ensuing eighteen months. Because we were initially interested in the dilemmas and inequities of paying for ART (Whyte et al. 2004), we tried to include people getting medicines on a fee basis, even though the rollout of free ART was already under way by the time we began. Around half of our informants had started out paying for the treatment, but most had shifted from fee to free by the time our study ended. The majority of the people we interviewed in late 2005 and early 2006 had initiated ART at least a year earlier. We heard about, and in some cases followed directly, their gains in health and resumption of work.

The inclusion of people who had been able to buy treatment at one point meant that our interlocutors turned out to be somewhat better educated and more likely to have wage employment than the average Ugandan. Of the forty-eight people we originally interviewed, nineteen had salaried jobs, while eight of the twenty-three we followed over a year and a half earned regular wages. All except four of the nineteen people on salary were state employees, a proportion that reflects their preponderance in the salariat. They included soldiers, teachers, health workers, a university lecturer, a railwayman, a prisons officer, and a Uganda Revenue Authority officer. As I will show, their situations contrasted in important ways with those of the majority of our informants. Like most people in Uganda, these latter were farmers (often called peasants in Ugandan English), small-scale business people, and manual laborers who were not on a regular payroll. In addition to "digging," they earned their livelihoods as brick makers, construction workers, market traders, shopkeepers, purveyors of cooked food and alcohol, and skilled craftsmen (tailor, electrician, metalworker).

The Kinds and Qualities of Work

In his discussion of the ways in which work was categorized and valued on the Kenya coast, David Parkin approached work as "productive tasks or activities which offer the individual control over his own and his family's destiny" (1979, 318). The concept of control allowed him to explain the greater value attached to monthly wage labor as opposed to casual labor or small business ventures, even when the latter yielded a higher income. Parkin's (1979, 322) informants felt that being able to count on a regular income allowed one to plan "not just one's immediate budget but one's very life," that is, life in the social sense. Casual labor, trade, or craft was less dependable in both amount and timing of earnings. Although you might do well one day, the next day could bring nothing. In Uganda, people often speak of those without regular employment as *gambling*, a term that captures the same quality of unreliability that Parkin underlined.

The focus on endeavors to control present and future circumstances is helpful for understanding the concerns of the first generation about work. Planning and control had particular temporal and spatial dimensions for them. They were conscious of changes in their bodies over time. Illness and, for many, the initial side effects of ARVs had diminished their strength and impaired their ability to work. People often spoke of becoming "useless," indicating that weakness was not only an individual bodily experience but also a social condition that inhibited them from contributing productively in their families and workplaces. In time, treatment enabled them to work again and thus to be "useful," though not always with the capacity they once had (Kaler et al. 2010, 7–9). But then another problem appeared; overexertion could exhaust them and make them fall sick again. The spatial and temporal fixing of treatment could collide with the requirements of work. Being on ART meant being tied to a program and reporting to that site at regular intervals to get medicinal supplies. Whereas the mobility of certain occupations had earlier been seen as a key factor in transmitting the virus, the era of ART made mobility another kind of problem. Some people had to accept being relatively immobilized, especially those on programs requiring clients to be a resident in a delimited catchment area (the CDC's Home-based AIDS Care and Mbuya Reach Out). Others had to move between the places where they obtained their drugs every month or two and the places where they worked or had families.

The second chance via treatment was an opportunity to work and our interlocutors were preoccupied with livelihood issues. As Russell and Seeley (2010, 376) argue, "narratives of work and resource mobilization are interpreted to be adaptive strategies that facilitated a transition to living with HIV as a chronic condition: they were people's 'quests' to regain control, create order, reduce dependence on others, and to feel 'normal' again." But our informants also emphasized the difficulties of maintaining control, keeping order, and being independent. Their situation differed from that of the Giriama people of whom Parkin wrote in the 1970s and to some extent also from that of the ART clients described by Russell and Seeley (2010), most of whom were subsistence farmers. While monthly wage labor had high value for some of the reasons adduced by Parkin, control over destiny was never guaranteed. Job assignments, transfers, workplace politics, failure or delay in wage payment, and fear of job loss undermined their confidence in being able to steer their lives. While such worries affected all employees, those on ART felt them more keenly than their HIV negative colleagues.

Following Parkin, we can distinguish salary jobs from other ways of earning cash. Ugandans mark the difference with the label *working class* to denote those fortunate enough to have a paycheck every month (not as in U.S. and British English, those who do unskilled or manual labor). The term is relative to the position of the speaker: more sophisticated people use it of white collar workers, while for others even an ordinary soldier is working class because he gets a salary. One of those we followed closely, John, had made his way up from porter to locomotive driver in the railways. My colleague in this project, David Kyaddondo, reckoned that many educated urbanites might not consider a railwayman "working class," but that people in his home village certainly would. To be working class is to have an address, that is, to be located in an organization. Being working class does not generally mean relying exclusively on a salary; almost everyone does more than one kind of work, including unpaid family labor. In fact, it is those with a monthly wage who can invest in small business ventures and farming or perhaps even property that can generate additional income.

In a major essay on millennial capitalism and the nation-state, Comaroff and Comaroff (2000, 305) discuss the apparent demise of a discourse on class and the revaluation of gambling, both on the market and in lotteries (295). Here too we see the shifts that re-centering brings to discussions of the state of the state. Ugandan government employees, and their compatriots, have formulated notions of *class* in a way that fits a political economy where most people have no salaried employment. The unemployed are gamblers by default, and gambling has only negative social value. Ugandan popular discourse is not about class in relation to the means of production, nor does it reflect class consciousness in the sense of articulated political interest.[9] Perhaps it implies class distinctions in terms of the ability to consume, though that is to put an altogether different light on Parkin's ability to control own and family destiny.

Self-Employment as Gambling

Mama Girl, a farmer and local councilor who shared a household with her co-widow, also a farmer, explained that they did not know where they would find the money for the next term's school fees. "We're just gambling," she said, in the same spirit that animates people in Francophone Africa when they say "On se débrouille" to indicate the unsure business of making one's way in a world short on stable institutions and workplaces (S. Whyte 2008). Life without a regular salary is a gamble for everyone. Losing trading capital because of sudden family needs, customers who fail to pay, crackdowns from the authorities, deceptions and failures on the part of associates: all these contingencies are well known to anyone working in the informal economy (which is almost everyone in some way or another).

But people who have been gravely ill, who feel their health is fragile, and who are uncertain about the immediate and more distant future feel especially vulnerable to the chanciness of livelihood endeavors. Bernard compared the difficulties of self-employment to his earlier salary job. He had worked twenty-two years for the National Insurance Corporation, but when the (old-style) para-statal was privatized in 2002, he was retrenched—

just before he started on ART. He recounted: "I started doing business but it wasn't easy because I was used to being an office person. I incurred a lot of thefts, the money I had invested decreased. I used to trade in radios, but these days I sell used clothes. I tried to do poultry rearing and failed."

Survival depended on others. Amid the chances of gambling, people time and again found help from their household and family members. When Jessica first started on ARVs and was feeling ill from side effects, she occasionally kept her daughter home from school to prepare the cooked food that earned them cash. Dominic, a former herdsman turned butcher, praised his hard-working wife, who grew what they needed to eat and even managed to sell some millet and groundnuts in order to buy sugar and salt. Most appreciated of all were the household members who earned a steady wage. The contrast between self-employment and earning a salary was clear in many of the homes we visited.

William was a builder; he found work where he could. At our second visit, he had nothing to do. He had been constructing a house for a man in Luwero, who was earning money from a tipper truck. When the truck was stolen (Luwero is on the road to Sudan where such trucks found a good market), the man could no longer hire William. So William depended on his wife, a primary school teacher. "If she were not working, I don't know what we would be eating now. I ask her 'Has the salary come?' When the salary delays, life becomes very difficult."

Herbert, shopkeeper in a small eastern Ugandan trading center, has a second wife who was a head teacher. Her salary helped to pay school fees for his various children. Once, when we visited, he was still weak after hospitalization. His wife had been interdicted (suspended) from work. "She came from work as usual but she had a letter. When I read it, I collapsed because I was not seeing any future with our children because she is the one paying school fees after me adding on a little from my shop. I found myself in hospital on drip for two days. I realized I am not a strong man. My wife laughed at me and asked how I could collapse just because of a job. But it was also because of corruption and tribalism. I had just given my wife 200,000 shillings to bribe the District Education Officer. He asked for it, but three weeks later he sent her a letter of interdiction anyhow. Aahh, when I thought about the money, my wife losing a job, I collapsed and found myself on drip in hospital." The heavy value that Herbert attached to his wife's salary and the workplace politics that led to her interdiction were themes in all the working-class lives we came to know. But before we consider the attractions and uncertainties of life on a government salary, we may review a special form of gambling associated with the provision of ART.

Volunteer Work as Hoping

The habitus of gambling is what Johnson-Hanks (2005) called "judicious opportunism." She argued that this alternative to rational action in pursuit of set goals is pronounced under the contingent conditions of contemporary African societies: "The challenge is not to formulate a plan and implement it regardless of what comes but to adapt to the moment, to be calm and supple, recognizing the difference between a promising and an unpromising offer. . . . Maintaining options is the central aim of action under judicious opportunism" (Johnson-Hanks 2005, 370). The advent of free ART and the coexisting congeries of material support projects brought new options for HIV positive people. There were jobs to be had for the clients of treatment programs such as Mbuya Reach Out in Kampala, which employed a team of Community AIDS and TB Treatment Supporters. And even where there was no clear cadre of HIV positive employees, there was widespread hope of getting some kind of paid position in the donor-funded project. Volunteer work was a way of positioning oneself. (Government employees also positioned themselves in relation to donor projects, but their situations were much more secure, of course, since they were already on contract.)

The principle of Greater Involvement of People with AIDS (GIPA), adopted at the 1994 Paris AIDS Summit, called for the participation of HIV positive people at all levels of policy making, administration, and implementation of AIDS activities. It has been most widely realized in the recruitment of "expert clients" as assistants in clinical and outreach work and as peer counselors for others who are positive or on treatment. Expert clients provide some relief to hard-pressed health workers, struggling with the enormous workload of treating so many people, although there are also tensions between professionals and volunteers over competence and responsibility (Kyakuwa 2009).

Educated people, who speak English, are chosen as volunteers. They are not paid for their time, but they receive allowances for attending workshops and sometimes for lunch and transport. One of our interlocutors was Jolly, running a small food kiosk, from a working-class family, with some secondary education. She was happy the last time we visited her, because she had been selected for training as a peer counselor at the national hospital clinic where she received treatment. It was volunteer work, "but they will be providing us with transport so I don't know," she said hopefully (Whyte et al. 2013). A friend of mine described how she spent every Thursday assisting at her district hospital AIDS clinic, weighing patients, doing paperwork, supplying medicines. She was paid nothing but attended seminars about once a month for which she received an allowance of a few thousand shillings. She had earlier had paid work with a World Vision AIDS project that had phased out; she was keeping her hand in, and maintaining her CV, in case other opportunities presented themselves.

Volunteering as "judicious opportunism" is not new in the health sector. The history of village health workers, community distributors of contraceptives or antimalarials, vaccination assistants in immunization campaigns, and the training of traditional birth attendants and traditional healers is a story of volunteer work. While the sponsors of these donor-funded programs expected people to give their time for the good of the community, those who volunteered were interested in the small allowances and other benefits (gum boots, T-shirts, medical equipment). They hoped to parlay their training and experience into an income. After the projects closed, some opened drug shops and small clinics; some got taken on as paid nursing aides at local government health centers. At the very least, they were often recruited again for the next project, with whatever allowances it might bring. The difference between earlier health volunteering and the current wave of "expert clients" is that a disease diagnosis is a prerequisite for positioning oneself. The livelihood concerns of the current generation of AIDS volunteers are particularly acute.

Qualities of Government Employment

In addition to the staff of donor-funded NGOs and nonprofit enterprises, the salariat includes those employed by private individuals and enterprises — agricultural, factory, domestic, and service workers. However, commercial agriculture and industry are relatively small, and the business sector cannot compare to that of neighboring Kenya. The majority of people on payrolls work for government.[10] The image of public service takes on meaning compared to alternatives. Not only were public employees better off than those who had to "gamble" for a livelihood, but they were also at an advantage compared to most other members of the salariat.

First and most importantly was the relative regularity of pay, the point that Parkin emphasized long ago. (In contrast, people working for private Ugandan businesses could go for months without salary, staying on in hope and because they knew that they would never collect anything at all if they quit—the growing business of private nursery, primary, and secondary schools was notorious in this regard.) For our interlocutors on ART, being paid every month was a blessing. A reliable salary was evident in body size. When Robinah went home for a visit some months after starting on ART, her neighbors were astounded at her transformation from skeleton to solid woman. Unable to believe that medicine had worked the miracle, they wondered if she had gotten a job. Around the same time there was an article in one of the national newspapers decrying potbellies in the police. Having a government salary made it easier to get credit from local shopkeepers. It was possible to plan for the recurring expenses of school fees or to get the bursar to allow the balance to be paid later. Employees could get advances on their salaries.

They still had money problems. For many, like the soldiers, the wages were low. Salaries were sometimes delayed, even though timeliness had improved immensely in recent years. For practically everyone, employment meant obligations to help members of their extended families who moved in with them or turned to them for help, contributing to the constant insufficiency of cash (Wendland [2010] describes the same pattern in Malawi). John, the railwayman, recalled with a sigh what it was like to get his first job as a railway porter and try to meet the expectations of family members dispersed all over the country. "You know, I had to take care of everybody—people everywhere—north, central, eastern." Despite all the demands, those with a regular income could sometimes put aside enough to invest in farming or a small business. Later in his career, John was able to purchase a grinding machine so his wife could run a milling business in their village. Dorothy, the prison officer, and her husband, a teacher, farmed groundnuts and kept some cows at their rural home.

Unlike everyone else in Uganda, government employees could hope for a pension upon retirement. (As in most African countries, there is no social security allowance for older people.) If they were retrenched, they received a severance package. If they died, their spouses received an insurance payment. Sometimes it was difficult to collect them, but at least public sector workers had the prospect of getting such benefits. Particularly the potential of one-time lump payments figured prominently for several of our interlocutors, who dreamed of the investments they could make. Herbert, who had collapsed upon hearing that his wife was interdicted, at an earlier point was encouraging her to resign and get her retirement benefits so they could go into business together. The prospect of a retrenchment nest egg was John's only comfort during the difficult months when Uganda Railways was being privatized and he was convinced he would be sacked. Like Bernard, who was retrenched when Uganda Life Insurance went private, he hoped to invest in a profitable business that would keep his family as the salary had done.

Two of the widows we followed benefited from the fact that their husbands had been relatively high-ranking civil servants. Cathy, a university-educated resident of Kampala, did not have to gamble to find school fees for her children every term, as did Mama Girl and her co-widow. Her husband had been a district official, and after his death, the administrator general's office kept an account for her and their children, from which educational costs were paid directly to the school. She was also given a one-time payment from which she completed a land purchase and started a small business trading in cloth. In spite of disagreements with the office administering the funds and suspicions of corruption, Cathy affirmed that the benefits she derived from her husband's government job placed her advantageously compared to others on her ART program. Mama Girl, the farmer and local councilor, had also received remuneration when her husband, a government officer, died. The money was given to her alone — 3.8 million shillings, a veritable fortune in rural Uganda. Her co-wife and her husband's brothers were bitter that she had used it on herself. She spent it partly on trips to TASO in the nearest town, but mainly on medicines from Swissgarde, a South African multilevel marketing firm that sells nutritional supplements at high prices. She claims that she would have died had it not been for that money and the medicine it bought.

Different government jobs carried different kinds of perks. Health workers and teachers in rural settings sometimes got staff housing. Prison officers, police, and soldiers were housed in police lines and barracks. John had a house on the same Kampala railway housing estate that Grillo (1973) had studied in the mid-1960s. Rent was deducted from his salary but he would never have been able to find comparable housing for the price on the open market. Other perks were less obvious and some were holdovers from the era of regimes. Prison officers could make use of prisoners' unpaid labor; Dorothy had a trusty who minded her cows and did other work around her house. Schoolteachers sometimes used pupils to run errands or help in their gardens. A head teacher could allocate, perhaps for a price, a certain number of places at the school. Soldiers used free land around the barracks to cultivate crops. A health worker I knew had a nursing aide sell snacks for her in the waiting room. Thus there is a parallel economy for civil servants—or perhaps it is less parallel than intertwined with the obvious one.

One of the essential qualities of government employment for those on ART is relative job security. The 2006 amendments to the Employment Act protect employees when they fall ill, irrespective of the type of sickness, and guarantee full salary for a total of thirty days sick leave for those on contract. After this period, keeping a job depends on specific policy and contract terms. Employers can terminate employees if they have been grounded for a period considered "long." Government employees are generally treated with greater leniency than private sector employees. A policewoman I know was sick and hardly able to work for half a year. When I asked her if she had registered herself on sick leave, she just laughed and said not yet. It was not until she actually started on ART that she took her sick leave. (Ironically she had finally returned to work when she missed roll call one day and was sanctioned for absenteeism.) Widespread absenteeism, the very characteristic that is criticized for making public service inefficient, is the quality that allows people weakened by HIV and side effects of ART to continue to collect their much needed salaries. Nevertheless, like other employees, civil servants on ART worry about keeping their jobs when they cannot perform adequately.

During the period before free availability of ART, some businesses paid for treatment for their essential workers.[11] As for government workers, the para-statal JCRC offered gratis treatment to health workers before the rollout of free treatment in 2004 to 2005, and several we interviewed had availed themselves of this possibility. (High ranking army officers presumably benefited as well, since the collaboration behind JCRC included the Ministry of Defense.) Teachers, ordinary soldiers, and police were left to scrape money together to buy drugs themselves if they could. At least they were in a better position to do so than the great majority without working-class advantages. The interdigitation of the nation-state embodied in its workers, and the congeries of foreign-funded projects, was very clear in this phase when some government health workers were "rescued" and others with a salary could purchase treatment. Later, as free treatment became more widely available, the ties were less obvious and more complicated but no less significant.

It was the case of John the railwayman that showed most dramatically how the changing role of the state affected those in its employ. John had been struggling to pay for his treatment and missed work frequently because of illness. He recounted that the board of the para-statal Uganda Railways Corporation (URC) had already made the decision to fire him when the government announced that employees should not be laid off because of ill health. Under a broader change of policy, the corporation began to pay for employees' ART at JCRC facilities. John recalled how he fell to his knees to thank the official who told him to fill in the forms that would allow him to be treated at URC expense. His troubles were not over. During the eighteen months we visited John, he was interdicted because he was held responsible for an accident and his salary was cut by half. At the same time he got the news that the URC was being privatized. The South African company that was taking over announced that staff would be reduced from 2,000 to 600. Being interdicted, he knew he had no chance of staying on. He would have to vacate his house and take his children studying in Kampala back to the inferior village school. The JCRC informed him that they were giving him the last dose of free drugs. He would have to buy them since his job was ending. Yet he was on an expensive second-line regimen that he could never afford, and so he decided to go back to his village and wait to die. With the severance package perhaps he could make an investment that would support his family. Miraculously, the new management decided to retain him and to continue covering all his medical expenses. John's life was contingent upon his employment, a dependence that swung him between relief and distress.

Workplace Politics

For all the advantages of government employment, the potential it offered for greater control over one's destiny was seldom secure. One of the dictionary definitions of the prefix *para* is faulty, irregular, and disordered. In this sense civil servants on ART lived in a kind of double para-state. Their health was faulty even after they improved on treatment and this made them more concerned about the possible irregularities of their working conditions. They imagined that among their colleagues and superiors were some who wished them ill. They feared being transferred or dismissed. At the very least they supposed that they would be passed by when opportunities arose for further training and promotion. Competition, suspicion, and manipulation are the flip side of the cooperation and mutual support that characterize civil service workplaces. Most people agree that irregular practices, sometimes called survival strategies or corruption, have increased exponentially since the days of the "original Uganda." All government employees know the underside of public service, but for those on ART the uncertainties and mistrust were more ominous.

Dorothy, the prison officer, spoke warmly of her fellow staff, who encouraged her through the painful side effects of her drug, Triomune. But she was also convinced that other colleagues were scheming against her. First she was to be transferred, which she attributed to the fact that her bosses wanted to give her job to people from their own tribe. When that threat passed, she was designated to go for training for three months at Luzira Prison, far from her home. She worried about how intensive it was going to be. "I hope it is not real army training! I don't think I can manage that training and they do not know that I am sick. I am also worried about how I will be getting my drugs because they cannot give them to someone else. You have to pick them up yourself." But when we asked why she did not simply tell the authorities that she was on medication, she replied: "You know, there are many people who want our jobs and some are those who had wanted me transferred from here. And in fact when they heard that I was going for further training, they were not happy about it. That is why I have to go."

Dorothy found confirmation of her mistrust when she discovered that she had been reported dead and struck off the payroll. "I went to our salary office to complain about not receiving my salary only to be told that they knew I had passed away and some could not believe seeing me, those who knew me! I was very shocked and I realized we live with murderers! I could not believe someone could just go to the office and do that to me." Two of the soldiers, Tom and Saddam, also found that their names had been deleted from the pay list because someone reported them sick and not active in the army. All three managed to get reinstated, but at considerable cost in paperwork, chasing from office to office, and going without salary for some months. Saddam was convinced that malice and corruption were to blame. Such problems were experienced by others in employment, but people on ART were especially dependent on regular income and were more deeply affected.

Unlike Dorothy, most employees told their immediate bosses about their illness and treatment. They needed to explain their absences from work and to request lighter duties. The soldiers to whom we spoke had all informed their superior officers, though none of them had managed to access free treatment through the army. All had started out paying for their drugs.

What they did achieve was some leniency in their assignments. They were placed at barracks close to medical facilities and they were not sent on extremely strenuous missions. Saddam was assigned to a barracks where there was a military hospital. The operations in which he participated were to pick up dead and wounded soldiers in southern Sudan and Karamoja and bring them back to the hospital. That was hard enough. But given that he and others who were on treatment at one time thought they would be demobilized because they were sickly, he felt he had to tough it out. "Even though I am weak and not feeling well, I have to go and lift those casualties, or else I would be considered noneffective. The conditions are very bad where we go out to get the bodies, but I always go with my medicines. Otherwise I have light duties." Saddam remarked that he could not be sent on any mission in the Congo because of his poor health.

Some of our informants were quite open in their workplaces about their status and treatment. Roscoe, one of the teachers, told us: "With me I am open, being a teacher. Even at school I have discussed the dangers of the virus. I talk to the upper classes where there are adolescents. I tell them I am a victim. At school there is no problem because I discussed it with them. They gave me leave when I was down. I also discussed with the parents' committees. The community—they maintain the relationship. They even come to visit me." Roscoe made a virtue of talking about being positive, as did Goretti, a nursing assistant. She told all her coworkers that she was sick and sung their praises for being so supportive. She worked as a counselor in the weekly HIV clinic, turning her positive status into a platform for helping others and, in the process, receiving encouragement from her colleagues. Yet such virtuosity was not typical. As we know from another study in Uganda, even nurses who counsel clients to be open about their status often do not wish their patients and fellow health workers to know that they themselves are positive (Kyakuwa 2009b).

Most people did not announce their status broadly at their workplace. They might tell a few close colleagues, but beyond those there was a feeling that you did not really know whether workmates were genuinely sympathetic. They did not want to be talked about; concern about "rumor mongering" and "backbiting" reflected uncertainty about the dispositions of others. Some were very careful about keeping their secret and were convinced that no one knew except their boss. Others had not actually told their colleagues, but thought they suspected it anyhow.

Why are people concerned about talk? Juma, who crossed the border to get his ARVs in Uganda but lived and worked in Kenya, asserted that stigmatization was great there and many people got laid off from their jobs when their employers realized they were positive. He thought that he himself would have been fired had not a friend pleaded for him with his boss. But our Ugandan informants were not primarily concerned that they would be fired because they were positive. John's threatened dismissal was not due to his serostatus; in fact he was rehired by the new management with full knowledge of his health record.

What people worried about was that HIV status could play into the workplace politics, upon which their prospects depended. They did not want to be thought of as less competent or less dependable colleagues because of their illness and need for treatment, nor did they want to have their every mistake or absence attributed to their serostatus. They were very sensitive to being overlooked for chances of further education or promotion, assuming that it was because they were positive. Major Charles said that while his superior officers accepted that he should not be transferred to remote places far from treatment sources, they discriminated against him by not selecting him for courses, which might have provided extra money and facilitated promotion in the ranks. Benjamin, a Uganda Revenue officer, did not want to ask for more leave, though his feet were so swollen from the side effects of his medicine that he could not put on shoes. He feared not dismissal but transfer to a place less convenient for treatment.

A medical intervention, ART, funded by foreign donors, allows people to perform their government jobs, which in turn facilitate their lives on ART. But there are tensions inherent in this salutary interplay. The territorial purview of the government may require its employees to be transferred, while the fixity of ART immobilizes them. There is an interesting inversion here: while the para-state of this collection's title is linked to deterritorialization (Ferguson 2006) and movable enclaves within and beyond national territory, those benefiting from ART are tied to sites of treatment. They need fixity, but government work may require mobility within administrative locations of national territory.

Moreover, the authority and competence of teachers, health workers, and administrators may match awkwardly with the position of patient or client in an AIDS clinic. While biopolitical interventions propose new forms of sociality and identity (Rabinow 1996; Rose and Novas 2005; Nguyen 2005), maintaining one's credibility and career possibilities as a government worker may require hiding or downplaying one's bio-identity as HIV positive.

In Uganda, as in many African countries, the government is a major employer. The shifting forms of the para-state, where foreign funds support activities and services within public agencies, have not changed that fact and may even have improved conditions for some government workers. Where even university graduates have trouble finding a job, and most people live by "gambling," the security of government work is enviable. For people struggling to make a life on ART, there are particular advantages to state employment. The obvious one is salary; in regularity and amount it might not measure up to the standards of the best jobs in donor-funded projects. But it far exceeds most of the wages in small private businesses, and a regular salary allows people to invest in other sources of income.

Moreover, a government job not only benefits the employee; it also provides a measure of security for other members of the family and household, as we have seen. Children of government workers often have better schooling opportunities. As adults they may have better chances of salaried employment, though not necessarily in government service. Many people with jobs in the private or nonprofit sector come from families of government employees, as in the family about which Meinert writes in this volume. Thus the working class reproduces itself, also in the current era when government work is so thoroughly entwined with externally funded projects and possibilities.

A government job provides status and position from which to obtain other opportunities. This was particularly clear in the case of government health workers, both those who were interlocutors in our ART study and others I have known over the years. Research projects and donor-funded health interventions recruit doctors, nurses, midwives, clinical officers, and laboratory technicians from government service to take on extra tasks for the duration of the project (S. Whyte 2011, 44). They retain their government posts and are even better qualified for the next project that appears. In Uganda many of these opportunities are associated with the response to AIDS, either in research or more commonly in interventions. Remarkably, the para-state of science provides twice over for many health workers — offering extra opportunities for earning and supplying the treatment that allows them to keep on working.

The concerns of government workers on ART provide another angle on the state of the state in the era of strong international biopolitical interventions. Like practically all HIV positive people, they are dependent on foreign organizations for their medicines. Government services would be even more debilitated without treatment for thousands of teachers, health workers, and policemen. In a sense, public services are reinvigorated by the life science intercessions of PEPFAR, the Global Fund, and other such organizations. But to stop at the bioscience understanding of survival is to ignore life and livelihood, just as an exclusive focus on the growing role of international research, expertise, and funding ignores the continuing significance of national government in the everyday lives of citizens as well as its employees.

Notes

1 Nearly three quarters of paid employees had education above a secondary level, while unpaid family workers tended to have only primary education or none at all. Men outnumbered women more than two to one in paid employment and self-employment (UBOS 2002, 26–29).

2 This chapter builds on material presented more fully in our "polygraph" *Second Chances* (S. Whyte 2014).

3 A civil servant explained to us with a wry smile: "They pretend to pay us and we pretend to work."

4 In early March 2011, the front page headlines of the government-controlled national newspaper trumpeted "Civil Servants' Salaries Paid." The story was that pay had been late by four days but had been deposited in employees' bank accounts at 1: 00 P.M. on the previous day. Also pensions, gratuities, and arrears were about to be paid. This was to counter widespread rumors that the government had used so much on ensuring victory in the recent elections that it could not cover salaries (*New Vision*, March 5, 2011). Still it was striking that a four-day delay could make headlines after what government employees had experienced in the 1980s.

5 While it is easy, and sometimes useful, to make sweeping narratives of historical transformation in the form of general periodizations of African state history, it is important to remember that each state had its own history requiring its own periodization. Uganda's history had different phases than its neighbors Kenya, Tanzania, Rwanda, and Sudan.

6 Semiautonomous bodies have been established increasingly since 2000. They are formally independent of government ministries and are often designated as *authorities*. They were meant to have primarily regulatory functions, but they take on implementation as well. Their employees are not restricted by civil service salary scales and often are better paid than colleagues in ministries. In fact, the

UBOS does not include them in figures for civil servants (UBOS 2011, 21). They have their own budgets, overseen by the auditor general, and can generate funds from fees as well as external donors.

7 A fourteen-year university cooperation funded by the Danish International Development Agency, DANIDA.

8 The team was composed of Hanne O. Mogensen, Lotte Meinert, Michael Whyte, Phoebe Kajubi, David Kyaddondo, Godfrey Etyang Siu, Jenipher Twebaze, and myself. I gratefully acknowledge their part in our common project. Appreciation goes also to the Danish Ministry of Foreign Affairs, which supported our collaboration through a grant for Enhancement of Research Capacity.

9 That such a notion of class interest existed from colonial times is documented in Grillo's (1974) study of the Railway African Union in Kampala. But as he emphasized, active trade unionists were a tiny minority of employees, and then, as now, the proportion of the labor force in waged work was small at 17 percent of African males in Uganda and Kenya (Grillo 1974, 11). Today the National Organization of Trade Unions counts under 200,000 members—about 10 percent of those eligible to join. As source of income, Norway's Labour Organization provides substantially more than union member dues (NOTU Annual Report 2010).

10 It is difficult to find reliable figures for government employment. One source estimated the army at 40,000 to 45,000 in 2007 (International Institute of Strategic Studies), while another put it at 50,000 to 70,000 (Tripp 2010, 141). The Uganda Police Force gave its strength at 38,000 for 2009 (UPF homepage); at the end of 2010 many more were recruited in anticipation of the national elections in February 2011. One source (Bogomolova et al. 2007) put pensionable teachers at 141,000 (but it is unclear whether this includes faculty at the five public universities and twenty-five public tertiary education institutions) and "civil servants" at 70,000 for 2003 to 2004. The latter figure presumably covers public administration: the many ministries, government agencies, and authorities, as well as the constantly growing number of districts. The National Organization of Trade Unions estimated 350,000 eligible members for the Union of Government Employees and Allied Workers, which includes mainly national and district administration (NOTU 2010).

11 A study completed in 2004 found that only ten of thirty-seven medium to large companies did so (Feeley 2004). Those who did tended to be "semiautonomous bodies" or large organizations, often multinationals, with a skilled labor force. The employees who were highly qualified and would be hardest to replace were the ones who benefited. Reports from other African countries also showed that differences in the value of workers to their employers were directly evident. (Whyte et al. 2004 special issue of AIDS on business and HIV UNGASS).

References

Barnett, Tony, and Piers Blaikie. 1992. *AIDS in Africa: Its Present and Future Impact*. New York: Guilford Press.

Barnett, Tony, and Alan Whiteside. 2002. *AIDS in the Twenty-first Century: Disease and Globalization*. Basingstoke, UK: Palgrave Macmillan.

Bogomolova, Tatyana, Gregorio Impavido, and Montserrat Pallares-Miralles. 2007. *An Assessment of Reform Options for the Public Service Pension Fund in Uganda*. World Bank.

Byakika-Tusiime, J., et al. 2005. "Adherence to HIV Antiretroviral Therapy in HIV+ Ugandan Patients Purchasing Therapy." *International Journal of STD and AIDS* 16: 38–41.

Comaroff, Jean, and John Comaroff. 2000. "Millenial Capitalism: First Thoughts on a Second Coming." *Public Culture* 12, no. 2: 291–343.

Epstein, Helen. 2007. *The Invisible Cure: Why We Are Losing the Fight Against AIDS in Africa*. New York: Picador.

Feeley, Rich, Paul Bukuliki, and Peter Cowley. 2004. *The Role of the Private Sector in Preventing and Treating HIV/AIDS in Uganda: An Assessment of Current Activities and the Outlook for Future Action*. Boston: Boston University Center for International Health and Development.

Grillo, R. D. 1973. *African Railwaymen: Solidarity and Opposition in an East African Labour Force*. Cambridge: Cambridge University Press.

Grillo, R. D. 1974. *Race, Class, and Militancy: An African Trade Union, 1939–1965*. New York: Chandler.

Hyden, Goran. 1995. "Bringing Voluntarism Back In." In *Service Provision under Stress in East Africa: The State, NGOs and People's Organizations in Kenya, Tanzania, and Uganda*, edited by J. Semboja and O. Therkildsen, 35–50. Copenhagen: Center for Development Research.

Iliffe, John. 2006. *The African AIDS Epidemic: A History*. Athens: Ohio University Press.

Jamal, Vali. 1991. "The Agrarian Context of the Ugandan Crisis." In *Changing Uganda*, edited by H. B. Hansen and M. Twaddle, 78–97. London: James Currey.

Johnson-Hanks, Jenifer. 2005. "When the Future Decides: Uncertainty and Intentional Action in Contemporary Cameroon." *Current Anthropology* 46, no. 3: 363–85.

Kabugo, Charles, et al. 2005. "Long-Term Experience Providing Antiretroviral Drugs in a Fee-for-Service Clinic in Uganda: Evidence of Extended Virologic and CD4+ Cell Count Responses." *Journal of Acquired Immune Deficiency Syndrome* 38, no. 5: 578–83.

Kaler, Amy, et al. 2010. "'Living by the Hoe' in the Age of Treatment: Perceptions of Household Well-Being after Antiretroviral Treatment among Family Members of Persons with AIDS." *AIDS Care* 22, no. 4: 509–19.

Kinsman, John. 2008. "Pragmatic Choices: Research, Politics and AIDS Control in Uganda." PhD diss., University of Amsterdam.

Kyakuwa, Margaret. 2009a. "More Hands in Complex ART Delivery? Experiences from the Expert Clients Initiative in Rural Uganda." *African Sociological Review* 13, no. 1: 143–67.

Kyakuwa, Margaret. 2009b. "Ethnographic Experiences of HIV-Positive Nurses in Managing Stigma at a Clinic in Rural Uganda." *African Journal of AIDS Research* 8, no. 3: 367–78.

Masquelier, Adeline. 2001. "Behind the Dispensary's Prosperous Façade: Imagining the State in Rural Niger." *Public Culture* 13, no. 2: 267–91.

Nabuguzi, Emmanuel. 1995. "Popular Initiatives in Service Provision in Uganda." In *Service Provision under Stress in East Africa: The State, NGOs and People's Organizations in Kenya, Tanzania, and Uganda*, edited by J. Semboja and O. Therkildsen, 192–208. Copenhagen: Center for Development Research.

Nguyen, Vinh-Kim. 2005. "Antiretroviral Globalism, Biopolitics, and Therapeutic Citizenship." In *Global Assemblages. Technology, Politics, and Ethics as Anthropological Problems*, edited by A. Ong and S. J. Collier, 124–44. Oxford: Blackwell.

Nguyen, Vinh-Kim. 2009. "Government-by-Exception: Enrolment and Experimentality in Mass HIV Treatment Programmes in Africa." *Social Theory and Health* 7: 196–217.

Nguyen, Vinh-Kim. 2010. *The Republic of Therapy: Triage and Sovereignty in West Africa's Time of AIDS*. Durham, NC: Duke University Press.

NOTU (National Organization of Trade Unions). 2010. *Annual Report 2010*. Kampala: National Organization of Trade Unions. http://www.notu.or.ug/down loads/NOTU-ANNUAL%202010.pdf.

Obbo, Christine. 1991. "Women, Children, and a 'Living Wage.'" In *Changing Uganda*, edited by H. B. Hansen and M. Twaddle, 98–112. London: James Currey.

Parkhurst, Justin O. 2005. "The Response to HIV/AIDS and the Construction of National Legitimacy: Lessons from Uganda." *Development and Change* 36, no. 3: 571–90.

Parkin, David. 1979. "The Categorization of Work: Cases from Coastal Kenya." In *Social Anthropology of Work*, edited by S. Wallman, 317–35. London: Academic Press.

Putzel, James. 2004. "The Politics of Action on AIDS: A Case Study of Uganda." *Public Administration and Development* 24: 19–30.

Rice, Andrew. 2009. *The Teeth May Smile but the Heart Does Not Forget: Murder and Memory in Uganda*. New York: Picador.

Rose, Nikolas, and Carlos Novas. 2005. "Biological Citizenship." In *Global Assemblages. Technology, Politics, and Ethics as Anthropological Problems*, edited by A. Ong and S. J. Collier, 439–63. Oxford: Blackwell.

Russell, Steven, and Janet Seeley. 2010. "The Transition to Living with HIV as a

Chronic Condition in Rural Uganda: Working to Create Order and Control When on Antiretroviral Therapy." *Social Science and Medicine* 70: 375–82.

Tripp, Aili Mari. 2010. *Museveni's Uganda: Paradoxes of Power in a Hybrid Regime*. Boulder, CO: Lynne Rienner.

Twaddle, Michael, and Holger Bernt Hansen. 1998. "The Changing State of Uganda." In *Developing Uganda*, edited by H. B. Hansen and M. Twaddle, 1–18. Oxford: James Currey.

UBOS (Uganda Bureau of Statistics). 2006. *The 2002 Uganda Population and Housing Census, Economic Characteristics*. Kampala: UBOS.

UBOS (Uganda Bureau of Statistics). 2012. *Statistical Abstract 2011*. Kampala: UBOS.

Whyte, Michael A. 1990. "The Process of Survival in Southeastern Uganda." In *Adaptive Strategies in African Arid Lands*, edited by M. Bovin and L. Manger, 121–45. Uppsala: Scandinavian Institute of African Studies.

Whyte, S. R., M. A. Whyte, Lotte Meinert, and Jenipher Twebaze. 2013. "Therapeutic Clientship: Belonging in Uganda's Mosaic of AIDS Projects." In *When People Come First: Anthropology and Social Innovation in Global Health*, edited by João Biehl and Adriana Petryna. Princeton, NJ: Princeton University Press.

Whyte, Susan Reynolds, et al. 2004. "Treating AIDS: Dilemmas of Unequal Access in Uganda." *Journal of Social Aspects of HIV/AIDS* 1, no. 1: 14–26.

Whyte, Susan Reynolds. 2008. "Discrimination: Afterthoughts on Crisis and Chronicity." *Ethnos* 73, no. 1: 97–100.

Whyte, Susan Reynolds. 2011. "Writing Knowledge and Acknowledgement: Possibilities in Medical Research." In *Evidence, Ethos, and Experiment: The Anthropology and History of Medical Research in Africa*, edited by Paul Wenzel Geissler, 29–56. Oxford: Berghahn Books.

Whyte, Susan Reynolds, ed. 2014. *Second Chances: Surviving AIDS in Uganda*. Durham, NC: Duke University Press.

PART IV

Affective Wholes

CHAPTER 7

Molecular and Municipal Politics:

Research and Regulation in Dakar

Branwyn Poleykett

In 2008 I arrived in Dakar to research official and clandestine sex work in the city. Senegal is one of the few former French colonies to have explicitly pursued the sanitary regulation of female commercial sex work after independence. While it appears that in many African countries there are scattered and informal policies of colonial and postcolonial regulation (see Jackson 2002; Shaw 1995), in Senegal the rights and responsibilities of official sex workers are codified and carefully observed. The law requires that providers of sexual services present themselves at regular intervals (officially every fifteen days, in practice, once a month) at a dedicated clinic, and that they submit to compulsory serological and gynecological examinations. Figures from 2004 show that there are 1,500 women registered at Dakar's state clinic, and just under 1,000 have been consulted at least twice in the previous year (Espirito Santo and Etheredge 2004). I was intrigued by the survival of this policy in twenty-first-century Dakar. Why was sanitary regulation—a form of governance often closely associated with authoritarian colonial rule— pursued in postcolonial Senegal, and under what guise was regulation now practiced in Dakar?

However, when I arrived at the state clinic and began to observe the everyday practices of regulation—registration, consultation, testing, organized and ad hoc care—I realized that the clinic had multiple and distinctively blended functions. The official sex workers registered at the Institute of Social Hygiene (IHS) had been enrolled in longitudinal research projects, and the records held by the state detailing the women's personal and medical details thus "constitute[d] official rosters from which prostitutes could be accessed for research purposes" (Espirito Santo and Etheredge 2004, 138). On one side of the clinic, state social workers, sage femmes, and nurses registered new women, dealt with the police, and made sure that women fulfilled the legal obligations attached to registration. On the other side of the clinic, two doctors employed by a biomedical research team provided high quality medical care and coordinated a longitudinal cohort study. As I conducted ethnographic fieldwork and oral history interviews with social workers and research doctors, I began to see how far these two functions overlapped in practice.

The background of the research at the state clinic is the discovery of HIV-2 in Senegal. In 1984 a Senegalese research scientist, Professor Souleymane Mboup, began to draw blood from hospital patients and registered sex workers looking for a reservoir of HIV in these populations. One of these blood samples, which he sent to colleagues at Harvard for testing, was found to be infected with a distinct type of HIV virus, eventually designated HIV-2. In 1985 an Inter-University Convention was signed between Harvard, the Université Cheikh Anta Diop in Dakar, and the Universities of Tours and Limoges in France. This collaboration resulted in the natural history of HIV-2, one of the longest studies of HIV-infected people in the world, and a considerable transfer of expertise, personnel, and laboratory equipment between Boston and Souleymane Mboup's laboratory at Dantec Hospital in Dakar. The natural history project was carried out among the population of official sex workers registered at Dakar's state clinic: a population that had long been seen as a "gold mine" for scientific research (Gilbert 2009).

Natural history studies of HIV map the "natural" (unimpeded by use of drugs to arrest the multiplication of the virus) course of disease from the point of infection, moving through diagnostic stages, and eventually to death. The Senegalese natural history project, known also as the "prostitute project," mapped the epidemiology and infectivity across ten different genetic HIV-1 subtypes, and compares HIV-1 subtypes to HIV-2 subtypes (Kanki et al. 1999). There have been few successful natural history studies conducted in Africa. Natural history studies require large numbers of people to consent to regular testing over a long period of time, usually longer than ten years (Jaffar et al. 2004). However, when natural history data is verified, it can correct widespread misapprehensions about the epidemiological specificity of the African epidemic, and it can be an invaluable tool in planning and executing prevention programs (Morgan and Whitworth 2001).

As I will explore further in this chapter, there are several reasons why the state clinic presented such "ideal" conditions for biomedical research and why the natural history research in Dakar succeeded where others on the African continent have failed. First, the registered women are comfortable with giving data. For example, Gilbert et al. (2003) note that "HIV-1 and HIV-2 serostatus data at each clinic visit were available from all sex workers. Information on nationality, age, date of cohort entry, and years of registered prostitution were available from greater than 99 percent of the sex workers." Second, HIV-2 — "the world's other HIV virus" (Gilbert 2003, 41) — has a distinctive epidemiology. The interval between infection with HIV-2 and death is significantly longer than in HIV-1 infected individuals, as HIV-2 produces more "long-term nonprogressors." This makes a cohort, including some HIV-2 infected individuals, a significant resource because "if scientists can unlock the mechanisms that allow these individuals to achieve viral control, it could represent a major step forward in the development of an HIV vaccine" (Gilbert 2003, 29).

I went to the state clinic to study *regulation*, the patching together of different policing, data gathering, and care practices to classify and work on poor women's sexual behavior. I found myself studying the complex relationship between state sanitary regulation and experimental science. How was biomedical research work integrated into this highly specific social and clinical space? How do the practices associated with biomedical research "spill out into mundane medical environments" (Petryna 2007, 290)? What happens in these complex spaces in which care, state bureaucracy, and biomedical research are shuffled into one another? Are these spaces crucibles for the organization and experience of a distinctive condition of experimentality, the history and effects of which it might be possible to trace (Davies 2010; Nguyen 2009; Ronnell 2005)?

Since the discovery of HIV-2 and the launch of the multilateral research project, the work of sanitary regulation and the work of research has been bound together at the state clinic through the persistent "boundary transgressions between biomedical experimentation and governance" (Rottenberg 2009, 424). There is no straightforward "delegation" of state power to the individuals associated with the trial. Nor does the trial attempt to directly reproduce or counterfeit state powers, detaching the "signature of the state" and adopting it as their own (Das 2004); rather, the porous boundary between regulation and research both makes possible and holds together experimental work, reshaping and working upon local relations of care. As I conducted ethnographic fieldwork at the clinic, I began to look "beyond authoritarian high modernism" as a means of understanding and interpreting regulatory practice and toward a "more general problematic of 'improvement' emerging from a governmental rationality focused on the welfare of populations" (Li 2005, 383) and effected through "prosaic" state practice (Painter 2006).

In this chapter I consider some of the changes that have taken place at the clinic as state sanitary regulation is influenced by and practiced through biomedical research. I discuss the strategic leveraging of resources for research, which helped to build capacity and to begin the process of making state regulation congruent with research objectives. I then pay close attention to the banal bureaucratic practices that predate the arrival of biomedical research but that also shift to accommodate research work and help to arrange and assemble the research subjects. I then examine the changes that have taken place at the clinic—the proliferation and alliances and the thickening of connectivity, a traffic between different actors that produces social relations based on consent and pleasure as well as on coercion and police work. Here I focus on how the forms of political organization and social solidarity engaged by registered women have helped to create, contour, and sustain an experimental cohort. Finally, I consider what kinds of ideas about experimental spaces might be read in the collaborative care work undertaken by state social workers and research scientists.

Regulation in Dakar

The current legal and medical arrangements for the regulation of official sex workers in Senegal have their roots in postwar France. On April 13, 1946, the bill known colloquially as the Loi Marthe Richard was promulgated simultaneously in France and in French West Africa. The bill purported to bring an end to the so-called French system of regulated prostitution and ordered that local authorities close down the *maisons de tolerance* or the legally recognized brothels. The central sanitary register of prostitutes was destroyed, marking a symbolic break with the old strategies of planning and policing. However, the Loi Marthe Richard was swiftly followed by the Loi du 24 Avril 1946, which required that women open a new *fichier sanitaire-social*, a file that would record women's details and their medical histories and would be held simultaneously at police stations and at special dedicated sexual health clinics. This covert maintenance of regulation under a new legal guise was out of step with the postwar human rights regime in Europe: as Alain Corbin (1990, 352) notes, "sanitarism . . . was already anachronistic when it was established in its ultimate form in 1946. It could not be maintained for long, and . . . the surveillance and marginalisation of the prostitute would have to be based on other arguments." In France this legislation was repealed in 1960, and France became one of the most vociferously abolitionist countries in the world. However, Senegal gained independence in 1960, and what was the "last gasp" of European state sanitarism, a hangover—as Alain Corbin argues—from the nineteenth century, was the beginning of a complex and thoroughly postcolonial story in Senegal.

The state clinic is still housed in the late colonial hospital, a dilapidated but still strikingly beautiful building built in the Sahelian style, which became fashionable after interest was sparked by the African pavilion at the colonial exposition in Marseilles in 1931. Thomas Shaw's (2006) study traces the peculiar combination of genuine admiration, artifice, and expediency that influenced the French adoption of the Islamic-influenced adobe architecture of the Sahel. After Fashoda and the First World War, the French authorities in Dakar moved to build an "imperial city," stung by allegations that the capital of French West Africa resembled a "dismal provincial town" (Betts 1985). As Raymond Betts (1985, 193) argues, architecture in Dakar was never neutral: "Because Dakar became the major city of Senegal, the colony in which the doctrine of assimilation was given its greatest publicity and most intensive practice, urban development, both spatial and social, was closely regarded and criticized." In the final decade of French rule the colonial authorities imported the West African vernacular style filtered through the imaginations of the curators of the colonial expositions and built three buildings in the Sahelian style: the cathedral, the maternity hospital, and the IHS. Of the three, the polyclinic is probably the most impressive and the most superficially "authentic"; as Thomas Shaw points out, the buttery terra cotta of the low exterior walls does resemble mud.

Postindependence, in 1960, some of the zeal with which the colonial authorities had executed the regulatory program ebbed away. However, interest in regulation remained and the law on prostitution was recodified in 1969. This postcolonial law drew heavily on the colonial legal framework (Becker and Collignon 1999), but also on the experiences of clinic staff who had visited urban health centers in Washington and Baltimore in the United States. The 1969 law reiterates some of the discursive emphasis on "equilibrium" so evident in sanitary statism—the emphasis is placed upon individual state employees to judiciously balance the "social" and the "medical."

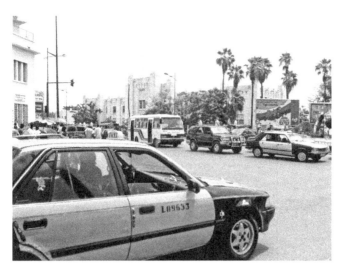

Figure 7.1. The clinic in the city. Photograph by Branwyn Poleykett, 2011.

The law argues that medical and legal authorities should always weigh the health costs against any moral or social benefit that might be involved in the policing of prostitution. In this way the 1969 law is a continuation of the colonial "sanitation syndrome" (Swanson 1977) that had characterized colonial regulation.

During the 1970s biomedical research was conducted with women registered at the state clinic; some of this research was funded by the USAID family planning program. The Senegalese team made a strong case for leveraging those funds for biomedical research into sexually transmitted infections. Dr. Ibra Ndoye, then head of the state clinic, now coordinator of the CNLS, stressed continuities in care, research, and intervention at the state clinic: "in the intervention there was always a mix of the sanitary and biological—because we tested [registered women] practically for free."

When the natural history project was launched, two doctors were "implanted" at the clinic to enhance the care provided to registered women and to oversee the enrollment and collection of data for the research program. The trial doctors arrived at the site in 1986 and have been continuously employed there since then. However, the collaboration with Harvard came to an end in 2001 and the Senegalese team members were placed in an invidious position. They were the custodians of a serological archive that could continue to be of paramount scientific importance. They also had developed trusting relationships with the official sex workers at the clinic, which they were not prepared to terminate. The state clinic could not simply shift back to the "old" system under which women's care was overseen by the nurses and social workers, but the resources of the state could not sustain the laboratory network and pay the salaries of the doctors who had been implanted by the natural history project. The commitment that they had made to distribute the social good of biomedical research through high quality care and trusting personal relationships had to be honored, but how? The team applied and won funding under the Comprehensive International Programme of Research on AIDS (CIPRA). Under the current arrangements the doctors' salaries are paid by CIPRA, allowing them to continue to do their work and to play the crucial role of mediators between the clinic and the laboratory.

Registration

From the beginning of the natural history trial until 1994, the research team had no clear and separate consent procedure for enrolling women—the research piggybacked on the registration and documentation procedures used by the social workers. Since 1994 consent procedures have changed, and the doctors handle the enrollment procedure and are responsible for ensuring that the women are fully informed about the research work. The enrollment is thus collapsed into the therapeutic encounter and is managed partly through the close and respectful relationships that the women have with the research physicians, although the doctors are clear that they treat all women regardless of decisions they make about participation in current or future research projects. Registration with the clinic, however, is the first point of contact between the women arriving to register and the clinic bureaucracy, and as such it is a key moment in establishing a relationship and beginning to unpack the women's experience, translating their lives into a set of local categories of risk. At the moment of registration, women are not only joining a community of sex workers—a community with its own spaces, its own memories, rituals of membership and conviviality—but they are also joining a pool of potential research subjects. In order to understand how the clinic became a research site and how longitudinal research has been carried out here so successfully, it is necessary to understand the circumstances of registration.

The potential social and personal cost of entering the state clinic as a registered sex worker is high. As one clinic worker puts it in Michelle Lewis Renaud's (1997) study of registered sex workers in Kaolack, Senegal, "being a prostitute is humbling but registering is humiliating, it's like signing up to be marginalised" (145). While women are legally entitled to deregister when they are no longer selling sex, in practice women report that this process is lengthy, invasive, and humiliating. Even when the women are deregistered the police keep their files open in the expectation that the women will lapse back into prostitution when their other economic activities fail (146). In tightly knit communities, women who have deregistered continue to experience anxiety about the security of information held at the clinics (Foley and Nguer 2010). Moreover there is a "clear connection between a police file and a health file" (Tandia 1998, 242), and some official sex workers claim that the police frequently use the information that they are required to give on registration to follow them and arrest them for soliciting (Bougazelli 2005, 10). Some sex workers claim to pay regular bribes to the police to avoid harassment (Foley and Nguer 2010, 331). There is certainly a high degree of cooperation between the police and the government clinics. If an official sex worker is stopped for soliciting, the police check the date of her last clinical appointment; if she has not been examined for some time, she will be detained and then escorted to the Institute of Social Hygiene. In other words, the line between licit and illicit practice is indistinct, and the police subject registered women to as much scrutiny as unregistered women.

Nevertheless, some women stress that they choose both to register and to keep coming back to the clinic. "We like it here," one woman told me. "If we didn't like it, we would all find somewhere else to go, we would all leave immediately." If "the story of healing is one of public power and private choice" (Feierman and Janzen 1992, 16), then *choosing* registration reflects women's exclusion from other spaces of biomedical care in the city and the trust that they place in the clinic's staff.

When women arrive to register, alone or accompanied by the police, the social workers have to be as explicit as possible about the legal implications of registration. They are also legally required to attempt to "dissuade" women from registering, which they usually do as they conduct the initial *enquête* or biographical interview. This responsibility to dissuade women from registration partly explains the brusque tone of the social workers' interactions with registered women. On several occasions, perhaps reading instinctive shock in my face, the head social worker corrected me impatiently: "We have to be firm with them; you don't understand what these women are like." However, the deep mutual respect and care that exists between registered women and the social workers that oversee the clinic is evident; the women know, for example, the names and ages of the registered women's children. The following exchange took place when a young Nigerian woman arrived to register at the clinic. It illustrates a particular relation of care that is expressed at this juncture (Brown 2010) and shows how the women begin to assemble their "sad story" (Agustin 2004) by answering questions and accounting for their presence at the clinic.

"Why have you left your country and come to my country?" the head social worker deadpans in mock grievance. The girl laughs and the second social worker chips in: "Nigeria is a rich country!"

"I don't know," the young girl replies, smiling a little uncertainly, and then adds mildly, "It's not our fault." She has been brought to the clinic by the police with two other young Nigerian women, part of a steady flow of women from Nigeria to Dakar—so many that the social workers have picked up a rudimentary pidgin. "There are people in Nigeria who said they could take us to Europe, they deceived us."

"You want to go to Europe!" the social workers crow.

"I will go, I will get to Europe," she says, still smiling and with her eyes cast politely down but quietly defiant.

"Do you know about AIDS, do you know how to protect yourself?"

"Yes."

"How do you protect yourself?"

"I use a condom."

"Every time?"

"Yes, every time."

"Do you have boyfriend, a nice Senegalese boyfriend? I can find you a nice Senegalese boyfriend."

"No," she laughs, "I don't want one. I don't want to get pregnant," she mimes the curve of a belly with her hand.

"Is your mother in life?" "Is your father in life?" She has one five-year-old son, left with her mother in Nigeria. The social worker takes her mother's and her father's names. The young woman watches anxiously as she fills one sheet with close, cramped notes and flips to the next page.

"This," she says, pointing at the file in front of her on the table, "this is to be a prostitute, you understand that?" The girl nods. "Why are you doing this?"

"I don't know."

"Can't you do anything else? If you go to Europe what will you do there?"

"Hairdressing."

"Hairdressing, is that all you know how to do?"

"Yes."

For this young Nigerian woman registration was a way of easing some of the pressures of working and seeking health care in a strange city, a city in which she has no intention of remaining. For other women registration is a calamitous life event, a decision only taken under intense and unbearable pressure. I was present at the registration of a Senegalese woman in her fifties. On the day of her registration, she arrived at the clinic at 6 a.m., partly to slip out of her neighborhood avoiding awkward questions and partly because the functioning of the clinic was, to her, entirely opaque and she wanted to make sure she did everything possible to conform to the demands of registration. "I have never been here before," she told me, rapping several times on the table to emphasize her point. "This isn't what I want, but I'm so tired. They told me that with a sanitary card it's easier, if you have trouble with the police you can show it to them. I have never been here before, I'm ashamed! Just give me to the carnet and I'll go."

On that day the woman was instructed to take an HIV test immediately and she nods her consent, but there is something that she has not understood. When she was told to return a month to the day she conceded cautiously, "Yes, if I have the time." When she is told that she must continue to return otherwise her sanitary card will be taken away and she will have more problems with the police, she shakes her head and clicks her tongue.

The social workers' office is tucked around the corner of the MST and dermatology block; it can be accessed by a discreet second entrance so that registered women can come to and fro without being observed. The clinic staff have worked hard to ensure a steady traffic of women, children, and men referred for dermatological complaints and have made sure that there is no obvious distinction between general consultations and the quiet corridor where sex workers' care is arranged. The trial doctor who left me at the door of the social workers' office—the room where the registrations take place and where women's data is held—stepped away respectfully describing the room as the "heart" of the clinic. Filing cabinets line the walls of the room, each containing individual files organized by year of registration. The first cabinet has drawers labeled 1970–1976, the second 1978–1980, after that there is one drawer for every year, each filled with familiar institutional-looking manila folders. On the far side of the room there is a larger cabinet with three drawers labeled *raflées* (picked up by the police), *decedées* (deceased), and *perdues de vues* (lost contact). There are three offenses for which a woman can be brought to the clinic by the police: soliciting, not having a sanitary card, and not attending medical appointments.

When a woman arrives to keep her monthly appointment, she pays a fee of 500 CFA for the consultation, collects her receipt, and comes to check in with the social workers. The social worker collects the woman's sanitary card, the auxiliary matches the date of registration on the card to the filing cabinets, picks out the file, drops the receipt and the card in the file, and drops it off with the nurse who will carry out whatever tests are required and a gynecological or serological examination and discuss any ongoing treatment or health problems. The nurse then fills in the *fiche de consultation*, which the social worker checks before stamping and dating the carnet. The consultations run on strict time cycles. Each woman should be consulted once a month; her first and then every other visit is a *visite complet*—with blood tests and gynecological examination. Alternate months are *visite simple*, consultations that allow the clinic staff to "check in" with the women, offer them more condoms, and make sure they are taking any prescribed medicine.

The card is the proof that the women are registered and are up to date with their consultations; they are required to carry this document at all times. The social workers complain that the women often lose their cards or forget it, or pretend to have lost them so that they can claim to be up to date with their consultations when they have missed appointments. This is a real headache for the clinic because they need to match the number on the card with the number on the file in order to be able to pull up the women's records. In order to dissuade women from forgetting or losing their cards, the clinic demands a police certificate certifying the loss of the carnet and charges the women 1000 CFA for a replacement. Even when the women remember the number on the card and want to be consulted they are refused. "How can we do a consultation without the card?" was the impatient reply when I asked why. The card is a legal document and the information it carries must correspond exactly to the care that a woman has received. The social workers and nurses are therefore reluctant to provide official care outside of the clinic's strict interior time cycles, but they go to great lengths to support registered women and their families when health or personal crises arise.

The file that is held at the IHS must contain up-to-date information, including the woman's name, mobile phone number, and address. It is very important, the head social worker explained, that the clinic has the exact address, because the women move around a lot and the clinic staff may need to do a home visit if they lose contact for a worrying period of time with a woman they perceive to be vulnerable. Indeed, a lot of the work that the social workers appear to do is constantly refining the address—which is by necessity descriptive, as Dakar has no postal service—and checking that the women's phone number is up to date, sometimes by putting it in to their own phones and making sure that her handset rings. When one of the women gives a number a little too quickly the social worker's suspicions are aroused. "Don't just make it up!" (*bul inventer de!*), she snaps; the woman repeats the number, slower this time. "Are you sure?" the social worker presses, until she is satisfied that the woman has given her the correct information. The social workers participate actively in preventing "loss to follow-up" by impressing upon the women that they must be conscientious about meeting their appointments and by conducting—or threatening to conduct—house visits. When I mentioned to the head social worker that there was a close and mutually dependent relationship between clinic bureaucracy and the organization of the research cohort she agreed: "It's us who have the addresses, not them." Some of the resources of the trial flowed through to the "other side" of the clinic in the form of a small amount of money, a *petite motivation* for the clinic staff to conduct home visits, which the social workers very much enjoy, as it allows them to get out into the city and be part of a more "hands-on" intervention. While this is not provided for under the resource allocation or within the remit of the state clinic, the social workers have used the research resources to explore creative work beyond their job descriptions and beyond the humdrum work of registering women and stamping their carnets.

It is not just this outreach work that links the daily practices of regulation to the work of creating and maintaining a research cohort. The social workers gather information in the form of a biographical story of risk and vulnerability, which is shared with the research physicians. Second, as they carry out the routine testing and physical inspection of the women, they prepare them for the testing associated with the research. The clinical "preparation" is similar to the process that Cussins (1996, 581) in a different context calls "anticipatory socio-naturalisation"; before the women consent to trial work they have already begun to understand the clinical itinerary upon which their care is contingent.

Paying attention to the "little things," the "numerous bureaucratic/logistical practices (which primarily shuffle paper), as opposed to theories about bureaucracy" (Thrift 2000, 382), shows up in scientific work in two important ways. First, it shows the many different kinds of work that happen in blended spaces of scientific production. Exploring the clinical hinterland of the trial shows not only the contingent and locally embedded work of science but also the banal processes through which research subjects are assembled and prepared for trial work. The registration biographies show how experimental populations are formed when women "choose" registration and how this choice is negotiated at the intersection of political economies and health crises (Petryna 2005; Rajan 2005). Second, this has the effect of exposing the work of largely female state employees who do the delicate and difficult work of balancing and mediating between regulation, trial work, and care. It is the activities of generally female and low paid nurses and social workers that transform women into "cooperative subjects for HIV/AIDS research" (Booth 2004, 7).

Cared for by the Test: Pleasure, Choice, and Proximity to the Laboratory

I have discussed the banal practices of registration that both begin to produce the women as sex workers, cluing them in as to how they can and should move through the institution, and begin the "un-blackboxing" (Cussins 1996) of their bodies and care, a process that will continue through the medical research process. I move now to briefly discuss two stories that reveal some of the pleasure of membership and clinic attendance.

The giving and testing of blood associated with registration and regulation is done separately from testing associated with the research function of the clinic. If the clinic's internal blood testing schedules overlap with the testing associated with the research, then the clinic staff tend to defer the compulsory blood test until the woman's next appointment. This is a gesture of care and respect for the women (*prélever ici, prélever la, c'est fatigant pour elles!*). The rituals of regular blood testing and the movement of blood samples around the clinic play a significant part in producing the state clinic as a distinctive space of care and intervention.

The most visible manifestation of the "microspatialities" of disease and care (Hinchcliffe 2001, 189) associated with biomedical research and the enhanced laboratory capacity that it has brought is the constant tracking to and fro of technicians carrying cool bags and moving blood samples out of the clinic and into the laboratory. Registered women do not, for the most part, find the idea of giving blood problematic or laborious; they are familiar with the itinerary of blood and swabs and appear to derive feelings of security and pleasure from this circulation. When asked what is special and desirable about the care they receive at the state clinic compared to other forms of care they might opt for, many women respond: "here you give blood." Another woman, when I asked why she "chose" registration at the state clinic as she sought out care, drew attention to the existence of a supportive NGO, Association Awa, and access to the laboratory: "here, there is Awa and close by there is the laboratory." For many of the women at the clinic, membership of Awa and proximity to the laboratory are the two poles of superior care associated with registration. The distribution of registered women's bodily proxies around the clinic and the laboratory is framed in a "warm" way; it is discussed as a process that secures the high quality of their care. Compliance with testing demonstrates belonging, understanding, and commitment to the clinic, but there is also pleasure in testing. As Beth Greenhough (2006, 448) argues, "the process of bodily commoditization is not just one of alienation . . . we might see in the process of becoming technically equivalent an expansion, rather than a reduction, of possibilities, connections and associations."

So although the social worker protested to me in the face of my tiresome questions about testing, trialing, and the experimental work of the clinic, "everything 'biological' is at the hospital laboratory and with the research team," that is not strictly true. As Jeannette Pols and Ingunn Moser (2009, 179) argue, drawing in technologies—often interpreted as the "cold" other to "warm" care—can allow researchers to formulate new questions about "what kind of affective social relations are enabled by medical technologies." Listening in a "realist mode" to the "events people report on" (Mol 2002, 15) exposes some of the less evident ways in which experiments are lived as social good and can show up in some of the humanist presuppositions that inhere in anthropologists' readings of technology and biomedicine in the lives of ordinary Africans.

Humanitarian Police Work: Awa and the State Clinic

The diagnosis of the first case of HIV-2 in Senegal and the establishment of a cohort trial at the IHS led to profound changes at the clinic. This diagnosis led to the arrival of a new experimental regime set up to investigate the viral specificity of the population of sex workers registered at the institute, enhancing its laboratory capacity, working on its epistemologies of intervention, adjusting its ethical terrain, and reorganizing its maps of expertise. A second and related change that has taken place has been the creation of Awa, a radical, sex worker–run association. Awa was founded in the clinic by the social workers and a group of registered women.

In the early 1990s members of Awa began to organize themselves around the prevention and diagnosis of the new virus. They were going out into bars and trying to solve the problem they had already diagnosed: women were resisting registration and staying away from the IHS unless they were taken there by force. The registered women adopted a different tactic, speaking frankly and persuasively to their unregistered peers and persuading them that the many rumors that circulated about the IHS were untrue or exaggerated. One leader, referred to respectfully as a doyenne of the clinic who had been working around the IHS for many years, reflecting on the changes at that time, observed that the police would bring unregistered women to the clinic, or women working with Awa would bring them (*polis moo ko indiwoon walla animatrices moo ko indi*).

In the last few years, Awa has moved out of the clinic and into offices close by and now works more widely with vulnerable women. However, Awa also maintains an intimate and somewhat problematic relationship with the IHS. In an interview the current director explained to me that because Awa was "born" in the state clinic, "we cannot go beyond the services provided by the state." However, she qualified this, saying "but we are also an NGO, and we have a vision, while the state just has an approach, which is purely based on public health principles."

The *anciennes* are maternal figures and slick advocates for Awa and for the clinic. Following the anciennes around the clinic and observing their interactions with other women, it is clear that the links between Awa and the clinic are decisive when they are persuading young women to register; in these interactions they specifically stress that Awa will pay their *ordonaanse* (prescriptions). One woman, when asked how she saw the clinic, responded: "It's good! Even the doctors! If you are a member of Awa they will help you as well. Everything in here [points to head] they can help, they help with money—when they write you a prescription, if you don't have the money, they will give you another piece of paper—that's the bill—you can take that to Awa." Moving between the Awa offices and the IHS with women who were going to collect money for their ordonaanse, it is clear that the functions of these two facilities are in practice closely related. Insofar as positive consent and enthusiasm for state sanitary policy exists, it seems to me to be sustained to a large extent by the advantages associated with the membership of Awa.

These two stories, one about the "warm" feelings associated with testing and the other concerned with sex workers' forms of organization and association, also illustrate some of the complex overlapping worlds at the clinic. These are two processes that help to create, contour, and sustain the experimental cohort. The membership of Awa helps to sustain these overlapping projects, making registration and consultation more palatable for women and contributing to the close and trusting relationships at the clinic. Here paying attention to the state serves to bring into sharp focus the multiple networks of welfare that sustain, define, and delineate its practices.

The profound interpenetration of experimental and regulatory practices is not only evident in the bureaucratic confusion and in the mixing and mingling of functions that are part of the daily practice of clinical work and more generally part of pragmatically mobilizing and maximizing resources in state spaces, where need constantly outstrips what is available for the social and medical response, but the confusion of care, experiment, and welfare is also present in the kinds of affect that tie women to the clinic, in the pleasurable rituals of belonging, in the production of experimental sites as clinical space marked by distinctive forms of care. The process of assembling, contouring, and maintaining the integrity of the research cohort is accomplished through registered women's own forms of organization and through the testing practices that mark it out as an exceptional space of care.

———————

There are clear affinities between the "containment" tactics of regulation and the conditions required by biomedical research in order that scientific work can be validated. The legal regulation of commercial sex work in Dakar has provided Senegalese scientists with access to a relatively stable population of sexually active women who are thoroughly socialized into providing blood samples and who are legally obliged to return at regular intervals for consultation and care. What is important for me is to draw out the consequences of these shifting relations of care at the state clinic.

Female commercial sex workers, seen as "unsanitary citizens," must "reproduce the official discourse bodily, by adapting hygienic practices and demonstrating subservience to medical authority" (Briggs 2004, 177); a policy with its roots in the colonial era, which treated these "public" women as proxies for the Senegalese population, has created the ideal conditions for biomedical research. This is a story that exposes the "unseemly affinities between experimental matters of fact, biopolitical modes of rationality, and historically specific forms of governance" (Power and Vasudevan 2007, 1791). The women registered at the IHS are a population made legible by institutional arrangements that have their roots in colonial sanitary policy, in local scientific recuperations of USAID-funded family planning programs, and in humanitarian intervention, and as such each of these interventions might be viewed with a profound degree of ambivalence. Is this not an example of the practices associated with the disciplining of the body, exposing the underlying congruencies between modern ideologies (Agamben 1998)? Moreover, in the process of making congruent the aims and rationales of regulation and research, have state and non-state actors not further entrenched the variegated citizenship (Ong 1999) that underpinned colonial sanitary policy?

In this chapter I have argued that the articulation between regulation and research at the IHS produces highly complex local, social, and care relations. The evolution of research and regulation at the state clinic is not a single project. These two bureaucratic forms do not come together as part of a concerted effort, and their interweaving is much more a product of care, obligation, reciprocity, curiosity, and creativity than cynical or opportunistic profiteering. Historicizing, localizing, and nuancing "experimentality" does not necessarily render less effective the political tools we have to critique and to intervene upon experimental regimes. Might we begin to nuance accounts of "experimentality" with stories about citizen patients moving between overlapping fields of historically constituted instrumentality, inhabiting and exploring different identities in each one? What kinds of agency might become visible in these moments and at these junctures? Answering the question Marilyn Strathern poses about the central problem of instrumentality, "How can we tell the difference between an extension or realization of human capacity and its perversion or subversion?" (Strathern 1991, 43), is not an easy task. However, as Cheah (2006, 1556) argues, the "humanity" of peoples vulnerable to exploitation and instrumentalization "comes into presence as a result of a complex and sensitive series of negotiations between the mobile, conflicting interests of different forces." Tracing the historical affinities and the material transgressions between experiment and governance at a single site offers insights into the multiple actors who have made up these interventions. These actors have collaboratively created a new kind of regulation that breaks with the practices of sanitary state policy while still bearing the traces of the state spaces and projects from which this new configuration emerged.

Note

1   Article 8, Décret No. 69–616 du Mai 1969 portant application de la loi no. 66–21 du 1ᵉʳ Février 1966.

References

Agamben, Giorgio. 1998. *Homo Sacer: Sovereign Power and Bare Life*. Palo Alto, CA: Stanford University Press.

Agustín, Laura. 2004. "Alternate Ethics, or: Telling Lies to Researchers." *Research for Sex Work* 7:6–7.

Becker, Charles, and Rene Collignon. 1999. "A History of Sexually Transmitted Diseases and AIDS in Senegal: Difficulties in Accounting for Social Logics in Health Policy." In *Histories of Sexually Transmitted Diseases and HIV/AIDS in Sub-Saharan Africa*, ed. Philip W. Setel, Milton J. Lewis, and Maryinez Lyons. Westport, CT: Greenwood Press.

Betts, Raymond F. 1985. "Dakar: Ville impériale, 1857–1960." In *Colonial Cities*, ed. R. J. Ross and G. J. Telkamp. Dordrecht, Netherlands: Martinus Nijhoff.

Booth, Karen M. 2004. *Local Women, Global Science: Fighting AIDS in Kenya*. Bloomington: Indiana University Press.

Bougazelli, Jérôme. 2006. "L'ambiguïté des textes sur la prostitution au Sénégal." In *Droit et Santé en Afrique: Actes du colloque international de Dakar, 28 Mars–1er Avril 2005*. Bordeaux: Les Etudes Hospitalières.

Briggs, Charles L. 2004. "Theorizing Modernity Conspiratorially: Science, Scale and the Political Economy of Public Discourse in Explanations of a Cholera Epidemic." *American Ethnologist* 31, no. 2: 164–87.

Brown, Hannah. 2010. "If We Sympathise with Them, They'll Relax: Fear/Respect and Medical Care in a Kenyan Hospital." *Medische Antropologie* 22, no. 1: 125–42.

Cheah, Pheng. 2006. "Humanity in the Field of Instrumentality." *PMLA* 121, no. 5: 1552–57.

Corbin, Alain. 1990. *Women for Hire: Prostitution and Sexuality in France after 1850*. Cambridge, MA: Harvard University Press.

Cussins, Charis. 1996. "Ontological Choreography: Agency through Objectification in Infertility Clinics." *Social Studies of Science* 26: 575–610.

Das, Veena. 2004. "The Signature of the State: The Paradox of Illegibility." In *Anthropology in the Margins of the State*, ed. Veena Das and Deborah Poole. Santa Fe, NM: School of American Research Press.

Davies, Gail. 2010. "Where Do Experiments End?" *Geoforum* 41:667–70.

Espirito Santo, Maria Eugênia, and Gina D. Etheredge. 2004. "And Then I Became a Prostitute . . . Some Aspects of Prostitution and Brothel Prostitutes in Dakar, Senegal." *Social Science Journal* 41, no. 1: 137–46.

Foley, Ellen, and Rokhaya Nguer. 2010. "Courting Success in HIV/AIDS Prevention: The Challenges of Addressing a Concentrated Epidemic in Senegal." *African Journal of AIDS Research* 9, no. 4: 325–36.

Gilbert, Peter B., W. Ian McKeague, Geoffrey Eisen, Christopher Mullins, Aissatou Gueye-Ndiaye, Souleymane Mboup, and Phyllis J. Kanki. 2003. "Comparison of HIV-1 and HIV-2 Infectivity from a Prospective Cohort Study in Senegal." *Statistics in Medicine* 22:573–93.

Gilbert, Hannah. 2010. "Spinning Blood into Gold: Science, Sex Work, and HIV-2 in Senegal." PhD diss., McGill University.

Greenhough, Beth. 2006. "Decontextualised? Dissociated? Detached? Mapping the Networks of Bio-Informatic Exchange." *Environment and Planning A* 38, no. 3: 445–63.

Hinchliffe, Steve. 2001. "Indeterminacy In-decisions—Science, Policy and Politics in the BSE (Bovine Spongiform Encephalopathy) Crisis." *Transactions of the Institute of British Geographers* 26, no. 2: 182–204.

Janzen, John M., and Steven Feierman. 1992. *The Social Basis of Health and Healing in Africa*. Berkeley: University of California Press.

Jackson, Lynette. 2002. "'When in the White Man's Town': Zimbabwean Women Remember Chibheura (Compulsory VD examinations)." In *Women in Colonial Africa: An Introduction*, ed. Jean Allman, Susan Geiger, and Nakanyike Musisi. Bloomington: Indiana University Press.

Jaffar, Shabbar, Alison D. Grant, Jimmy Whitworth, Peter G. Smith, and Hilton Whittle. 2004. "The Natural History of HIV-1 and HIV-2 Infections in Adults in Africa: A Literature Review." *Bulletin of the World Health Organisation* 82, no. 6: 462–69.

Kanki, Phillis J. 1999. "Human Immunodeficiency Virus Type 2 (HIV-2)." *AIDS Review* 1, no. 20: 101–8.

Li, Tania Murray. 2005. "Beyond 'the State' and Failed Schemes." *American Anthropologist* 107, no. 3: 383–94.

Mol, Annemarie. 2002. *The Body Multiple: Ontology in Medical Practice*. Durham, NC: Duke University Press.

Mol, Annemarie, Ingunn Moser, and Jeannette Pols. 2010. *Care in Practice: On Tinkering in Clinics, Homes and Farms*. Bielefeld, Germany: Transcript Verlag.

Morgan, Dilys, and Jimmy A. G. Whitworth. 2001. "The Natural History of HIV-1 Infection in Africa." *Nature Medicine* 7:143–45.

Nguyen, Vinh-Kim. 2009. "Government by Exception: Enrollment and Experimentality in Mass HIV Treatment Programmes in Africa." *Social Theory and Health* 7:196–217.

Painter, Joe. 2006. "Prosaic Geographies of Stateness." *Political Geography* 25:752–74.

Petryna, Adriana. 2005. "Ethical Variability: Drug Development and Globalizing Clinical Trials." *American Ethnologist* 32, no. 2: 183–97.

Petryna, Adriana. 2007. "Experimentality: On the Global Mobility and Regulation of Human Subjects Research." *PoLAR* 30, no. 2: 288–384.

Pols, Jeanette, and Ingunn Moser. 2009. "Cold Technologies Versus Warm Care? On Affective and Social Relations with and through Care Technologies." *Alter, European Journal of Disability* 3:159–78.

Powell, Richard C., and Alexander Vasudevan. 2007. "Geographies of Experiment." *Environment and Planning A* 39, no. 8: 1790–93.

Renaud, Michelle Lewis. 1997. *Women at the Crossroads: A Prostitute Community's Response to AIDS in Urban Senegal*. Amsterdam: Gordon and Breach.

Ronnell, Avital. 2003. "Proving Grounds: On Nietzsche and the Test Drive." *MLN* 118, no. 3: 653–69.

Rottenberg, Richard. 2009. "Social and Public Experiments and New Figurations of Science and Politics in Postcolonial Africa." *Postcolonial Studies* 12, no. 4: 423–40.

Shaw, Caroline. 1995. *Colonial Inscriptions: Race, Sex and Class in Kenya*. Minneapolis: University of Minnesota Press.

Shaw, Thomas M. 2006. *Irony and Illusion in the Architecture of Imperial Dakar*. Lampeter, Wales: Edwin Mellon Press.

Strathern, Marilyn. 1991. *Partial Connections*. Savage, MD: Rowman and Littlefield.

Sunder Rajan, Kaushik. 2005. "Subjects of Speculation: Emergent Life Sciences and Market Logics in the United States and India." *American Anthropologist* 107:19–30.

Swanson, Maynard. 1977. "The Sanitation Syndrome: Bubonic Plague and Urban Native Policy in the Cape Colony, 1900–1909." *Journal of African History* 18, no. 3: 387–410.

Tandia, Oumar. 1998. "Prostitution in Senegal." In *Global Sex Workers: Rights, Resistance and Redefinition*, ed. Kamala Kempadoo and Jo Doezema. New York: Routledge.

Thrift, Nigel. 2000. "It's the Little Things." In *Geopolitical Traditions: A Century of Geopolitical Thought*, ed. Klaus Dodds and David Atkinson. New York: Routledge.

Travers, K., S. Mboup, R. Marlink, A. Gueye-Nidaye et al. 1995. "Natural Protection against HIV-1 Provided by HIV-2." *Science* 268, no. 5217: 1612–15.

CHAPTER 8

The Work of the Virus: Cutting and
Creating Relations in an ART Project
Lotte Meinert

This chapter describes the encounter between a major internationally funded
medical antiretroviral therapy (ART) research project (herewith, the Project)
and a large polygynous extended family (herewith, the Family) in a rural
area in East Africa.[1]

The wider context of the meeting of scientific research and lived realities in East Africa may be thought of as multiple relations between the HIV
virus and international science, state and government, citizens, individuals,
and bodies, kinship and social networks and ARV medicine. In this chapter
I explore various layers of these relationships and effects of the encounter
between the Project and the Family. The chapter describes how the Project
has affected and changed relationships within the Family unit as well as relations between families and others in the local community. The analytical focus is on the cutting and creation of relationships between members,
networks, and wholes: the virus as part of individual bodies and as part
of research projects, individuals as members of families, science projects,
and "the state." These different networks are founded and held together by
associated values and ethics of larger wholes, in this case of kinship, bioscience, and modernity. Individuals navigating these networks may cut or
create links, leaving old networks for new ones altogether based on inclination, opportunity, and denunciation. I have been inspired to think about
the encounter between the virus, the Family, the Project, and the medicine
via actor-network theory (Law 2003; Latour 2005) and Marilyn Strathern's
(1996) ideas about "cutting" as well. What I attempt to give a glimpse of
here is what happens when the virus works, not primarily at a biological
level but more so at a social level: when family members in existing rural networks are propelled into, and choose to do, HIV work and to be gatekeepers

and brokers of access to a channel of ART, or "miracle medicine," made available by a global actor in medical science.

Mindful of the fallacy that holds, that research projects only have intended effects for the time of their implementation, I explore how the Project, its medical technology, and the individualistic ethic of benefits and obligations contributed to subtle and obvious changes in relations, and ideas about relations, between families and public health care. Some members of families found new employment as "workers of the virus," while others have become part of the research Project as objects of study. In research terminology they have become *clients* and their biological children have become *client-children*; their husbands or wives have been defined as *clients-partners*. The strict Project definitions of the nuclear family fit poorly with lived realities but have been made to determine who will be included and excluded from the study and its potential benefits. Family members who have been employed by the Project include a daughter, employed as a counselor to clients and their nuclear families, and a son, engaged as a fieldworker delivering ART medicine to clients. These Project employees have been equipped with embassy identity tags, motorcycles, helmets, and other pieces of equipment, which make them visibly different from their relatives. They have gone through training and have signed contracts promising to adhere to Project regulations and codes of conduct. Other Family members have applied for jobs in the research Project, but they did not get these positions. Some relatives work in the public health care system and experience their work and working conditions being altered by the presence of the research Project from that perspective.

The families' various kinds of involvement in the Project have redefined relationships between family members in various ways. Generational, gender, and kinship-based hierarchies are challenged and sometimes suspended and new hierarchies are emerging. New and old conflicts have erupted in the family and community, and alliances are created, reemphasized, or bracketed. Actors are making new cuts and links in their social networks based on principles of social organization (see Strathern 1996) other than the usual ones. The ART medicine being delivered by the fieldworkers to clients once a week has become a powerful point of reference for families, researchers, fieldworkers, and counselors. For the clients, access to the medicine and the regular ingestion of ART has become not only a matter of life and death but also a material matter and social matter tying them to a physical place and linking them in a specific way to other people. For the researchers, the clients' compliance with the medication is essential for the creation of valid scientific knowledge. For counselors and fieldworkers, ensuring the clients' compliance to the Project is important for positive job evaluation and job safeguarding.

The medicine has obviously become a central reference in the network between the people, who invest enormous expectations and intensive work in the therapy. What I want to focus on here is the dynamics of abandonment and creation through cutting and linking of networks by kin, fieldworkers, counselors, and researchers as they negotiate the making of research and subjectivities around ART.

The Family

I first met the Family in 1996. I was looking for a place to stay with my family while doing fieldwork, and we were directed to Mzee, who is a respected, elderly "big man" of the area.[2] Mzee is now retired but has had a long history in government work, including senior ministerial positions in former regimes. There is a family tradition of being involved with government, colonial administration, and the Catholic mission. Mzee's father was trained by the Catholic missionaries and later became a prominent chief in the area, and several of Mzee's brothers have held administrative positions in government bodies. Mzee has three wives, who all live in the home together in a relatively peaceful polygynous union, with some of the youngest of their in total twenty-seven children, a dozen grandchildren, a few great-grandchildren, and many other family members, helpers, visitors, and friends. My comparatively very small family and I ended up staying in the house of the eldest son, not far from the Family compound. We gradually learned how this large polygynous family worked as a network of units. Some of the younger children in the Family were sent to stay with older brothers and sisters in other parts of the country to do their schooling, to help out in the household, and to keep the relationships alive. One of the older sisters connected several of her younger siblings to job positions where she was working. The older sisters and brothers who earned a salary paid school fees for some of the younger siblings. Some family members were closer than others, which at times created tensions but seldom manifested in open conflict. Mzee was, in his discreet way, constantly monitoring relationships and trying to iron out uneven textures. Everybody respected Mzee as head and patron of the extended family, felt obliged to contribute to the family, and expected protection and inclusion in return. Some Family members accused each other of stealing, others were jealous when somebody had success, and there was relatively constant but harmless gossiping. Most of the children in the Family were well educated; all had finished at least the first part of secondary school and a few had continued to university, where they had obtained bachelor degrees. But the majority had problems finding a job, despite decent exam results, and despite Mzee's and other family members' connections. Only one of the sons in the family had managed to get a job in a government position. Most of the other family members describe themselves as "looking for a job" or "self-employed," as eldest son said with a brilliant white smile, disguising numerous frustrated attempts to run a business. After little over a year, my family and I moved away from the area, but I keep visiting the Family when doing other fieldwork in the area and we stay in touch by phone.

The Virus: Pre-ART Times

Ever since the first burial I attended in pre-ART times (1997) in one of the compounds neighboring the Family, I became painfully aware of the importance of the virus as an actant in local networks—a very effective, omnipresent, and implicit actant. My inquiries about the cause of death of the young woman who was being buried were clearly embarrassing and quieted cleverly by one of the Family brothers escorting me to the burial. During these years one could only mention AIDS in careful ways in order not to hurt or "convict" anybody (see Whyte 1997). One had to be especially careful when talking to two of the sisters in the Family. The first sister I will call the Counselor. Her husband had died from what was suspected to be AIDS back in the early 1990s, and she had become an active member of the major HIV/AIDS counseling NGO in the country. There was quiet speculation, but nobody spoke aloud about fears of her also being infected. She never mentioned her HIV status herself. Instead Family members spoke appreciatively about how well she managed to support her children and all the work she did in the AIDS support NGO, helping members deal with their losses, test results, inheritance issues, and other difficulties. Through her NGO work, the Counselor made new connections in the local area. She was visiting widows and widowers and recording their stories and losses, connecting them to the NGO and opening possibilities of food support, legal support, and other kinds of help. While moving around with the Counselor in a small NGO car, it became clear to me that she was well known and respected in the area. Almost everyone we passed on the road greeted her, and when we reached the family we were supposed to visit, several people came to make appointments with her to come and see their families or to meet privately in her office. After seven years of work and presence, she had with dedication and determination built a local network of people living with AIDS in this area.

Although the Counselor was gaining local recognition for "doing the work of the virus," earning money through this and building a network, the virus kept cutting and devastating networks rather than building new connections and links. The Family had a harsh experience of this, like many other families in the area, when one of their grown and married daughters returned home thin, vulnerable, and depressed. Her husband's family had sent her back to her paternal home when they realized that she was "sickly" (an often-used euphemism for having AIDS). Mzee was furious with his son-in-law and the family-in-law, because they returned his daughter in this state, without explanation, and without escort. She herself chose the strategy of "just keeping quiet" and did not mention much about the conflict with her family-in-law. I stumbled into the conflict unknowingly, when I sent a letter on behalf of a woman in the village to an organization, which I did not know the son-in-law was working for. The reply I received on behalf of the woman was inappropriately impertinent and harsh in its tone, copied to a long list of authorities. I was shocked and puzzled about this reaction to a minor request, and I asked Mzee to take a look at the letters. When Mzee saw the signature of his son-in-law and read the harsh words, he was clearly offended and told me not to worry because, between the lines, the letter actually was addressed to the Family and not to me and the woman. He explained that this was "the fool who had ruined his daughter" and who was now trying to attack the Family. This daughter was admitted in different hospitals several times and almost all Family members were involved in taking care of her by staying with her in hospital, cooking for her, bathing her, paying her medical bills, buying her passion fruit juice and food she appreciated. However, she was deteriorating quickly, and despite receiving the best available medical care at that point in time—the pre-ART era—she inevitably passed away. A message was sent to the family-in-law regarding the burial. As she was married and bridewealth had been at least partly paid, she was supposed to be buried in the compound of her in-laws. However, Mzee chose not to acknowledge this and announced that she would be buried at home, thereby cutting off the opportunity for the family-in-law to show that they were a responsible and proper family. Only a minimal delegation of in-laws turned up at the burial, and even after that the air between the families remained cold and polluted due to the unresolved question of who brought the virus into the marriage and families (see Whyte 2005).

The virus was destructive at all levels in society, even though it also created jobs for some and an economy around AIDS was beginning to develop. The hospitals were overburdened with AIDS patients, and understaffed with health personnel, who were also affected by AIDS themselves and facing impossible care tasks. All institutions were affected in one way or the other. I remember the outcry at the local primary school when official government rules were passed regarding participation in burials in order to limit absenteeism from work. Families buried their dead at a rate nobody had experienced before. Some families were falling apart and the hopelessness of AIDS combined with serious poverty increased cases of domestic violence, alcoholism, and theft. However, most families managed the burden of caring for the sick, looking after orphans, and somehow making ends meet. There was a peculiar mix of resilience, reconciliation, and resignation that people expressed when they talked about the HIV virus as "our disease" and the "illness of our times." Still, in the pre-ART AIDS era, the societal picture painted by the virus was horrifying and hopeless.

The "Miracle Medicine," 2002

Also hopeless were the expressions of the Family parents when another daughter came home, with her one-year-old son, breaking the shocking news that her husband had suddenly died from AIDS and that she herself was HIV positive. "We were still grieving for [our late daughter] and it felt like the cement on her grave had barely dried, when we received [this daughter]," one of the mothers lamented tiredly. Yet, in the meantime, ART medicine had started coming into the country and was available at a clinic in the capital city. The Counselor sister, through her work in the AIDS NGO, was aware of this and tried to assure the Family that they would be able to keep this daughter alive if she received the medicine. Mzee and the mothers had not heard much about ART and were not convinced about this new "miracle medicine," having just lost one of their daughters. But as the new patient got worse, they agreed to admit her to the clinic in the capital city. "If your child is sick, you don't have a choice; you have to try everything possible, even if you cannot afford it," Mzee said. The cost of the medicine was extremely high at that time, not to mention the required laboratory tests that had to accompany and monitor the efficiency of the medicine. Again all family members had to contribute to the care and the medical bills of their sister, which did create some turbulence and strain in the family network, as some were willing to spend all their savings, while others only contributed small amounts and were considered stingy. Still others did not manage to "find any money at all." As soon as the daughter was medically stabilized she was taken home, and one of the family members would go every second week to buy medicine for her from the far-away clinic (a day's journey). The medical expenses became a constant burden and reason for quarrels in the family. Although everybody did their best to avoid having the sick daughter hear any quarrels, lest she would be discouraged from taking the medicine, she was clearly aware of the problems that the cost of her treatment caused. She also experienced some side effects of the medication (mainly dizziness and headache) and said to the Family that she had agreed with the doctor to take a "medicine holiday." After the so-called holiday she probably never took the medicine again, due to the side effects, the cost of the medicine, and the problems this caused. One day she fell and broke her leg. The fracture would not heal, and according to Mzee, this made her lose hope that she would ever be able to live a normal life again. After one year she was buried next to her sibling. The miracle of the medicine did not happen.

The Powerful ART Project of 2003: Opportunities and New Ways

The year 2003 became a year of changes for the Family and others with HIV patients in their care in the area. A large study on ART was initiated in the district. The organization conducting the study had already carried out a study on infection prophylaxis among HIV positive people in collaboration with the AIDS NGO in the district. This larger, new ART study brought grand possibilities. The Project was probably not fully aware of the public signals it sent (it made quite a splash) and the expectations it raised when it put up a new air-conditioned Project building within the district hospital compound. Despite its—for the public—suggestive location, the new building was not really for patients. After all, the Project was set up to study the provision of ART in homes. Instead the new building was to be used for computers, files, and researchers.

Jobs as counselors, fieldworkers, mechanics, secretaries, cleaners, and data-entry clerks were advertised. Tenders for cars, motorcycles, construction work, office equipment, and so on were given out. Mzee commented that this Project might actually change the economy of the place, as "these people are really strong." He explained that if one or two Family members could get a foot into the project, the whole Family would benefit. Being a former senior government employee, Mzee always commented on the "new ways" of "projects" with some reservation, because "they come and go before you find out what they do," but he pragmatically advised his children to apply for jobs in such projects because these were the only real opportunities. The projects he knew and referred to were developmental and aid-related. As we will see, this type of scientific research project was unprecedented in the area and came with scientific rigor and financial clout. Given its mission and focus, it was foremost concerned with high quality data collection and "proper science." Its priorities differed from the usual development projects.

As it turned out, in this case the Family would find out what the project was doing—some of its members would participate in the doing. Several Family members tried and some did get a foot into the project, but through different doors: some through the employment door and others through the client door. The Counselor sister was employed as a Project counselor on a three-year contract. Another brother from the Family, with developmental NGO experience, was employed as a Fieldworker on a one-year contract that was continually extended. When reflecting upon why and how they got the jobs, both the sister and brother maintained that they were selected in the rigid employment process by the Project because they had the right work experience with NGOs and papers to prove this, not because of who they knew, which is considered the usual way of getting a job in the area. The Counselor sister and Fieldworker brother were sent by the Project to do courses and trainings in the capital city before starting the actual work. They were given embassy identity tags; each had a motorcycle, helmet, and other equipment. The Counselor sister's salary increased more than ten-fold compared to what she earned in her NGO job. Other Family members were less fortunate: one of the sisters who had just finished her bachelor degree applied, but she did not get a position. She did not have relevant working experience. Another brother, who had also been working with an NGO earlier, applied but did not get the job. He felt that the reason he didn't get the job was because he didn't know the right people, and he kept being slightly offended that the brother and sister who got into the Project could not "organize something for him." The Counselor sister was furious about this, and told her brother that "these days you need papers—knowing someone does not help—you need real papers." The eldest brother, who is a mechanic, applied for different jobs and tenders in the Project, but he was not successful either. When I tried to console those who did not get a job by saying that the Project only offered short-term contracts anyway, and that they would be better off getting a proper government position somewhere, they did not appear to agree. Even if it was just a short-term perspective, Project salaries were much higher than government ones, and you would not have to "chase your check" as many government employees had to. The job of the Counselor sister was to visit the patients and families and advise them regarding compliance, hygiene, social, psychological, and sexual issues. In principle the counselors were supposed to "mainly listen" to the patients and their families. In practice the counselors had an hour-long questionnaire to fill in regarding the mentioned issues and very little time and attention was available for whatever other problems the clients would want to discuss. The ethos of scientific rigor in the Project somehow seemed to trickle down into the relationship between the Counselor and her clients, even though this was not intended and even though she had rather confidential relationships with some of the clients from her earlier work.

At the time, the Project was only planned for a three-year period. When it started enrolling clients based on a stringent set of criteria for inclusion, things started moving quickly. The "inclusion" criteria in fact, quite in accordance with the scientific objectives of the exercise, excluded many. To be included, the client had to be a long-term member of the AIDS NGO most active in the area, have a CD4 count below 250,[3] and had to live and sleep seven days a week in the surveyed household. The latter criterion makes a lot of sense for a longitudinal study, and perhaps for a bedridden, weak patient it is a non-issue. Still, it proved to be problematic for some patients.

As mentioned, the Counselor sister who had worked in the AIDS NGO for seven years had advised many Family members, friends, and neighbors in the area who were HIV positive to become members. These now met the first formal Project criteria and many were included in the study. To give some examples: a male member of the Family's extensive network of in-laws was enrolled as one of the first clients. A neighbor and clan-mate was enrolled, but was unfortunately one of the few clients in the study who passed away, shortly after enrollment. A cousin was enrolled and became one of the success stories of the Project. A male neighbor from one of the other relatively rich families was enrolled together with his wife. A Family daughter was also enrolled in the study, but she died before the project started handing out medicine. Thus, Family members, in-laws, clan-mates, others from the Family's social peer group, and those in proximity networks were invoked to contribute to the formation of the research Project network. A significant segment of the Counselor sister's original network-based voluntarism and self-help was transposed to become a part of a research network founded on extractive research principles and counseling geared toward fulfilling sample integrity requirements instead of the life aspirations of clients in the broadest sense.

The Creation of Client Subjectivities

The Project term *clients* became part of the Project lingo to signal the "in-group." They were given information about the purpose of study: to find out about the best and most affordable way to provide ARV therapy to poor rural populations. They were told about three "arms" in the study. One arm of clients would be given information about the progress of their CD4 counts and viral loads, another arm of clients would not be given this information and neither would their doctors (double-blind), and in the third arm only the doctors would know clients' results (single-blind).

Clients were called for meetings at the newly built Project office in the district hospital, where they were given information about the research project. Those who were too sick to come to the Project office were given the information at home or in hospital. Every client was told that the research would go on for three years, that they had to comply with the medicine regime, and that they were to stay in their homes seven days a week, otherwise they would be removed from the study. The term *client* may as well have been coined as *client-body* to more overtly reflect the biomedical preoccupation of the research. In real life, the person would, as we will see, aspire to work and have social interaction that included physical and social mobility. This was an ethical dilemma that counselors and fieldworkers had to negotiate on a daily basis, because to get access to medicine, the client had to give up the fundamental freedom of movement.

To formalize the Project-client relation (and in adherence to international research standards), all clients had to sign informed consent forms: two-page-long statements in English in very small print. These papers contained the quintessence of the ethics of scientific research and the associated legal-individualistic relation of benefits and obligations between Project and client. In the poor rural context, this contract probably had more symbolic significance than informational value. National staff such as the Counselor sister and the Fieldworker brother had important roles to play in culturally translating the informed consent forms and its real-life implications. I heard the Fieldworker brother explain the forms in simple local language to one of the clients' teenage children before she was tested for HIV. I was impressed—as far as my own local language skills allow it—with the patient and detailed translation and interpretation he did. He explained the purpose of the study and all the conditions it entailed. Still, when I asked participants in the study about the purpose of the Project, they said it was mostly "to give people medicine." I only recall one of the clients I talked to who actually understood that she was part of a study and that the main purpose of receiving the medicine and all the medical care and support was the creation of science. This participant proudly said: "I have signed ALL the papers in the project, dedicated my whole body to [the Project]. Even when I die they can study my blood, my bones, everything." In this context it was quite a remarkable decision and statement because it was believed that burial and its rituals are highly important for the continuation of life in the family she would leave behind. Thus, implicit in her choice to dedicate her body to science might also be a criticism of her family and how she felt they had neglected her when she was dying from AIDS.

In each household of a client, Project personnel came to register and test all nuclear family members for HIV: husbands, wives, and biological children. If any of these were HIV positive, or became HIV positive during the study, they were also included. If they were to benefit from the Project (and its use of medicines of different kinds), they had to sign informed consent forms and commit to staying in the household for the duration of the Project. Other HIV positive persons in the area who did not live up to inclusion criteria for the Project or who were not family members could not get into the Project. Marrying a client, as we will see, was one of the possible loopholes for gaining access to medicine.

A male client from the Counselor sister's village network did not comply with the Project's medical prescriptions. He kept drinking alcohol and smoking cigarettes, he did not eat properly, and he sometimes forgot to take the medicine. His health was not improving the way it should have. The doctors at the Project were worried about his health, and the Counselor sister went there several times to counsel him and his wife about taking the drugs, stopping the drinking and smoking, and eating properly. On some occasions she did not find him at home, as he should have been, according to the Project regulations, and other times she found him very drunk in a bar in the trading center. In these cases, she had to report his "noncompliance" to the Project office. Assumedly, this case reflected badly on her counseling skills. The client said that he was threatened with removal from the study (de facto denying him access to the ART) if he did not follow the Project rules. He got angry and went to the Project office to complain about his counselor:

> I told those people that I would not accept her way of talking—demanding that I be at home whenever she came to counsel me. I had to go to my gardens to work! Who was she to demand, anyway? I told those people that I did not even need a counselor, and what was causing most of my problems was having a counselor! What I need from them is only the medicine, I don't need the talking and I can even get my own transport to pick up the medicine, they don't need to deliver at my home every week, demanding that I be at home.

The Project decided to assign a new counselor, who perhaps did not visit him quite as often and who reportedly "talked in a different way" (and perhaps not as much). This client eventually stopped drinking and began to take the medicine as prescribed. The Counselor sister was still upset with him after "giving up on him." "He is a very difficult person, he is not advisable at all—he will not listen to anything you say. He just shuts up completely and looks at you in a very fierce way. That case was so difficult for me. It even made me look as if I was not doing my job properly. I kept going there and bounced, I kept talking to him, but he did not change and yet he is from my village." It seems that "being from my village," that is, from a close social network, put some obligation on the client to behave in a way that made the Counselor look good. Gratitude with some humility and appreciation seemed called for, not recalcitrance and, worse, successfully bypassing the Counselor in the Project network hierarchy.

A cousin sister of the Counselor and the Fieldworker had been enrolled in the project from the very start and had a very different kind of relationship with her counselors and fieldworkers: "Those people in the Project just love me, because I am a real success case. I started with only 13 *askaris* [askari means "guard" in Kiswahili and is used as a local reference to CD4 cells; see Meinert et al. 2009]. I had resistant TB, but now I have gained over 25 kilograms and I am very good. The way they have talked to me to encourage me to take the medicine, to eat well, talking about stigma, talking about the future, talking about my worries. They have become my real, real friends."

The creation of friendships and new kinds of nurturing bonds through ART and working relationships within the Project were remarkable. Over time the everyday working terms of the counselors and fieldworkers changed. In the beginning, the clients were referred to as "index-persons." After some time the term was changed to client, which was done partly to adopt a less technical and more familiar language and partly because this was more in line with counseling terminology. This change of terminology also reflects the social process of creating specific subjectivities in the Project positions of patrons and clients. These positions were not only created by the Project and forced upon people, but they were also very actively appropriated and re-created by the clients and the local employees. The Counselor sister worked in her home area where her clan members lived. When she visited the homes where clients lived, aunts and uncles and other distant family members asked her to include them in the Project or requested other forms of help. They did not believe her when she tried to explain that she did not have the power to include new members in the Project, and that she was not supposed to give presents to clients. Her clan members found her "proud" and said she had forgotten how to treat family. They expected her to be their patron in all respects now that she had a "big job" in the Project, but she could only look after the Project's clients in a very restricted way. After a number of conflicts, the Counselor sister was moved to work outside her home area. The Counselor sister found a way of helping—and also cutting off, abandoning, and quieting—some people from her home area by offering monetary loans. Officially this was not part of the Project, but the clan members regarded it as part of the Project because it was made possible by the Counselor's salary from the Project. This further established the patron-client relationship between the Project and families.

At one point the Counselor gave a loan to a brother-in-law involved in the Project as a client for a brick-making project. This loan merged kinship and Project networks: it was a double link between the two people involved. But the brother-in-law's venture was not successful. Neighbors said that the brother-in-law spent the money gambling, and he never paid back the money to the Counselor. The brother-in-law told me that he fell sick every time he saw the Counselor, because he feared what she might do if he did not manage to pay back the money: "You see my life now depends on this medicine, so I cannot afford to mess up that connection." He was not sure if the Counselor could actually cut him off from the project, so that he would not receive his medicine. Irrespective of that, he was still worried about maintaining a good connection to the Project through the Counselor sister. The overlaying networks of science and kin had increased the agency of the Counselor within the kinship network. As an in-law and a woman, she would be less likely to be able to cut a link if it were based on kinship only; as a Counselor, the brother-in-law feared she could invoke the tough guidelines of client behavior of the Project (which could, however, not be done). As it turned out, there were no consequences.[4]

"Our People"

By employing the Counselor sister, the Project gained access to her network as well as her considerable individual skills and experience. Being a gatekeeper and broker of access to the "miracle medicine" significantly increased her social recognition locally and thus her social agency in the kinship network. As I will explore in more depth below, the Counselor's professional empowerment and identification with the individualistic ethics underlying the Project became part of a drive to cut free from the morality associated with patrilineal family networks. Her Fieldworker brother chose an approach that was more intermediate in nature. His identification with the ethics of the Project was pragmatic. The individual tough justice approach of the Project could be a shield against claims to "special treatment" by Family and other network members. At the same time, his mode of interaction focused on mediating local and Project ethics through the models of explanation he used.

I went with the Fieldworker on his motorbike to visit some of his Project clients. His job was mainly to deliver weekly packages of medicine to clients. As we drove through the landscape he pointed out homesteads that were also included in the Project, saying "these are our people, and those are also our people, this one was one of the first, she is now a grandmother [using a kinship vocabulary] in the project" (see Geissler et al. 2008). When explaining the different arms of the Project (the open, single-blind, and double-blind groups) to the clients, he used the metaphor of different clans, who each have their clan animal that they can't eat, touch, or even mention.

The visits in the homes of his clients were in some respects carried out like family visits. Children would first come and greet us, bring chairs for us to sit on in the shade of a tree, all family members would come to greet us; there would be an exchange of local news (mainly about burials) and in some cases we were offered a drink. He would hand over the medicine; the client or a relative would thank him and sign for it. Exchanges seemed very much to be done in the spirit of reciprocity. The Project gives medicine — the clients give their compliance with Project rules and access to do "science" on their bodies and lives. However, as mentioned earlier, it is seldom clear how clients understand the value of what they give in return for the medicine (see Leach and Fairhead 2007). Some of the clients, like the cousin sister and the man who was difficult to counsel, felt the value of what they had to give up: mobility, drinking, and sexual relations in order to become the new kinds of subjectivities needed in the Project, disciplined, hygienic, well-fed home-bodies loyal to the Project.

On some occasions the Fieldworker brother had to conduct an interview with a client based on a questionnaire, in other places he had to do HIV tests on clients' family members, to see if they were eligible to be included in the Project. He explained that he had not had many problems with people from his home, that is, clan members, expecting help of different kinds, but sometimes he brought them some passion fruits, sugar, or what they asked for. "It is not as bad for fieldworkers as for counselors," he said.

> People know that you just come to deliver the medicine, but you don't talk so deep to them about their problems as the counselors do. People know that you are not the one to decide, but you can always take their request. . . . In the beginning the most difficult part was to make home people understand that they could not ride on the motorbike with me to town if they had a problem. Project rules are very strict: you are not supposed to carry any passenger on the motorbike. If you are seen with a passenger you lose your job. It is the same if you lose medicine: one fieldworker lost a package of medicine on his trip, and he was fired. There is no way of bending the rules of this Project. So if you find one of your family members sick, badly off, needs to go to hospital, you just have to say sorry there is no way on this motorbike. Sometimes I go to town and pay for a special hire to go and pick them up. At least in that way you can try to help. But people are now used — they know that this Project is very strict and none of the motorbikes can take passengers.

Other research projects, like the malaria vaccine trial in the Gambia, described by Geissler et al. (2008), have had to change transport regulations in order to develop good relations with the trial community. In this ART study, the transport regulations, as well as inclusion and exclusion criteria, were possibly kept so rigid because the Project perceived the "gift" it was giving to the trial community: medicine and survival. Therefore, the Project demanded what they saw as sufficient return from clients: full-time access to study their bodies and lives for three years (and this was later extended to six years).

The Pragmatics of Life

A brother-in-law to the Counselor sister and Fieldworker was also included in the study from the beginning. His wife was also HIV positive, but she was not included because her CD4 count was still high. She never complained about that but had adopted the pervasive NGO discourse about "living positively" almost in a religious way, and she was patiently waiting to be included in the ART project, "when she was ready." Meanwhile she had appropriated the positive identity as a very active member of an NGO drama group, which traveled around the district to perform and inform about AIDS. She earned enough money to sustain the family by doing this and had gained control over her life and family. Her husband, the brother-in-law, was uncomfortable with the situation. He was envious because he would prefer himself to be the one providing for and being in control of the family, and he was jealous about his wife interacting with other men in the drama group.

About two years into the Project he suspected that his wife was having an affair with another man in the drama group and became very upset. As a member of another AIDS NGO, the Post-Test Club, he started seeing an HIV-positive woman. His wife heard rumors that her husband had taken a new wife, who was pregnant with his child. She was furious and moved to her father's home for some months. Having adopted the "living positively ideology," she said she was worried about reinfection and about having another child to care for when they were all infected, "I work hard to buy good food for my husband, to plan for the children's schooling, and meanwhile he is in the bar with another woman. Now if he marries this woman, she will also be included in Project, and if her CD4 count is below [250] she will be given medicine. Maybe he wants to punish me for something I have not done. I have not been unfaithful to him, and I will not become bitter because of what he is trying to do. I am living positively—I plan for myself and for my children."

The man did not marry the new wife officially (he would need family support for this) but he was aware — and the potential wife was probably aware — that if they married, this connection would carry her into the Project. Indeed this loophole existed, but reportedly discouraging clients from having new relationships and pregnancies was common Project practice.

Wholes and Their Members: Science and State, Clients and Citizens

Thus far, the Project has been described in a way that most local people saw it: job opportunities leading to differentiations between those who got jobs and those who failed; those who could meet poorly understood outside rules (that is, those who became clients) and those who did not. People, inevitably, started living *with* instead of living *for* the Project. The Project's attempts to control movement and delineate fixed nuclear families, which would stay in permanent and stable homes, proved to be largely untenable. Family members were moving in and out of homes, and some members moved to town and requested not to have their medicine brought to their new homes, saying that they preferred to pick the medicine up themselves from the Project office. The relationship between the clients and the Project was planned to be regulated and ruled by informed consent forms and agreements. But these were obviously more relevant in other legal settings than in the rural setting. The actual relationships were negotiated pragmatically with fieldworkers and counselors as important middlemen.

The relationships were transformed from neutral science — subject relationships — to a kind of patron-client relationship, which involved more complex protection, caring, and obligation than originally planned for, and then a kind of dynamic relationship where clients and Project employees continually tried to negotiate conditions and did not take all Project rules as final decisions.

From the perspective of the Project, the district-wide study was set up to find ways of providing ART inexpensively to poor rural population segments and to provide care at peoples' homes. One of the aims was to evaluate clinical monitoring versus laboratory monitoring of AIDS patients, as this could bring down the cost of ART significantly. The Project was, by design, set up in parallel to the government health system. When we asked one of the Project's international doctors why they did not work through the government health system, he asked us back provokingly, "Which health system?," evoking the Africa as a weak state narrative and indicating that the government health system was malfunctioning and not worth investing in. If clients got sick, they were asked to either send a message to the Project and then a doctor or nurse would come to see them at home and deliver medicine there or they could come to the district hospital. If they had to be admitted to the hospital, they were given the equivalent of US$1.50 a day for food. In serious cases the Project doctors would take over the treatment of the patient, as in the case of the cousin, who was admitted to the hospital for several months with resistant tuberculosis. She was given a private room in the ward and had a wheelchair and other small privileges compared to the other patients in the hospital. The nurses in the hospital were well aware of the "food money" received by the Project patients, and they would often ask the Project patients to pay for their medical treatment or simply to give some of the money to the nurses. One of the doctors working at the district hospital when the Project started said that he was proud that it had chosen to work together with his hospital and that he was looking forward to the collaboration and saw a bright future for the hospital. After one year of "collaboration," he was clearly less optimistic. "The work of [the Project] is very good," he said, "but it makes the work we do at the hospital look bad. Our patients look at the Project clients who get money, medicine, attention, and ask us why they cannot have that level of care. But we don't have the resources and our best staff have left and been employed by the Project." In the beginning the difference between the Project and the hospital was visibly very striking because the Project building was a newly built and bright white wing, sparsely inhabited by researchers and few patients, surrounded by new vehicles and motorcycles. It stood out next to the hospital wings that were dilapidated after many years of intensive use, having very little resources and being crowded with patients in the wards and relatives doing laundry and cooking outside the wards. After a couple of years, the Project sponsored a new paint job for the hospital, which helped to even out the visible difference between the Project and the government hospital. Yet the differences between the research Project and the government health system remain profound. Evidently, this is deliberate and a matter of choice. It would be possible, in principle, to adjust the Project should one want to lessen the detachment from the government health system. Other ART projects in the country, which are less science-oriented and more preoccupied with sustainability, have made an effort to be integrated with the government health services. However, this was not the pursuit of the Project. The differences between state-run health systems and "international" research projects are rooted in fundamentally dissimilar ideas about "wholes" and their constituent parts or "members."

The larger whole of the (old) health system is "the state" and government with its idea and hope of becoming "the providing state" that coordinates services for citizens and protects and defends its citizens. Citizens, in turn, are expected to adopt an identity as members of the state and are obliged to contribute to the development of the country. As members they are responsible to the whole, members pay tax to the state, and have rights to vote for politicians to head this whole. The Project refers foremost to its international root organization and the larger "global" whole, which congeals around ART medicine, associated international research and the donor community, and the pharmaceutical industry—called "science." The members created by this whole are clients, who in some respects are in time-limited patron-client relationships with their projects. They depend on the patron for inclusion in the whole, and for the provision of medicine, and hence for survival. In return the clients are obliged to remain loyal to the rules and needs of the patron and have to take on the identity as clients. In the words of Nguyen (2004), the members of this new whole are "therapeutic citizens,"[5] who are treated according to biosciences' ethical guidelines; they have rights to say "no" to the medicine or to be kept alive by the medicine and health care provided by the Project. The new whole relies on its members in a very specific and limited way, mainly as medicine-naïve bodies, who comply with medication regimes. The new whole does not expect— or accept—further involvement with its client members in terms of social interaction, economic productivity, or political engagement. The whole associated with this ART research also does not operate with a very long time horizon and does not consider it its responsibility to deal with the members as complex and complete human beings, but it chooses to focus on them as bodies, which are meant to be kept alive for a period of time. The Project through its medical provisions and informed consent documents presents a stark choice to people: gain access to life-prolonging medicine and accept the conditions of being a client or die from your HIV infection. Nobody who was asked—as far as I was informed—declined to be a client.

Cutting and Linking, Destruction and Creation

Networks are the pathways that connect members to larger wholes. Links are continuously developed and established, actors are made to act by many others (Latour 2005), and connections can also be cut and the flow of energy in a network may be withheld (Strathern 1996). The process of networking is inherently and simultaneously constituted by acts of cutting and linking—destructive and creative at the same time. The effects of the HIV virus have been extremely destructive, killing individuals, ripping families apart, demolishing institutions, yet at the same time the virus has created a whole new economy, with job opportunities and thus possible survival for individuals and families, and established new and strong institutions.

The Project described in this chapter attempted to stop the cyclical social cutting and linking in order to be able to turn the knowledge created by the Project into controlled and precise science. As a client in the Project you and your benefitting family members became tied to your homestead geographically. Your family ties had been established and officially signed for and could not be renegotiated—except by marriage and birth of new children. Biological or married family could make claims to treatment by pointing to the official family record, which had been established by the Project. The client did not have the right to cut off family members from having the benefits from the project. Those rights were established by Project regulations.

When you were an employee in the Project doing the powerful "work of the virus," you were able to cut the connection to your family and homestead or parts of the family if you wanted to create new networks of friends and colleagues to make up for the lost family network—or you could choose to have a very limited social network and accept the terms of your new economic and social possibilities. As a family member to an employee you might be disappointed if you expected to be easily included in the research Project, but as a family member to an employee you might enjoy some of the wealth of the employee being distributed in the family network or you might find yourself cut off from the person who had gotten employment, perhaps because you became or could potentially become an economic burden.

A more general point is that projects always introduce new kinds of relationships, creating fruitful connections as well as conflicts that reach beyond the scope and purpose of the project itself. With research projects, as with other forms of social change, people see possibilities of discarding and establishing networks based on new forms of social organization (Strathern

1996). In the case of this specific ART research Project, the same factors that formed a project-internal perspective, contributing to efficacy in achieving set results and targets (good research and office facilities, professionally managed and controlled, well-remunerated staff), also set it apart in the life experience of the Family members, clients, and the local community. Association with the Project's power became an explanation for why cutting and linking happened.

Notes

I would like to acknowledge the Living with ART research group under the TORCH project, especially Susan Reynolds Whyte for her continuous interest and encouragement. Even though this chapter is based on a different set of data, some of the analysis has grown out of our common work. Many thanks to my colleague Bjarke Nielsen for his insistence and assistance in discussing this material in the light of actor-network theory. The discussion continues! I would also like to thank P. Wenzel Geissler warmly for his enthusiasm and encouragement.

1   I wrote this chapter with great affection for the people who shared and taught me about the complications of this encounter and other issues. I have chosen to respect their privacy and not use real names or make specific geographical references or project descriptions in order to avoid contributing to further conflicts. Instead I refer to the persons by the roles they have in the Family or the ones they assumed in the Project.

2   *Mzee* is the respectful title of an elderly man.

3   Having a CD4 count below 250 is an indication of a seriously lowered immune system.

4   For a more thorough discussion of therapeutic clientship, see Whyte et al. (2011).

5   "Therapeutic citizenship is a biopolitical citizenship, a system of claims and ethical projects that arise out of the conjugation of techniques used to govern populations and manage individual bodies. The notion of therapeutic citizenship points to the growing transnational influence of biomedical knowledge and practice in the government of human and non-human affairs" (Nguyen 2004, 126).

References

Geissler, P. Wenzel, Ann Kelly, Robert Pool, and Babatunde Imokhuede. 2008. "'He Is Now Like a Brother, I Can Even Give Him Some Blood'—Relational Ethics and Material Exchanges in a Malaria Vaccine 'Trial Community' in The Gambia." *Social Science and Medicine* 67:696–707.

Geissler, P. Wenzel, and Ruth J. Prince. 2010. *The Land Is Dying: Contingency, Creativity and Conflict in Western Kenya*. Oxford: Berghahn.

Latour, Bruno. 2005. *Reassembling the Social*. Oxford: Oxford University Press.

Law, John. 2003. "Notes on the Theory of Actor Network: Ordering, Strategy, and Heterogeneity." Centre for Science Studies, Lancaster University. http://lancs .ac.uk/fass/sociology/papers/law-ordering-and-obdurancy.

Leach, Melissa, and James Fairhead. 2007. *Vaccine Anxieties: Global Science, Child Health and Society*. London: Earthscan.

Meinert, Lotte, Hanne Mogensen, and Jenipher Twebaze. 2009. "Tests for Life Chances: CD4 Miracles and Obstacles in Uganda." *Anthropology and Medicine* 16, no. 2: 195–209.

Nguyen, Vinh-Kim. 2004. "Antiretroviral Globalism, Biopolitics, and Therapeutic Citizenship." In *Global Assemblages: Technology, Politics and Ethics as Anthropological Problems*, ed. Aihwa Ong and Stephen J. Collier. Boston: Wiley-Blackwell.

Strathern, Marilyn. 1996. "Cutting the Network." *Journal of the Royal Anthropological Institute* 2, no. 3: 517–35.

Whyte, Susan R. 1997. *Questioning Misfortune: The Pragmatics of Uncertainty in Eastern Uganda*. Cambridge: Cambridge University Press.

Whyte, Susan R. 2005. "Going Home? Burial and Belonging in the Era of AIDS." *Africa* 75, no. 2: 154–72.

Whyte, Susan R., Michael Whyte, Lotte Meinert, and Jenipher Twebaze. 2011. "Therapeutic Clientship: Belonging in Uganda's Mosaic of AIDS Projects." In *When People Come First: Anthropology and Social Innovation in Global Health*, ed. João Biehl and Adriana Petryna. Durham, NC: Duke University Press.

PART V

Struggling Nation

CHAPTER 9

The Blue Warriors: Ecology,

Participation, and Public Health

in Malaria Control Experiments

Uli Beisel

The Blue Warriors: Insecticide Spraying against Malaria in Ghana

At 7:30 A.M. in June 2008, 116 men in blue overalls hop onto the back of pickup trucks and leave the compound of a gold-mining company in Ghana. It's a peculiar image, a fleet of dark blue pickups with eight men each swarm out to fulfil their daily mission. The pickups, which belong to the gold-mining company, have the following words painted on their sides: Community Malaria Control Programme. After a ten-minute drive, the workday begins, and teams spread out into the settlement. It's always two men going together. One person is responsible for the preparation of the rooms; he asks the inhabitants of the houses for entry permission, covers the furniture and belongings of people with white sheets, and fills in a short statistical form. The second person in the team is mostly unrecognizable: he not only wears his blue overalls but also a helmet and protective mask over his face. The spraying pump hanging over his shoulder only heightens the scary impression he makes. And then the spraying begins: within a few minutes the inside walls of all the rooms in a habitation get carefully covered with a thin layer of insecticide that sticks on the walls for up to six months. The operation's aim is to kill *Anopheles* mosquitoes and prevent malaria in the city.

This is how a normal work day begins for the 116 sprayers of a multinational gold-mining company's malaria control program in a city of 200,000 inhabitants in Ghana. The mine implements this project as part of their corporate social responsibility activities (CSR).[1] The program has been active since 2005 and has, according to company data, reduced malaria incidences by 75 percent in the city (Global Fund 2010). This corporate project triggered a major public-private partnership (PPP) between the

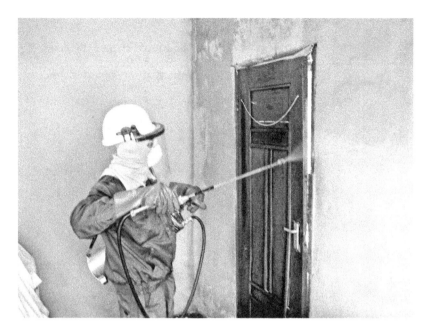

Figure 9.1. Sprayer at work.

gold-mining company, the Global Fund for HIV/AIDS, Tuberculosis, and Malaria (Global Fund), and the Ghanaian Ministry of Health. In 2007–2008 the partners applied at the Global Fund for a five-year US$158 million grant to conduct malaria control activities in forty districts in Ghana. The Global Fund approved the grant in late 2008, and since January 2011 the gold mine and the Ghanaian government are cooperating on a large-scale insecticide spraying campaign. The new project is modeled after the initial corporate social responsibility project, and the gold-mining company is the principal recipient of the grant as well as responsible for the project's implementation. This makes the company the first recipient in the private sector of a major Global Fund grant in Africa (Global Fund 2010).

This chapter is concerned with the origins of this new para-statal initiative in Ghana.[2] It maps out the scientific design and public engagement strategies of the gold-mining company's initial malaria control program; a citywide CSR project that is being extended to the currently largest national Ghanaian malaria control project. In the following pages, I explore the implications of this shift from citywide to national malaria control and from corporate project to publicly funded health care. I propose that the gold-mining company's initial project takes the form of a "real-world experiment" (Krohn and Weyer 1994; Szerzynski 2006). It is argued that, in the age of insecticide resistance, malaria control activities have become necessarily experimental; interventions are not only routinely monitored but also have to be modified and adapted in order to stay effective. The project moves continuously between science and public health intervention, as well as between laboratory and field. This need for scientific monitoring of resistance in mosquito populations and the consequential adaptation of control strategies contradicts the idea of insecticide spraying as a public health intervention that is based on sound scientific evidence. Instead the project becomes explicitly experimental, with less predictable effectivity and outcomes. Understanding the project as a real-world experiment underlines the uncertainty that is attached to insecticide spraying against malaria today. This, I suggest, not only renders the malaria control project a scientific and ecological experiment but also makes it visible as a "social and public experiment" (Rottenburg 2009).

In a second step, this chapter analyzes the extension of the initial corporate project into a new national-level spraying initiative. This transformation entails projecting the experimental landscape from city to nation. Furthermore, the new project converts a CSR project into a complex, parastatal arrangement between international donor, multinational company, and the Ghanaian state. This new partnership approach reconfigures the relation between state and corporate, between public and private sector. The project is not one or the other but a combination of both; situated somewhere in between a CSR initiative and a public health project—it becomes para-statal. James Ferguson has suggested that such shifted power relations can be understood as "transnational topographies of power," with "political entities that may be better conceptualized as not 'below' the state but as integral parts of a new transnational apparatus of governmentality. This new apparatus does not replace the older system of nation-states . . . but overlays it and coexists with it" (Ferguson 2006, 103). In this way of thinking, transnational donors or multinational companies become "horizontal contemporaries of the state" that shape and blur the distinction between public and private as well as between state and civil. However, there is a need to specify the concrete roles of governments, corporations, and the public in such partnerships. In line with the broader argument of this edited volume, this chapter conceptualizes such emerging configurations as *para-statal*, underlining the continuing albeit changing engagement of state agencies in the complex relations between transnational donors and state and private business in this Ghanaian malaria control project. By looking to the corporate precursor of one of those emerging transnational or para-statal partnerships, this chapter specifies how transnational, private, and state and public actors come together in shaping a malaria control project in practice. The following sections introduce the case study and the project's scientific logic and design and develop an analysis of the relation between ecology and public engagement that prevails in the project. The last section discusses the extension of the project from city to nation and reflects on the relation between private, state, and public actors raised by the project and its role in Ghanaian malaria control today.

The Gold Mine's CSR Malaria Project

SCIENTIFIC CORPORATE MALARIA CONTROL

In 2006, when the project was inaugurated by the then president of Ghana, John Kufuor, he termed the spray men *blue warriors*—a term referring to both the blue overalls of the men and their mission: the fight against malaria. Ryan, the manager of the program, likes the term and smilingly adds that the team even built a flag stand for him, as a signpost to his former career in the military. The entomologist of the project also comments on Ryan's former profession: "You know lots of malaria control was done by the military, the Panama Canal and so on. It's all military stuff."

Indeed, one could describe the project as located somewhere between a military intervention and a scientific experiment. A scientific experiment with meticulously planned logistics that is: for instance, in the headquarters one finds a big table with an aerial photograph of the city. With the help of this picture the city is divided into spraying areas, which are allocated to different teams and sprayed at different times. The spray teams are carefully composed and supervised: There are 116 sprayers, and the smallest working units are two-man teams, who partner in the house-to-house spraying. Those two-man teams belong to sixteen-man teams per designated spraying area. Each team has a team leader, and the team leaders are in turn supervised by the head of operations, who coordinates the different units. On top of the pyramid are the deputy director and the director of the Malaria Control Centre, who are also regularly in the spraying areas to supervise and support the work.

The sprayers are employed as untrained staff; they receive spraying training from the Malaria Control Centre itself. Behind the buildings of the center the project manager shows me a wall: "Here is the wall of pain," he jokes. "This is where we practice the spraying." Before every round of spraying—once every five to six months—the men have to undergo a spraying course, where their technique is practiced. All sprayers are full-time employees of the company but only on temporary contracts. Sprayers are usually employed for one spraying cycle of five to six months, which is followed by a break of one to two months. The workers are not employed in the break, and while in practice most sprayers are reemployed in the next spraying cycle, the company is not required to do so. This puts the employees in a precarious position, and as one of the sprayers, Yaw, told me, it makes it difficult to express criticisms and demand for workers' rights. For instance, Yaw fears that carrying the heavy insecticide pump on his shoulder every day might one day have health consequences for him. Because of the short contracts, however, he does not feel able to speak out on this issue. Yaw fears that if he did, he would simply not be employed again for the next round of spraying.

In terms of malaria control, the project concentrates mainly on vector control, but the overall strategy is broader, encompassing the following four key elements: vector control (via indoor residual spraying [IRS] but also larviciding of breeding sites); surveillance and monitoring of malaria rates and case numbers; improved disease management (diagnosis and treatment); as well as information, education, communication, and health promotion. In order to adapt to potentially arising insecticide resistance, the company conducts rigorous scientific "surveillance, monitoring, and research," uses rotating insecticides, applies regular larviciding, and removes found larvae by hand (GMC 2007). Potential resistance is also why a scientific—or to be more specific, an entomological—component has such a prominent place in this CSR malaria control project. In order to counteract rising resistance quickly and keep the intervention effective, the project has to incorporate research into the intervention.

Thus, in addition to the sprayers, the company employs an entomologist, who is not only the head of the laboratory and insectary but also coordinates eighteen members of staff, who are employed for the mosquito collections that happen every second night. The project maintains nine sentinel sites in the city plus three control sites outside the sprayed area. Sentinel sites are used to monitor the mosquito populations, and every second night, two men per site expose their legs in each sentinel site and function as "human landing catches" to attract mosquitoes and then carefully collect the caught mosquitoes in cups (Kelly 2011).[3] The cups are ordered in hourly progression so as to determine how many mosquitoes were caught when, and this enables the entomologist to reconstruct the biting cycle. The caught mosquitoes are further transported to the insectary, where they are counted, analyzed for insecticide resistance, and finally frozen for future reference.

In addition to the caught mosquitoes, the insectary hosts a live mosquito colony, which is used to conduct bioassays every month. This means the team puts fifteen to twenty-five mosquitoes in one cone that is attached to a sprayed wall and assesses the "knock-down rates"; that is, they count how many mosquitoes die after how many minutes. This proves the continuing effectivity of an insecticide or alerts the team to emerging resistance quickly. All these labor-intensive activities make the team intimately familiar with the mosquito population of the city; they know which species of mosquitoes live where, in which densities, how these populations developed over time, and if resistances arise and where.

But the research and monitoring team is not only concerned with mosquitoes; it also monitors parasites. The team takes blood samples from the city's human population, both from within the sprayed community and outside. And the results sometimes even shock the team itself: outside of the city the malaria parasite prevalence has been as high as 50 percent in random checks of non-ill people.[4] The results of the analyses feed directly into decisions about insecticide selection, larviciding, and the intervention strategy more generally. The research is conducted by the entomologist and his team, supervised by two renowned South African entomologists, and documented in several peer-reviewed scientific papers.[5] Furthermore, the project operates standard operational procedures and is certified under ISO 14001 for their environmental management. Thus, the company has invested much into the project; they have not only employed over 120 people but also built a local malaria center with a well-equipped insectary and laboratory. As documented above, this means that the company not only conducts operational research but also integrates scientific, entomological, and medical research into their CSR intervention. As the project manager explains to me, such a research-based approach is important to the ethos of the project, the constant movement of data from the field, lab experiments, and an adaptable intervention strategy is necessary to act on changes in mosquito and parasite micro-ecologies. Being sensitive to the local specifics of the mosquito and parasite population becomes crucial to the success of a malaria control intervention in the age of resistance. The project manager underlines the importance of being familiar with the locality: "Some organi-

zations bring in experts, who don't know what is happening. You have to be here and be patient to see and understand. I have got time, I'm in no rush."

INDOOR RESIDUAL SPRAYING AND
SHIFTING MOSQUITO ECOLOGIES

With insecticide spraying, the discussed project relies on a technique with a long and complex history in malaria control. In the 1940s the discovery of DDT as a cheap and effective insecticide against *Anopheles* mosquitoes revolutionized malaria vector control. Insecticide spraying with DDT was the main control tool—and in many ways enabled—the WHO's first global malaria eradication program from 1956 to 1969. The campaign was the first concerted and large-scale effort at eradicating malaria worldwide, albeit with only mixed success that ultimately led to its early abandonment after only fourteen years. From the beginning of the eradication campaign, time was considered to be of the essence, as malariologists knew insecticide resistance against DDT was going to emerge sooner or later (Packard 2006, 155). The battle against malaria with DDT needed to be quick and tough, and this might be one of the reasons why sub-Saharan Africa was excluded from the eradication program from its inception (Malowany 2000). The global eradication campaign was never truly global, as it excluded the continent with the highest disease burden; today Africa still shoulders 91 percent of malaria's death toll (WHO 2008, viii).[6]

When the WHO eradication program ended in 1969, resistance against DDT had already spread widely. In addition, a public controversy on the toxicity of DDT and its potential effects on human and environmental health, which was mainly triggered by Rachel Carson's book *Silent Spring* (1962), led to a DDT ban in the United States and later a worldwide ban (EPA 1972). The result was that DDT and insecticide spraying lost popularity. However, the last decades have seen a resurgence of malaria, which is presumed to have been triggered partly by (drug and insecticide) resistance, as well as by massive decreases in funding for malaria control after the eradication campaign ended. In urgent need for more effective antimalarial measures, the WHO brought insecticide spraying back on the agenda in 2006 (WHO 2006). And this time spraying mainly concentrates on Africa; today in many sub-Saharan African countries IRS—with DDT as well as with other insecticides—is common practice.

IRS aims at diminishing the local mosquito population to a degree that will significantly hamper the transmission of malaria. Reducing a mosquito population is, however, challenging: one *Anopheles* mosquito on average lives ten to fourteen days and lays between 50 and 200 eggs per oviposition, which enables populations to evolve and reproduce quickly (Service and Townson 2002, 68). Furthermore, currently around 430 species of *Anopheles* are known, of which around 70 are malaria vectors (59). The different species can be distinguished with regard to differences in breeding place preference, out- and indoor biting and resting, human and animal blood preference, and preferred biting times. Such differences matter when it comes to vector control: if one influences the conditions of habitats, the ecological niche of the different species changes and most likely also the population structures. For instance, increased outdoor biting would render IRS inefficient, and genetic differences across species can determine resistances to insecticides. Thus, in order to plan effective control interventions, one needs to both have a good idea about the different mosquito populations in the given locality and track their behavior and development.

Triggered by insecticide use not only in public health but also in agriculture, insecticide resistances have solidly settled into the sub-Saharan African landscapes over the last fifty years. This destabilizes the success and effectivity of established control strategies, such as IRS. As we saw in the previous section, the gold-mining company's project responds to the threat of emerging resistance with rigorous scientific "surveillance, monitoring, and research" of the mosquito population and uses rotating insecticides (GMC 2007). However, the repertoire of insecticides that are both effective and toxicologically safe is limited. At the present time only twelve insecticides from four classes are recommended for IRS (WHO, 2006). The four classes of insecticides target only two neurological sites, meaning that genetic mutations that make mosquitoes tolerant of the insecticides are similar and cross-resistance between insecticides is common (Enayati and Hemingway 2010). This not only attests to mosquitoes' evolutionary dynamism and adaptive capacities but also means that insecticide resistance in *Anopheles* mosquitoes poses a constant—and still growing—challenge to spraying initiatives today. Rather than leading to an increased openness in the search for locally suitable, innovative malaria control strategies, resistance has so far been answered mainly by a "more of the same" strategy. Evolutionary pressure is routinely answered by research and development investments that search for alternative insecticides, not alternative strategies. We will come back to this point, but first the next section sets out the role of the human "beneficiaries" in the project design.

Beside the implementation of spraying and entomological research, the project has a third component—"community liaison." Five members of staff "go after" the spray men, as the team leader Rachid puts it. If the sprayers do not find people in a house or if people refuse to get their house sprayed, Rachid's men go and check. "Often," Rachid says, "it is enough to educate people on where malaria comes from and inform them about the symptoms. Mostly, people don't think it is caused by mosquitoes; if someone dies early, it is believed to be witchcraft. When people learn, they often let the spray men spray." Rachid also organizes local committees in the municipality and meetings with the workers' union. The project has bought airtime at a local radio station twice a week in order to discuss the project and answer questions. Rachid and his team do a great job and the community relations seem to be working well; the 95 percent coverage rate of the spraying is testament to this.

However, what also helps are the subtleties of public advertisement. The spraying is announced in the city via public posters. One sentence on the poster is to be noted: "Every house must be sprayed." Legally this is not the case, not every house must be sprayed. The company can (and does) require residents of company houses to allow the spraying, but it has no power over private housing in the municipality. But the sentence plays with the fact that people might not know this and that they might not feel able to resist the power of the company, which is the main provider of formal employment in the city as well as the region.

The poster featured in figure 9.2 could be read as a subtle coercion mechanism. However, the public engagement process of the project cannot justifiably be reduced to this sentence, as Rachid's team is in constant dialogue with the community. But, and this is crucial, the relations with the community focus on education about malaria and on convincing people that the project is needed. The underlying assumption is that people do not understand the correct scientific cause of malaria and they do not know how to prevent it, and so the project focuses on education by drawing on behavior change communication tools. As Rachid put it: "when people learn, they often let the spray men spray."

But while considerable effort is made to bring the public "on board" and inform them about why the project is useful, the overall strategy of the intervention was designed without public involvement. One of my inter-

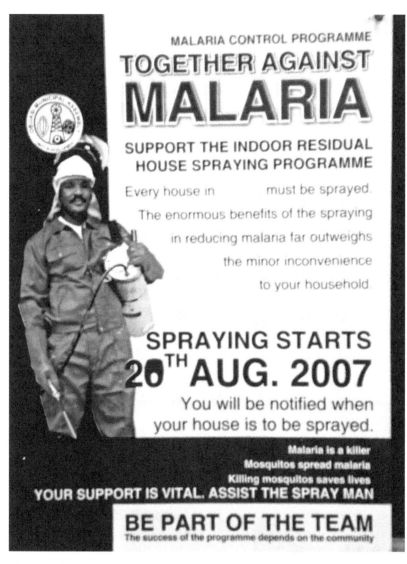

Figure 9.2. Spraying advertisement, 2007.

viewees from a local mining watchdog NGO remarked that the "beneficia-ries" of the project never had a say in the overall design of the experiment. While one can report adverse reactions or dislike of the smell of a particular insecticide, or refuse to take part in the spraying, he stated that no public in-quiry on the potential content and nature of the project had been conducted before the intervention started. To him, the company's choice to concentrate their activities on malaria ignores long-standing demands of the community to cover abandoned mining pits as part of the company's corporate responsibility.[7] Accordingly, my interviewee says that to him the philosophy of the project is wrong. It does not acknowledge that the company's practices might have increased the number of mosquito breeding places, and to him a responsive and responsible CSR project would have started with the question, "What led to breeding grounds?" He argues that the project has taken the wrong starting point and thereby marginalized local demands as well as expertise. In short, the public in the project becomes the passive recipient of malaria and its control, while the project team is seen as working toward a malaria-free city, thus becoming the active shapers of an emerging healthier cityscape.

Indoor Residual Spraying as a Real-World Experiment

CITIZEN SCIENCE

The trope that people do not understand what is at stake in science is familiar. Since the 1980s the relations between science and society received considerable attention in U.S.-European debates, both in the public sphere and academia. Scientific innovations such as nuclear energy or genetically modified organisms have been subjected to intense public debate. In many cases citizens' protests were understood to be the result of their "misunderstanding science." This approach to science-society relations was termed a *deficit model*, since it assumes the public to be ignorant about science. However, it has been shown that empirically a division between rational experts and an emotional public is not convincing, and an educational approach to public engagement with science not only often misses the public's concerns but also is an "unproductive and even counterproductive" way to frame the debate (Irwin and Wynne 1996, 219).[8] Irwin and Wynne argue that science needs to engage with "its own epistemological limitations" and open the debate up to different onto-epistemic framings and positionings (219).

As a consequence, fostering broad citizen participation has become an important component for science policy. While the results of such initiatives have been generally mixed and brought to light paradoxes and problems of a public participation paradigm (Cooke and Kothari 2001; Singh 2008), they arguably succeeded in destabilizing the primacy of scientific knowledge in societal decision making, underlining "that science can gain democratic public legitimacy only if it recognizes its own need to understand itself in relation to these other cultures, and to learn respectfully to negotiate with and to accommodate to them, rather than dismiss them as vacuous, untrustworthy, and emotive" (Leach et al. 2005, 9).

Public engagement processes with science as well as citizens' protest could also be understood as a reaction to what Krohn and Weyer (1994) characterize as an "experimental society," arguing that science increasingly conducts "real-world experiments" or, in the words of Szerszynski (2005), that the world has become a "laboratory without walls." The authors argue that experiments are not taking place in a "carefully isolated space" anymore; the boundary between experiment and world gets dissolved.[9] The concept of a real-world experiment enables us to distinguish between science mainly performed in the laboratory and scientific practices that move between field and laboratory or between "landscapes and labscapes" (Kohler 2002).

Importantly, mixing experimental and field practices changes the relationship between science, its research objects, and the public or, put differently, it modifies the definition of research "subject and object" (Stengers 2000, 130). As Szerszynski (2005, 192) has shown in his analysis of field trials with genetically modified crops: "In the laboratory without walls each 'datum' is also potentially a real-world risk event, bleeding out from the experimental context into wider society, so too do societal actions present themselves as data, as findings." Szerszynski argues that all public acts relating to a field trial are part of the experiment, including, for instance, people who destroy fields in protest. To him this underlines the need to rethink the ethics of engaging the public in real-world experiments. Public engagement processes would need to acknowledge the experimental character of their intervention and give space for people to engage actively. My case study of the malaria control project pushes these arguments further and invites us to integrate the shifting nature of ecology into the equation. What happens to our notion of public engagement if we understand IRS as a real-world experiment with the shifting ecologies of malaria rather than a public health intervention (as it would be generally conceived)?

INDOOR RESIDUAL SPRAYING AS A REAL-WORLD EXPERIMENT
I argue that the Ghanaian spraying initiative takes the form of a real-world experiment, because it is characterized by constant movement between laboratory and field (in this case the city where the spraying is conducted). IRS in the age of insecticide resistance cannot be reduced to the application

of a proven strategy but requires constant monitoring, surveillance, and adaptation. The project's strategies have to be subjected to "reality checks" continuously and render the interventions experimental: reaction and development of mosquitoes and parasites are observed, and the intervention strategies are modified and adapted accordingly. Knowledge moves between laboratory and field and between mosquitoes (which are generating knowledge about maneuvering their world) and scientists (who in turn create knowledge about how humans might best maneuver the world, avoiding mosquitoes and disease).

Those practices make one feature of the field sciences visible that is carefully removed in research solely based on laboratory techniques, namely "irreducible uncertainty" (Stengers 2000, 144). The specifics of place complicate the field sciences: "what one terrain allows us to affirm, another terrain can contradict" (Stengers 2000, 140). As a result, the boundaries between what is inside and outside of an experiment are more difficult to maintain. Accordingly, Szerzynski (2005) argues we have to understand "outsiders" as "insiders" in real-world experiments. To him, people who protest against an experiment are not intruding but belong to the experiment; they are a form of "data" (Szerzynski 2005, 192).[10]

This suggests an opening up of our understanding of experiments, and for giving more people (and things) the opportunity to take part in and define the terms of experiments. We could say that through monitoring and adaptation mechanisms the IRS project is already designed in a way that expects "things," in this case mosquitoes, to react to the experiment's intervention. However, at the end of the day, the IRS project still aims at keeping the mosquitoes as silent and passive as possible and hence keeping them in an object position. The IRS project allows the object to ask questions back; however, it does not foster the questioning of the overall socio-ecological strategy: What if the all-out, military-style war against mosquitoes and parasites is futile? Would modifying the conditions of how mosquitoes, parasites, and people live together be more effective than getting lost in a game of attack and counterstrike?

Similarly, the project's public engagement mainly focuses on education and learning. The need to achieve measurable success makes public health education tools such as "behavior change communication" a popular choice for IRS public engagement processes—it literally forms the path of least resistance. The project is herewith firmly anchored within a public health strategy of malaria that focuses on technological interventions, delivered with the help of public information and education (Kelly and Beisel 2011). Montgomery et al. (2010, 4) characterize the neglect of wide-ranging public engagement and broader sociocultural context as a "hallmark of public health approaches to malaria." Public health strategies in malaria control traditionally focus on top-down behavior change communication and information, education, communication.

However, such techniques were developed for public health interventions that were presumed to be based on sound and stable health knowledge. As has been shown, no stable facts exist in the age of insecticide resistance. IRS interventions today are real-world experiments, which are always in movement because the behavior of mosquitoes, parasites, and humans cannot be held stable. The objects of the experiment respond in unexpected ways, and this is why monitoring and surveillance need to be an integral part of IRS strategies. But ecological requirements of malaria control interventions sit uncomfortably with attempts to make democratic decisions about spraying. Especially in stable high transmission areas, success of IRS has always been notoriously hard to sustain, because mosquito population numbers bounce back quickly. For instance, the Garki spraying project in 1970s Nigeria was not able to break the malaria transmission cycle with IRS, and it famously watched malaria move quickly back into the sprayed area. Only two years after the spraying ceased, malaria rates were back at pre-project levels (Molineaux et al. 1980; Packard 2007).

Accordingly, high coverage rates of IRS are necessary in order to reduce the mosquito densities in a locality to sufficiently interrupt transmission (Kolaczinski et al. 2007). If coverage is only partial, spraying will be likely to reduce the mosquito density in covered places, but the overall effect in the bigger area (such as in a municipality as discussed here) would remain small. Second, if IRS coverage is patchy, the likelihood that one only repels the mosquitoes to areas with no IRS coverage, or where people refused the spraying, is high.

It is unclear, however, if high coverage rates would be achievable when a thorough public education and deliberation process is conducted before the intervention. In this context it is important to recall the contested history of insecticide spraying in the 1960s, which was characterized by one of the first worldwide and high-profile environmental controversies, triggered through the book *Silent Spring* by Rachel Carson (1962). Ultimately, the campaign led to the ban of DDT in most UN countries (U.S. EPA 1972; Ghana EPA 2006). Furthermore, comparatively high costs of spraying make it questionable that, after a thorough public deliberation process, IRS would achieve coverage rates of 80 percent.

Presently, top-down public health education tools are the standard choice for IRS public engagement processes. Public health education in this context means to inform and educate the public about the project and its (beneficial) effects in order to increase acceptance. Public engagement does not mean that the public has a say in the how questions of spraying or malaria control in general. However, as has been pointed out above, such techniques were developed for public health interventions that are based on sound and stable health knowledge. The process is based on the assumption that the intervention is proven to be beneficial to the public. And herewith we are at the second border-crossing of the IRS project: It is not only a combined lab and field intervention but also a scientific experiment and a public health intervention. As I have discussed above, there are no stable facts in the age of insecticide resistance—it is a constant game of intervention and response. This makes success and failure more elusive, and while malaria cases will decrease through spraying, it is more questionable if this reduction will be sustainable.

While the exclusion of citizens in decision-making processes is hardly new, I suggest that looking at the interactions between science, ecology, and democracy enables us to nuance this point further. The emergence of resistance destabilizes the success of the intervention strategy. While this could be seen as a chance to open up malaria control to alternative visions, it has led to more closure. Akin to how participation can create paradoxical effects of less involvement (Cooke and Kothari 2001), or how development projects become an antipolitics machine (Ferguson 1994), the emergence of insecticide resistance leads to cementing IRS and behavior change and communication strategies further into the standard repertoire of malaria control. The emergence and persistence of insecticide resistance has not triggered a thorough questioning of the predominant malaria control strategies and a search for more broadly conceived alternatives. Failure has led to closure, rather than to openness.

I suggest, thus, that understanding IRS as a real-world experiment would work toward a different mode of engagement: instead of focusing on rotating insecticides and educating people with behavior change education, the project could understand IRS as an experiment with more than one active experimenter and with inherently uncertain results. This means understanding the malaria control project not only as a scientific and ecological experiment but also as a "social and public experiment" (Rottenburg 2009). Such a reading of real-world experiments and experimentality does not characterize experiments as uncertain in order to highlight the dangers inherent. On the contrary, it suggests that recognizing and understanding science-based public health interventions as uncertain experiments in shifting malaria ecologies brings with it opportunities for public engagement, civic negotiation, and decision making. In complex real-world experiments scientists, mosquitoes, and the public alike are participants and shapers in an experiment that is conducted together with, instead of on, them. But how do the dynamics of science, ecology, and democracy in this corporate malaria control project relate to the wider para-statal constellations in malaria control in Ghana?

GOING NATIONAL: CORPORATE SOCIAL
RESPONSIBILITY MEETS PUBLIC HEALTH

Building on the concept and design of the earlier described corporate social responsibility project, a new major health initiative has just been launched in Ghana. The project conducts malaria control activities in forty districts in Ghana and is funded by the Global Fund with US$158 million over five years. As mentioned in the opening to this chapter, the two major partners in this project are the Ghanaian National Malaria Control Programme (NMCP) and the gold-mining company. The project is due to "cover forty districts with indoor residual spraying (IRS) by the end of 2013, with at least 90 percent of all houses sprayed per community" (GF 2008, 43). Even though the project covers other malaria control interventions too, IRS is the most important strategy of the project with an allocated US$122 million for spraying (77). The gold-mining company has been selected as the principal recipient for the IRS component and administers by far the biggest share of the funding (25). The grant acquisition was a success not only for the Ghanaian state but also for the company: it has become the first private company in Africa to receive a Global Fund grant. This signifies that the company's malaria control approach has received national and international recognition, as the design of the project will be based on their initial project (44). The deep influence of the private partner in this partnership can also be seen in the decision about where to locate the project geographically. Not only malaria transmission patterns or the demands of public health had to be taken into account but also crucially the interests of the private partner. Two-thirds of the districts covered by the project are located in the north of Ghana, where malaria is rife; however, one-third are in southwestern

Ghana, the area where the gold-mining company operates. This discrepancy between malaria transmission and project location shows that the interests of public health had to be combined with the interests of the private partner in the proposal.

––––––––––

Effectively, a multinational gold-mining company will lead what is currently the biggest public health project on malaria in Ghana—transforming public health into a para-statal project. With the CSR precursor project in mind, what lessons could be drawn for the new PPP health project? First, by extending the project over forty districts in Ghana the socio-ecological malaria experiment spreads too. The Global Fund project will follow the model of the CSR project and, by doing so, extend the uneasy relationship between spraying intervention, ecology, and democracy. The funding bid outlines that community sensitization and information is to proceed as follows: "The various 'Behaviour Change Communication' and 'Information, Education, Communication' approaches will use the available mass media, billboards, drama, art and theatre in order to deliver the relevant messages" (GF 2008, 49). Public engagement will focus on public health education. However, as I have argued, education as public engagement is inadequate, since the uncertainties involved in the spraying project cannot be seen as potential side effects but rather are an integral part of IRS in the age of insecticide resistance. IRS has to be seen as a real-world experiment transforming people and things, which would usually be considered as outsiders or beneficiaries, (unwittingly) into participants. An educational approach does not capture this complex relationship between experiment and its publics. Nevertheless, the public engagement strategy of the PPP project replicates the ethos of experimenting on the communities instead of experimenting with. Staying true to the uncertainty and working toward experimenting with would mean to transcend educational strategies, and to respectfully negotiate the design of an intervention, not only its implementation.

Second, as we have seen, the design of the CSR project emerged out of the interests of the company. Rather than focusing the project on the demands of the community (covering abandoned mining pits), the project focused on the company's chosen topic (malaria) and intervention strategy (IRS). Controlling malaria is not only contributing to the company's efficiency (through less sick days) but also might be cheaper than covering abandoned mining pits. Similarly, the PPP project based its decision on where to focus its project geographically not only on malaria transmission patterns or the demands of public health but also taking the interests of the private partner into account.

Thus, not only are the boundaries between laboratory and field blurred through IRS but so are the boundaries between state and private companies' involvement in health care. The PPP cannot afford to exclusively base their decision on the public interest, and much of the power in this new PPP lies with the gold-mining company. The company is the principal recipient of the funding from the Global Fund, and tasked with the financial management of the project (GF 2010).[11] In addition, the company is the principal implementer of the project and has designed the intervention, which is based on the corporate precursor project (GF 2008). In short, this project might better be called a private-public, rather than a public-private, partnership; as the project not only originated from a corporate CSR project but also continues to be interwoven with the gold-mining company and its interests. I opened this chapter with James Ferguson's suggestion that the new, "transnational apparatus of governmentality . . . does not replace the older system of nation-states . . . but overlays it and coexists with it" (2006, 103). This seems appropriate for the case of the Ghanaian spraying project: while the cooperation with the gold-mining company has in some ways replaced the state (such as in project design and implementation), it also depends on the state. The endorsement of the National Malaria Control Programme gives the project legitimacy to qualify as public health project and thus made the application to the Global Fund possible. In this sense some control is retained by the state, turning the project into a para-statal arrangement. However, the dominance of the corporate actor in financial and practical terms also shows that the imaginaries of this new para-statal constellation are markedly different from older state approaches to public health. Working with multinational companies not only enables the state to benefit from what the company's infrastructure may be able to offer Ghanaian malaria control but also complicates the negotiation between state, private, and public interests. As I suggested above, in particular the relationship of the project to the wider public and democratic decision making is ambiguous, and the project implementation strategy is characterized by a lack of genuine engagement with the public, the assumed beneficiaries. This raises the question of whether the public might more generally turn out to be the one-actor-too-many at the fragile negotiation table constituting para-statal partnerships? These complex dynamics deserve careful analytical attention as the Ghanaian spraying project unfolds and as global health as well as local health care provision in Africa is increasingly marked by para-statal science-business collaborations.

Notes

1 The gold-mining company is a major multinational mining company and one of the oldest in Ghana—founded and first commercially exploited by the British under colonial rule. The mine is therefore implicated in a history of mining enclaves in sub-Saharan Africa (Ferguson 2006), and it is tied into the complex political economy and geography of cheap labor on the one side and its (attempted) preservation through colonial and postcolonial corporate health initiatives on the other (e.g., Packard 1989; Rajak 2010). Most of these corporate health schemes focus on the companies' workforce and often imply intimate surveillance of workers' bodies and highly problematic inclusion and exclusion mechanisms (Packard 1989; Rajak 2010). The project this chapter engages with differs somewhat in this particular aspect, as the insecticide spraying targets the whole city. Nevertheless, as we will see in the following pages, the company's business gains are of primary importance to the project and its justification, creating a somewhat uneasy relation to the state and the broader public (see Rajak 2010).

2 This chapter draws on two ethnographic research visits to the gold-mining company's initial project in 2008. The visits were part of a broader ethnographic research project on malaria control initiatives in Ghana that I conducted in 2007–8. I wish to thank all research participants in Ghana, who have been very generous in sharing their time and knowledge with me.

3 *Human landing catch* is the technical term for an entomological technique to collect mosquitoes. Ann Kelly (2011) has elaborated in more depth on this technique and the labor involved in collecting mosquitoes.

4 These high prevalence rates of parasites in non-ill people are characteristic for stable high transmission areas, where people and parasites routinely cohabitate without necessarily developing malaria (see Owusu-Agyei et al. 2009).

5 In order to guarantee anonymity for my research participants, these papers cannot be referenced here.

6 This does not mean, however, that there was no insecticide spraying against mosquito transmitted diseases in sub-Saharan Africa in the beginning of the twentieth century. There was extensive DDT spraying against Tsetse flies to prevent sleeping sickness in East Africa (Hoppe 2003). Furthermore, several pilot projects and two major spraying initiatives (with insecticides other than DDT) against malaria got conducted in sub-Saharan Africa: the Pare-Taveta Scheme, 1954–59, in Tanzania-Kenya (Dobson et al. 2000; Wellcome Witness 1999) and

the Garki Project, 1969–76, in northern Nigeria (Molineaux and Gramiccia 1980). However, both showed that even though spraying reduced malaria mortality and morbidity considerably, it was not possible to break the transmission cycle. Once spraying stopped, malaria cases quickly reverted to prespraying levels.

7 Abandoned open pits constitute a serious health hazard for the population, and additionally they can create breeding spots for mosquitoes. However, covering pits in an environmentally friendly and sustainable way is an expensive enterprise. To my interview partner, this might be the reason why the company has chosen to not focus on this but on malaria prevention instead. In addition, focusing on a subject that goes beyond mitigating the mine's direct influence on the community makes for a wider conceived social responsibility project.

8 This is not to be read as a dismissal of science and its importance, but it highlights problems emerging from an unquestioned authority of science (Irwin and Wynne 1996, 8–9).

9 However, knowledge production has never happened outside of society, but always in constant negotiation with political and social processes (Pestre 2003). For instance, Bonneuil (2008, 281) in a study on late colonial and postcolonial Africa argues that "after the 1930s, development came to be seen as an experiment and Africa as a laboratory. This shift from 'governing, thanks to the light of science' to 'governing as an experimental activity' is an essential feature of the emergence of a development regime in Africa." Thus, Krohn and Weyer's diagnosis of an "experimental society" has to be seen as an integral feature of science rather than a new process.

10 Stengers (2003, 133) would probably like Szersynski's argument, since she also would not want to abolish the distinction between object and subject in experiments completely but to approach in a way that "modifies its meaning: it is recognized not as a right, but as a vector of risk, an operator of 'decentering.' It does not attribute to the subject the right to know an object, but to the object the power (to be constructed) to put the subject to the test."

11 In addition, the involvement of the company in the PPP might well mean a reduction in costs for their CSR project. The company has agreed to contribute US$1.7 million over five years to the Global Fund project, to be delivered in (already existing) equipment, expertise, and infrastructure. This would mean a substantial cost reduction for the mine, which in 2008 alone spent US$1.4 million on their CSR malaria control program.

References

Bonneuil, C. 2000. "Development as Experiment: Science and State Building in Late Colonial and Postcolonial Africa, 1930–1970." *Osiris* 15:258–81.

Carson, R. 1962. *Silent Spring*. Boston: Houghton Mifflin.

Cooke, B., and U. Kothari. 2001. *Participation: The New Tyranny?* London: Zed Books.

Dobson, M. J., M. Malowany, and B. Snow. 2000. "Malaria Control in East Africa: The Kampala Conference and the Pare-Taveta Scheme; a Meeting of Common and High Ground." *Parassitologia* 42:149–66.

Enayati, A., and J. Hemingway. 2010. "Malaria Management: Past, Present, and Future." *Annual Review of Entomology* 55:569–91.

Ferguson, J. 1994. *The Anti-Politics Machine: "Development," Depoliticization, and Bureaucratic Power in Lesotho.* Minneapolis: University of Minnesota Press.

Ferguson, J. 2005. "Seeing Like an Oil Company: Space, Security, and Global Capital in Neoliberal Africa." *American Anthropologist* 107:377–82.

Ferguson, J. 2006. *Global Shadows: Africa in the Neoliberal World Order.* Durham, NC: Duke University Press.

Global Fund. 2004. *A Force for Change: The Global Fund to Fight AIDS, Tuberculosis and Malaria.* Accessed February 12, 2007. http://www.theglobalfund.org/en /publications.

Global Fund. 2008. "Proposal Form Round 8—Malaria." Accessed January 13, 2009. http://www.theglobalfund.org/programs/grant/?compid=1678&lang=en& CountryId=GHN.

Global Fund. 2010. *Partnering for Global Health: The Global Fund and the Private Sector.* Accessed December 9, 2010. http://www.theglobalfund.org/en/privatesector /?lang=en.

GMC. 2007. *Country Report Ghana 07.* Available on request.

Hoppe, K. A. 2003. *Lords of the Fly: Sleeping Sickness Control in British East Africa, 1900–1960.* Westport, CT: Praeger.

Irwin, A., and B. Wynne. 1996. *Misunderstanding Science? The Public Reconstruction of Science and Technology.* Cambridge: Cambridge University Press.

Kelly, A. H. 2011. "Will He Be There? Mediating Malaria, Immobilizing Science." *Journal of Cultural Economy* 4, no. 1: 65–79.

Kelly, A. H., and U. Beisel. 2011. "Neglected Malarias: The Frontlines and Back Alleys of Global Health." *BioSocieties* 6, no. 1: 71–87.

Kohler, R. 2002. *Landscapes and Labscapes: Exploring the Lab-Field Border in Biology.* Chicago: University of Chicago Press.

Krohn, W., and J. Weyer. 1994. "Society as a Laboratory: The Social Risks of Experimental Research." *Science and Public Policy* 21, no. 3: 173–83.

Leach, M., I. Scoones, and B. Wynne. 2005. *Science and Citizens: Globalization and the Challenge of Engagement.* London: Zed Books.

Malowany, M. 2000. "Unfinished Agendas: Writing the History of Medicine of Sub-Saharan Africa." *African Affairs* 99:325–49.

Molineaux, L., and G. Gramiccia. 1980. *The Garki Project: Research on the Epidemiology and Control of Malaria in the Sudan Savanna of West Africa.* Geneva: World Health Organization.

Packard, R. M. 1989. *White Plague, Black Labour: Tuberculosis and the Political Economy of Health and Disease in South Africa*. Berkeley: University of California Press.

Packard, R. M. 2007. *The Making of a Tropical Disease: A Short History of Malaria*. Baltimore: Johns Hopkins University Press.

Pestre, D. 2003. "Regimes of Knowledge Production in Society: Towards a More Political and Social Reading." *Minerva* 41, no. 3: 245–61.

Rajak, D. 2010. "'HIV/AIDS Is Our Business': The Moral Economy of Treatment in a Transnational Mining Company." *Journal of the Royal Anthropological Institute* 1, no. 16: 551–71.

Service, M. W., and H. Townson. 2002. "The Anopheles Vector." In *Essential Malariology*, ed. D. A. Warrell and H. M. Gilles, 59–84. London: Arnold.

Singh, J. 2008. "The UK Nanojury as 'Upstream' Public Engagement." *Participatory Learning and Action* 58, no. 1: 27–32.

Stengers, I. 2000. *The Invention of Modern Science*. Minneapolis: University of Minnesota Press.

Szerszynski, B. 2005. "Beating the Unbound: Political Theatre in the Laboratory without Walls." In *Performing Nature: Explorations in Ecology and the Arts*, ed. G. Giannachi and N. Stewart, 181–97. Frankfurt: Peter Lang.

U.S. Environmental Protection Agency USA (U.S. EPA). 1972. "DDT Ban Takes Effect." Accessed August 17, 2007. http://www.epa.gov/history/topics/ddt/01.htm.

Wellcome Witnesses to Twentieth Century Medicine. 1999. *British Contributions to Medical Research and Education in Africa After the Second World War*. Accessed August 8, 2007. http://www.ucl.ac.uk/histmed/publications/wellcome_witnesses_c20th_med.

WHO. 2006. *Indoor Residual Spraying. Use of Indoor Residual Spraying for Scaling Up Global Malaria Control and Elimination*. Accessed June 10, 2007. http://www.who.int/topics/malaria/en/.

WHO. 2008. *World Malaria Report 2008*. Geneva: WHO.

CHAPTER 10

The Territory of Medical Research:

Experimentation in Africa's Smallest State

Ann H. Kelly

In view, however, of the small size of the Gambia, its comparatively simple (though none-theless pressing) problems . . . there would seem to be a strong argument for considering it as a case for the application of an overall research program.

—Raymond Firth, "Social Problems and Research in British West Africa"

A needle of swamp and arid savannah, the Gambia is the smallest country in Africa. It is a nation of riverbanks, running roughly two hundred miles east from the Atlantic Ocean and, at its widest, only thirty miles across. The Gambia is enveloped by Senegal and, though the British briefly pursued a policy of integration, its political sovereignty has remained unchallenged since it gained independence in 1964. The Gambia's relative political stability has been a draw for foreign aid; however, it remains one of the poorest countries in the world (UNDP 2010). It is also one of the most researched: the UK Medical Research Council (MRC), whose laboratories and field stations occupy sites on the north and south banks of the Gambia River, has funded and hosted international scientists for the better part of a century. Experiments conducted with Gambian populations have yielded key insights about nutrition, agronomy, and infectious and vector-borne diseases, transforming the field of tropical medicine (Geissler et al. 2008; Malowany 2001). The majority of that work has focused on malaria. Clinical studies conducted in the Gambia on the effectiveness of bed nets, pharmaceuticals, vaccines, and residual sprays form the basis for many current global policies on prevention and treatment (e.g., McGregor 1982; Snow et al. 1988; Conway 2007). "What the nation may lack in size and economic clout," said Tom Paulson in the *Seattle Post-Intelligencer* on March 23, 2001, "it makes up for as Africa's research laboratory."

The Gambia presents a provocative case study in how size mediates the impact of scientific inquiry on state sovereignty. This chapter, like others in this volume, is concerned with the shifting intersections of research and government under distinct political-economic configurations. Drawing together research conducted under a colonial administration with that undertaken today, it examines how nationhood, expert knowledge, and public health are articulated through past and current forms of experimentation. Further, I take up the issue of how scientific activity animates governmental practice as a question of scale, mapping the cross coordinates of science and development specific to this small nation. Like Raymond Firth in the epigraph that opens this chapter, I am interested in how Gambia's territorial dimensions impact the programs of research carried out in the country.

So what are the distinct administrative features of a microstate? In his analysis of state formation in Africa, Jeffrey Herbst (2000) claims that African politics labor under the strain of an excess of land. Unlike the traditional political analyses of European state formation, which link national development to conflict with neighboring states over the expansion of frontiers (e.g., Tilly 1990), Herbst suggests that while territorial conquest is clearly fundamental to the colonial enterprise, European investment in Africa prioritized securing access to labor rather than expanding control over land. With the exception of a few settler colonies, colonial influence petered out a short distance from capitals, established primarily to facilitate international commerce. The Gambia, for instance, was only ever a colony along its coast, where expatriate traders and officers resided. The rest of the country, inhabited primarily if not entirely by Africans, was a protectorate governed indirectly through village chiefs (Gray 1940). Herbst reads this systematic neglect of the rural areas into current African instabilities. The problem, he suggests, is not one of belligerent neighbors: state boundaries, though arbitrary in light of precolonial politics, have remained undisputed since independence. Rather, he argues, it is precisely this peaceful coexistence that has weakened the African state. Without the threat of invasion, there is little incentive to systemize taxation (which, in Europe, had served to underwrite warfare and, later, welfare), establish political infrastructures, or occupy frontier areas. Propped by foreign aid, governmental power pools at the core and dissipates at the periphery, a situation that breeds internal division and civil conflict. It is for these reasons that Herbst (2000, 140) believes "African conditions privilege nations that are relatively small." The smaller the state, the easier and less costly it is to consolidate administrative capacity.

With regards to the Gambia, Herbst's analysis is compelling, if only to help us understand how this poor tract of land avoided being absorbed into better-resourced and more-developed Senegal. One could argue that the combination of high population density and regional tensions worked to reinforce sovereignty; the very real prospect of becoming Senegalese catalyzed Gambian national identity (Welch and Claude 1966).[1] However, like any small economy, the Gambia is highly susceptible to external influences; according to the historians Arnold Hughes and David Perfect (2006, 277), "Gambia's lilliputian size and global marginality . . . mean that small crumbs from a donor's table could be sizeable." The Gambia's history as a site of research underscores the dramatic impact of foreign institutions on the microstate. After almost seventy years of location-based research, the MRC is now one of Gambia's largest employers (Beckerleg, Austin, and Weaver 1994; MRC Annual Report 2007). Though the institution is careful to demarcate its activities from governmental practice, it ostensibly functions as a parastatal body.[2] Enrolled as experimental subjects or employed on projects as assistants or menial laborers, Gambians have benefited from, and come to depend upon, the economic and health care opportunities provided by transnational scientific activities (Geissler and Molyneux 2008; Kelly et al. 2010). Rather than a vehicle for political consolidation, Gambia's compactness has rendered it available for foreign intervention. "Africa's laboratory" points to the limitations of an analysis that links state capacity to its size without due consideration to the role of transnational actors.

The experimental appeal of the Gambia's smallness has shifted over the years. During the colonial era, the country offered an ideal landscape to pilot new technologies and techniques of cultivation because their effects were clearly legible (Reynolds and Tansey 2001, 21). Among a delimited community and within a manageable landscape, experimental interventions produced immediate impacts that could be convincingly projected on a national scale. As opposed to the large, geographically diverse, and diffusely inhabited Tanzania (once described by a German colonial administrator "as a poor place for European experiments" [Bernhard Dernburg quoted in Iliffe 1969, 81]), the Gambia's size meant that research could be controlled and contained — scientifically, politically, and financially. As Sir Hillary Blood, the governor of the Gambia from 1942 to 1947, remarked in support of the nomination of a female nutritional assistant to the Colonial Office: "on account of its small size, Gambia could be regarded as a very suitable place for experimental appointments" (quoted in Berry 1998, 22).

The continuing significance of the MRC laboratories in the Gambia for global public health research is in large part due to the comprehensiveness of studies undertaken under its auspices. Sir Ian McGregor, the MRC's first scientific director, spent over thirty years producing a detailed demographic profile of the entire resident population of four coastal villages. The data revealed the long-term impact of malaria on community health and has provided the baseline for research into malaria morbidity and mortality, acquired immunity, and the potential effectiveness of disease control interventions.[3] That experimental value has allowed a shift in the scientific rationale for research in the country, from the developmental schemes piloted during the colonial period, which generated insights of relevance to the governance of colonial territories, toward that whose critical unit of scale is not the nation-state.[4] The Gambia has long operated as the tropics in miniature, offering a setting from which to generate public health policy for global application.

I track that evolving sociopolitical significance of research in the Gambia across two central sections. First, I begin by describing a late colonial project—described by its coordinators as the Gambia Experiment—intended to dramatically improve the health and standard of living of Genieri, a village on the south bank of the river, through mechanized rice cultivation of the surrounding swamplands. While the modernization of village life was central to the project's justification, the experimental protocol eschewed social transformation, emphasizing instead a prolonged process of so-called grafting of new agricultural practices and technology to village society. Of particular interest are the conflicting ideas held by the research team and the British Colonial Service about the scale of the experiment and what these views implied about the experiment's overall objective. Ultimately, these conflicting visions brought the project to a halt, but not before Genieri had undergone considerable transformation as a site of both agricultural and scientific knowledge production.

I then describe an experiment that took place between 2004 and 2007, just east of Genieri, which also sought to improve community health through a large-scale reworking of the Gambian swamps. Out of step with the current emphasis of global malaria control policy on the distribution of bed nets and home treatment, the Larval Control Project (LCP) drew connections between agricultural practices, intensive community collaboration, and improved health, echoing the rationale of the Genieri project conducted sixty years earlier. Further, like the processes of grafting agricultural practice trialed by the Gambia Experiment, large-scale larval control was ultimately deemed not viable in the Gambia, reflecting a similar misalignment between the scale of the project and that of the health problem it sought to address. The extension of the LCP's experimental practices to other aspects of village life reveals, however, the ways in which contemporary scientific activity animates development and how the social capacity of research may be different from that of experiments conducted in the past.

In discussing these two experimental projects my aim is not to draw a direct comparison but rather to demonstrate the different ways in which Gambian populations have become objects of governmental practice and biomedical knowledge. In the conclusion I will bring these empirical insights to bear on the MRC's recent decision to shift funding out of the Gambia and consider how this policy redraws the boundaries between experiment and social improvement, science and the state.

The Gambia Experiment

In 1946 many people who were living in a world dislocated by six years of war and struggling to get back to normal saw the necessity for change in Africa. The Gambia Experiment was a small attempt to make such change to persuade a village to take a gigantic step into the twentieth century.

—Veronica Berry, *The Gambia Experiment*

The oldest of Great Britain's possessions, the Gambia's initial value to the empire was as a trading post.[5] But long before Bathurst (the capital city now called Banjul) became a Crown colony, the River Gambia was entangled in the world economy. Since the fifteenth century, the Portuguese had maintained lucrative commercial relations with the riverside kingdoms, exchanging crops, cloth, and metalware for hides, ivory, and, eventually, slaves (Gray 1940).[6] Two centuries later, the Gambia had developed links with the British, French, and Dutch, who vied with the Portuguese for the exclusive right to trade in the estuary. In 1817 the British formalized their claim, establishing a garrison and battery to protect their merchant vessels and suppress the slave trade (Gailey 1964). Poor in natural resources, the Gambia's income was exclusively derived from re-exported goods. British mercantile interests in Bathurst did not extend beyond its function as an entrepôt until the London-based firm Foster and Smith recognized the profit-making potential of peanuts: in 1831 they built a mill in London to crush peanuts and render their oil, catalyzing a global market for the crop. By 1860, the Gambia had become the world leader in peanut production, exporting over 10,000 tons of peanuts to Europe and the United States (Wright 2010, 127–41).

While lucrative as a cash crop, peanuts did not provide a stable basis for a national economy. The rapid expansion of peanut cultivation came at the expense of other forms of agricultural production. Because they were harvested at the same time as other staples (such as rice, sorghum, and millet), growing peanuts meant farmers produced little else. By the mid-nineteenth century, demand for rice increased dramatically, while domestic production almost disappeared (Carney and Watts 1991). Farmers were able to buy rice on credit from British and French merchant houses, but at exorbitant interest rates. Thus, even when peanuts prices were high, farmers could barely afford the food they no longer grew. A poor yield or a drop-off in market prices plunged rural areas into debt. When Bathurst became an official colony in 1893, the British government also advanced rice to farmers, much of which was exported from Germany, who controlled a considerable portion of the East Asian market. With the outbreak of the First World War, this commercial arrangement was no longer viable and the Gambia was plunged into crisis (Wright 2009, 171).[7] As shipping to the colonies came to a halt and the oil industry was put on hold, peanut demand plummeted. Following the price collapse of the 1930s, the situation in the Gambia reached its nadir; the escalation of rural debt, food shortages, and the depreciation of the franc deepened the colony's dependence on the global groundnut market, which under the specter of another world war was increasingly volatile (Gray 1940, 487).[8]

In 1939 the British government passed the Colonial Development and Welfare Act to redress these economic vulnerabilities shared by the majority of British colonial subjects.[9] Radically expanding the scope of previous legislation, the act established an annual allowance of five and half million pounds for development projects and colonial research. This financial commitment to the colonies represented a sea change in British imperial governance.[10] Before the wars, the British pursued a policy of stringent self-reliance; colonial budgets were not to exceed the revenue they generated, and financial support was only extended for military matters, commercial infrastructure, or dire circumstances.[11] A political about-face, the 1939 act provided for large-scale investments in agriculture, education, public health and, further, for research in these areas (Havinden and Meredith 1993, 215–24). Though the Gambia was not a major recipient of welfare funds, government officials were awarded grants to pilot development schemes and collect socioeconomic and medical data. In 1944 the Gambia became the site of the Human Nutritional Research Unit (HNRU), an institution intended to intermediate between basic research and applications in the tropics by linking the London School of Hygiene and Tropical Medicine, the Hospital of Tropical Diseases, and the Colonial Office (Burgess 1956). Margaret Haswell (1975, 91), an agronomist who, under the auspices of the HNRU, conducted extensive research in the Gambia, explains the rationale: "Gambia was originally chosen by the Human Nutrition Research Unit of the Colonial Medical Research Council as a suitable area for research into the present problems and the development potential of rural peoples of the tropics because it offered a microcosm of conditions which were in fact widely prevalent in larger and less manageable areas."

The most pressing of these "present problems"—so clearly rendered in miniature—were food insecurity and malnutrition. The compounded effect of the Gambia's sandy soil, volatile climatic conditions, and groundnut monoculture made the country a particularly "suitable laboratory for nutritional inquiries" (Haswell 1975, xiii). Further, land in the Gambia seemed to be available in abundance: only approximately 25,000 out of a total of 334,000 acres of the tidal flood plain were exploited for rice production (Webb 1992, 553). The Gambia Experiment was the first large-scale nutrition study oriented toward national application. Combining expertise in anthropology, agronomy, nutrition, and medicine with technical knowledge of modern agricultural methods, its central objective was to transform the nutrition and living standards of a single village by increasing the acreage of swampland under cultivation. The project developed out of a proposal made to the Colonial Office by Benjamin Stanley Platt, the newly appointed director of the HNRU, who had conducted extensive nutritional surveys in the Gambia, Malawi, and Tanzania during the Second World War. A doctor by training with a penchant for fieldwork, Platt emphasized the potential of native resources to address public health problems; his multisectorial surveys not only attended to levels of malnutrition but also to local foods, taboos, cultivation practices, and gastronomic customs. With the funds made available by the Colonial Development and Welfare Act, Platt saw the potential for "digging into the fundamentals of African domestic economy" with the purpose of "utilizing the immense potentialities of this chronically indigent territory" (cited in Berry 1998, 25–26).

In 1946 Genieri, a Mandinka village located 110 miles up the river from

Bathurst, was chosen as the site for the Gambia Experiment. At the time, the population of Genieri numbered 460 and suffered from a high mortality rate; almost half the children born in the village died before reaching the age of ten. Positioned on a sandy ridge and overlooking a tidal swamp, Genieri spanned 2,800 acres of land, only about 10 percent of which was used for growing the main dietary staple, rice. As groundnuts were regarded the domain of men, rice was cultivated exclusively by women, a gender division that, combined with "the use of primitive tools and the failure to use manures," the Colonial Office claimed "resulted in low productivity" (cited in Berry 1998, 224). The results of an initial survey conducted by Platt confirmed that Genieri's epidemiological profile and inadequate food supply "was representative of the majority of rural villages in African colonies," and as a "fairly compact political, social and to some extent economic unit," it was identified as an advantageous site for controlled experimentation, a veritable "sociological laboratory" (cited in Berry 1998, 171). Genieri's location was also strategic: in the nearest town, Jenoi, the Department of Agriculture had established a field station to conduct experiments on salt-resistant strains of rice.[12] The relative isolation of the village from the urban economy of the coast and the proximity of agricultural expertise would enable experimenters to pilot "a pattern which can be copied in setting up other mechanized units on a production basis in communities in Gambia and indeed throughout West Africa" (H. A. Harding quoted in Berry 1998, 39). The challenge then, at least according to the Colonial Office, was to ensure the experiment modeled "the actual conditions which might obtain in the subsequent units" (H. A. Harding quoted in Berry 1998, 39).

The experimental protocol outlined two distinct yet interrelated initiatives. In the first years, an interdisciplinary Field Working Party, under the direction of William Berry[13]—a nutritionist who had previously worked under Platt—and in connection to the HNRU, would conduct general surveys on Genieri residents' state of health, levels of food consumption, and farming practices. Agricultural studies would describe the features of Genieri's climate and soil composition; ethnographic investigations would examine the local forms of social cohesion, land ownership, education and food consumption; finally clinical research would study the prevalence of anemia and parasitic and infectious diseases, as well as conditions associated with malnutrition (for example, potbelly), the height and weight of children, the daily calorie expenditure of domestic and agricultural work, and the strength and endurance of laborers.[14] Following this survey work, the Department of

Agriculture, under the direction of the Colonial Office, would conduct trials on the application of "mechanization" into village life, using tractors, plows, harrows, fertilizers, and irrigation to reclaim the low-lying salt marshes, first for cultivating rice and eventually to introduce a wide range of crops.[15] After a period of three years, these two sets of knowledge were to be "fused," comparing the cost of the interventions, the changes in caloric intake of the workers, and the overall improvements in health.

In technical terms, the experiment was not radical. "There are no special problems here," Berry wrote in a report to the Colonial Office, "the large scale cultivation of 'bottom lands' or fens by mechanical means is standard in both English and American agricultural practice and in both countries is an essential means of realizing the high potential fertility of the soils" (quoted in Berry 1998, 25).[16] The Gambia Experiment's particular challenge was, according to Berry, "the grafting of agricultural innovations onto African Society," introducing previously tested methods onto a landscape that was already farmed: "it must be clearly understood that our problem is not the technical one of working out the best machines and fertilizers; that will be done by other bodies, in Tanganyika and some of the West African Colonies. There, unoccupied land will be farmed as estates, and immigrants, leaving their own village societies, will be molded into new ones formed largely around the concerns of the estate. Our problems are those of using lands already farmed and a society already established. . . . Ours is not an agricultural demonstration plot, it is a human experiment" (quoted in Berry 1998, 54).

With society as its subject, the success of the Gambia Experiment hung not upon the immediate efficiency of the methods but rather upon the degree to which a modern agricultural system could be grafted onto Genieri village. In proposals and reports to the Colonial Office, Berry emphasized the gradual processes of molding the attitudes of farmers and of enabling the residents of Genieri to improve their standard of living on their own terms. Though the agricultural methods were preformulated, the experimental protocol organized that activity in such a way as "to give the local people confidence in their ability to control their environment" (Haswell 1953, 74). In the first year of the experiment, volunteer villagers were given practical courses in agricultural science and machine operations and also in reading, writing, arithmetic, and biology. This pedagogical process was complemented by finely grained research into local customs and methods of farming: as Margaret Haswell (1953, 72) observed, "they seem much more prepared to advance if what they do not know can be explained in terms of what they do know." To influence agricultural practice, generating data on increased crop yields was not enough. The value of modern technologies would ultimately be adjudicated by farmers and thus had to be demonstrated within the social organization of existing practices (Henke 2002). Further, the credibility of those demonstrations—whether or not farmers would continue to accommodate novel practices after the experiment ended—depended upon the degree to which farmers trusted the experimenters. To encourage those relationships, the Field Working Party built a clinic in the village and supplied free rations of rice for volunteers. In exchange the villagers provided supplementary land on the perimeter of their tillage areas to extend the acreage covered by the experiment.

This collaborative experimental process of grafting technologies onto Genieri society was ultimately intended to ensure the sustainability of the intervention on trial. On the whole, colonial development in the Gambia (and elsewhere in Africa) pursued the model of a plantation economy, increasing the production of cash crops by turning African farmers into paid laborers. The Gambia Experiment, in contrast, sought to improve production by retaining and reinforcing the collective features of village life and, in so doing, "avoid the social disintegration that is an inevitable consequence of advancement" (cited in Berry 1998, 225). Moreover, as the economic benefits of these new technologies would accrue to the village as a whole, the scheme would presumably pay for itself. When the agricultural equipment was introduced to the village at the start of the second year, the research community was confident in the project's methodology. In their annual report for 1947 to 1948, the London School of Hygiene and Tropical Medicine relayed the promising work in Genieri: "It seems likely that the villagers, having already recognized the value to them of improvements in production brought about by mechanical means will wish to put the money towards the purchase of equipment for themselves" (cited in Berry 1998, 224–25).

Initially, that optimism was vindicated; after the first two years of the Gambia Experiment, both the health of the village and its agricultural output had improved; in 1948 returns on labor increased by over 50 percent (Haswell 1953, 79). However, at the end of its second year, the future of the Gambia Experiment was becoming increasingly uncertain. The problem that had plagued the project from the outset was whether it was to be considered research or development. Though Berry insisted that the Gambia Experiment constituted "research in application," he recognized that its emphasis on social improvement suggested that it must do so "not, as many might perhaps prefer it, with minimum disturbance, but with the maximum of genuinely beneficial change" (cited in Berry 1998, 51). While the Field Working Party maintained that nutritional concerns—that is, the enhancement and diversification of food supply—should remain the experiment's central focus, from the point of view of the Colonial Office "beneficial change" had to be measured in economic output: "I quite appreciate that at the present the methods of cultivation are entirely experimental . . . [but] it is clear that if such mechanized cultivation is to be multiplied, it must be on an economic basis since neither His Majesty's Government nor the local Governments can afford to subsidise the loss on a large number of units" (H. A. Harding quoted in Berry 1998, 39).

Rather quickly it became clear that the increase in rice production would never offset the costs of installing and maintaining the new machinery. First, the reclaimed acreage covered by the experiment was too small. As Margaret Haswell (1953, 78) reflected years later, the mechanical requirements to drain and irrigate the swamps for rice cultivation were "out of all proportion to the scale of the project." Under Platt's direction, Berry had attempted to maintain the experiment's wide remit, requesting that in addition to harrows, ploughs, and drills to drain the rice that also sifters and diesel engines for milling and parboiling cereal grains be introduced. "No work," he wrote to the Colonial Office, "has, however, been done, either in the Unit or elsewhere, on the technology of the preparation of native meals and flours from various millets and sorghum" (cited in Berry 1998, 241). The value of demonstrating the health impact of agricultural mechanization did not solve, however, the fundamental problem "that the Genieri experiment is too costly to repeat on extensive scales."[17] Following the advice of the Colonial Office, the focus shifted to increasing the production of ground-nuts, simpler to cultivate and more likely to generate profit.

This change of protocol might have been anticipated. When Platt initially proposed the Gambia Experiment in 1946, the governor of the colony had expressed anxiety that the experiment might too closely overlap "high-priority" schemes planned by the Colonial Development Corporation (CDC). In contrast to the ideological impulse of the Colonial Welfare and Development Act, the central purpose of the CDC was to launch development schemes that would generate profit for Britain. In 1946, its first year of operation, the CDC launched several projects in the Gambia, including a poultry farm on the coast and a large-scale mechanized project to clear rice lands and harvest rice mechanically just up river from Genieri.[18] As questions were raised about the economic feasibility of the Gambia Experiment, the Colonial Office insisted on altering the project's experimental protocol to better support the work carried out by the CDC. Critically, the experimental groundnut plots would have to be much larger; the experiment was extended beyond Genieri to Jomarr, a village that was "more rectangular in shape" (cited in Berry 1998, 160) and thus more convenient to divide into experimental plots. To accommodate the scale of production, a number of villages in the vicinity of Genieri would have to be aggregated and redistributed into economic units: "the villages would be in groups of 20, with headquarters for each group for mechanical workshops and technical administrative and social service area" (cited in Berry 1998, 216).

The plans to restructure Genieri proved to be the breaking point for the Gambia Experiment. No longer an investigation in "grafting" technology—"done in such a way that village society is not disrupted"—it became the pilot of a plantation. Berry and other members of the team resigned and the experiment was ended in December 1950.[19] The agricultural work continued under the direction of the governor and the Department of Agriculture, who demarcated two large blocks of land for mechanization, one communally cultivated by villagers and the other dependent on paid labor, both of which were deemed a failure just a year later. Despite the use of machinery, the application of fertilizers, and draft animals, crop yields had not increased significantly. Moreover, farmers, who had become increasingly "contract-minded," seemed incapable of taking a long-term view of the experiments. In his report, the director of the Department of Agriculture expressed shock that the villagers' only response to his detailed explanations of the method and purposes of mechanization was to ask, "will there be any more contracts for clearing next season?" (cited in Berry 1998, 161).[20]

In his analysis of colonial policy following the Second World War, Christophe Bonneuil (1999, 2000) reads the emphasis on experimentation as a strategic rhetoric that helped the colonial state achieve greater control over its territory and justified the money lost when large-scale development schemes ended in failure. Regardless of their agricultural impact, experiments in mechanization, swamp drainage, and resettlement made villages more amenable for surveillance and intervention: they generated unmediated data on the population and, in so doing, shifted the object of governmental control from the community to the household heads. Throughout the 1950s and early 1960s, approximately 10,000 additional hectares of swamp were reclaimed for rice production in the Gambia to relatively limited economic success (Webb 1992). These vertical, technocratic experiments transformed Gambian agrarian society into a series of individualized units that, ironically, would serve as the basis for "grassroots" development projects in the 1980s and 1990s (Sumberg 1998).

The pragmatic possibilities of experimentation for the Colonial Office, and later the independent Gambian state, did not undermine the potential of the Gambia for basic scientific research. On the contrary, following the collapse of the Gambia Experiment, Platt, in his position as director of the HNRU, negotiated further funding for a research laboratory at Fajara. With an expanded brief, the newly named MRC Laboratories, the Gambia, planned to conduct "not only research in tropical medicine but also in general medical problems, some of which can more easily be studied in the Gambia where many cases can be seen of diseases which are rare [in the UK]" (Platt quoted in Berry 1998, 199).[21] One of the first overseas basic research facilities, the MRC Laboratories in the Gambia was designed to conduct fundamental research in biochemistry and virology. In the years that followed, it would provide significant contributions to international science, while partly abandoning the task of directly applying that knowledge.[22] As the MRC unit grew, exploring topics from anemia to liver disease and establishing new field stations up river, its approach to tropical medicine came to be referred to as "medicine in the tropics" (Tansey and Reynolds 2001, 37). The implication of that shift away from site-specific or "applied" problems was that the MRC could operate independently from governmental interests whether represented by the Colonial Office or, later, the Gambian state.

In hindsight, the biopolitical orientation of the Gambia Experiment—to bring scientific knowledge to bear on the organization and life of the population—was exceptional for research undertaken in the country.[23] After independence, the Gambian government experimented with both small- and large-scale swamp development and irrigation schemes to increase the productivity of rice growers (Carney 2008; Carney and Watts 1991). But these projects had no point of contact with the extensive research (nutritional or otherwise) conducted under the auspices of the MRC and were designed and implemented with foreign assistance—provided alternatively by the Taiwanese government, the World Bank, and the People's Republic of China. The MRC, meanwhile, has continued to operate independently from the government, though owing to its long institutional presence and the sheer size of its operations it has had a considerable impact on the health and wealth of the population. Its interactions with public institutions—such as hospitals, health centers, and universities—have depended on the scope of particular experiments and involved periodic support. The tenor of the MRC's view of its relationship to the Gambian government has remained consistent with how it was initially described in its 1957 report: "The African population is cooperative and the Government has warmly welcomed the presence of a research project, which makes an important impact on the life of a small community. Relations on all sides are cordial, to the benefit of all concerned" (cited in Reynolds and Tansey 2001, 21).

The following section gives those relations empirical texture by describing an MRC trial conducted in the vicinity of Genieri almost sixty years after the village first became an experimental site. Though by no means as "applied" as the Gambia Experiment, the Larval Control Project (LCP) piloted a policy of environmental management and thus aimed to establish links between research protocol and local practice—in other words, to "graft" a new technology onto the particular features of the experimental locality. Like the Gambia Experiment, the LCP's intervention was deemed inappropriate for its setting; the scale of the problem investigated could not be sustained by the scope of a scientific study. The LCP's fate, and that of the upcountry field station from which it was conducted, reveals what has changed in the relationship between science and government in the postcolonial Gambian context but also what ideas about the role and reach of research activity have remained constant over the past seventy years.

A Laboratory Landscape

Our study is unique in that it covers such a large area over an extended time period in contrast to the majority of published ecology studies, which were small-scale in space and time. . . . [But] using simple, low-cost technology is not an intervention that works everywhere, careful consideration needs to be given to the habitat characteristics responsible for the proliferation of malaria vectors.

—Majambere et al., "Is Mosquito Larval Source Management Appropriate for Reducing Malaria in Areas of Extensive Flooding in The Gambia?"

In an air-conditioned conference room at the Bill and Melinda Gates–funded Centre for Innovation against Malaria (CIAM), Lamin Jarju presented the findings of his masters of science thesis to an audience of donors, scientists, policy makers, and health practitioners.[24] A former data entry clerk at the MRC upcountry field station in Farafenni, Lamin had been selected to pursue a course in entomology at Durham University (UK) as part of a capacity building scheme built into a large-scale malaria control study funded by the U.S. National Institute of Health (NIH). The LCP, conducted between 2003 and 2008, aimed to reduce the incidence of malaria through the application of microbial larvicides to the landward edges of upcountry floodplains. Lamin's research explored one aspect of larval control: the impact of concrete bulwarks (or bunds) intended to prevent soil erosion and flooding on mosquito breeding grounds. Constructed in the early 1980s, the network of bunds was one of several agricultural projects funded by the International Foundation for Agricultural Development (IFAD), a UN investment scheme that granted direct support to communities by bypassing state bureaucracy.[25] Over the course of a year, Lamin had traveled across the country, undertaking the arduous task of collecting and analyzing samples from the water pooled around the embankments. His findings revealed that while reducing the salinity of low lying fields, the bunds also served as ideal breeding grounds for *Anopheles gambiae*, the most common malaria vector (Jarju 2008). Lamin concluded his talk with an admonition to the attending governmental ministers: "Healthy nation breeds wealthy nation: the Gambia's future depends on agricultural policy and malaria control working hand in hand."[26]

Lamin's rephrasing of a quintessentially modern governmentality is provocative.[27] Considering the MRC's remit to generate scientific insights of international relevance and the role of foreign bodies in agrarian reform, calibrating Gambian health and wealth hardly seem affairs of the state (e.g., Hansen and Stepputat 2001; Sharma and Gupta 2006). The trajectory of malaria research in the Gambia underscores that disjuncture between expert knowledge and national concerns. One of the more intractable public health problems, malaria intersects with housing, urban infrastructure, and rural development—the disease is a matter of governmental capacity (Suffian 2007). However, since the 1950s, global health policies have worked to disentangle malaria control from social and economic progress. Albeit in different ways, mid-century and contemporary eradication campaigns emphasize innovation in prevention, privileging the transfer of technology over building local capacity (Kelly and Beisel 2011).

Returning to a strategy neglected for the better part of the century, the LCP's investigative focus on environment management was a massive undertaking. A public health anachronism, the project aimed to situate malaria control within the specific ecological setting of upcountry Gambia. Because larval habitats are transient and unpredictable, the LCP required exhaustive and continual surveys of the experimental site, an area of approximately four hundred square kilometers along the north and south banks of the river (Majambere et al. 2007). In 2004, two years before the application of larvicide was to begin, the principal investigator, Steve Lindsay—a professor of vector biology at Durham University—hired four technicians from the National Malaria Control Programme (NMCP) and, in a small pilot area bordering the MRC's upcountry Farafenni field station, trained them to recognize larval habitats, identify mosquitoes, and use compasses and handheld Global Positioning Systems (GPS).

To gather baseline entomological data, the intervention area was divided into four zones, roughly one hundred square kilometers each, and surveyed continuously during the rainy seasons of 2004 and 2005. With villages located from one to eight kilometers from the river, the zones encompassed a wide range of micro-ecologies, including grassland, stream fringe, rice fields, and mangrove forest. Over the course of two years, monthly visits were made to each of 1,076 semipermanent water bodies identified during surveys. On these visits, the surveyors were asked to describe water bodies (noting temperature, pH, salinity, depth, and surrounding vegetation), to sample habitats for the presence of larvae, and occasionally to catch fish and frogs so that the contents of their guts could be examined at the lab.

When spraying began, surveillance intensified. The LCP used a species-specific, nonresidual microbial insecticide, Bti. While highly effective in killing mosquito larvae, Bti passes quickly through the ecosystem and must be reapplied on a weekly basis; spraying, therefore, required considerable and consistent manpower. Rather than hire fieldworkers from the coast, Silas Majambere and Margaret Pinder, the LCP's implementing scientists, recruited sixty Gambians residing in each of the four LCP intervention zones. After a month of training, the group was broken into teams of three to four spray men each led by a NMCP supervisor. Five days a week, from seven in the morning until one in the afternoon, the team would walk abreast, across two kilometers-long transepts, spreading Bti from the buckets strapped to their necks.

The advantage of enrolling residents as spray men was their familiarity with the landscape. The challenge was reorienting that awareness for the purposes of larval control—as Steve put it, "learning to see the breeding grounds from the swamp." Initially, this proved difficult. *Anophelese* mosquitoes typically breed in sunlit pools that require no greater depth than a footprint filled with rain. Further, there was a great deal of acreage to cover; finding all the potential habitats required meticulous and intensive attention. Further, because this was an experiment and not a program, these men were not hired for their services but compensated for their volunteered participation. While the money was good—roughly 150 dalasi or US$5 a day—the participatory emphasis of the project made it difficult to enforce rigorous quality controls or to replace people who seemed less up to the job. The arduous task of traversing large swaths of muddy landscape, carrying buckets, larvae dippers, maps, and heavy spray packs was exacerbated during the rainy season. When the routine application of larvicide was most critical, the swamp pools were at their greatest depth. The spray men, who, for the most part, could not swim, were reluctant to wade into water above their knees. To identify any habitats that might have been missed, Steve enlisted officers from the NMCP to conduct random spot checks of water bodies in the days following weekly application.

Recruiting spray men locally was risky. Indeed, when it became clear that larval control would not work in this environment, the spray men's lack of experience was cited as one of the contributing factors (Majambere et al. 2010). However, participation was central to the LCP's methodology. Rather than merely trialing intervention, the experiment was designed to produce knowledge about a specific policy; it was a pilot study for incipient government programs. What was on trial was a community-led system of management: could the training of local spray men be eventually extended to a nationwide, state-led disease control program? Like the Gambia Experiment, the LCP aimed to preempt the problem of sustainability by grafting the method to the context of intervention and thus generate social and technical links between the test setting to a future government intervention (Lezaun and Millo 2006).

Also like the Gambia Experiment, the LCP was a public health project: the value of its intervention was linked to its clinical effectiveness. To demonstrate the impact of larval control on the incidence of malaria, the LCP team enrolled eight hundred adults and two thousand children, aged six months to ten. In addition to a biannual collection of blood samples, a nurse and a fieldworker were stationed in each zone to monitor the participants' health, record all cases of malaria, and provide on-site care at any hour. Village health workers (VHWs) were a critical component in this surveillance strategy.[28] Initiated by the WHO's Alma Ata Declaration (1978), VHWs were intended to offer an administrative bridge between government structures and citizens (Gilson et al. 1989). In the Gambia VHWs are selected by village development committees, a volunteer body intended to encourage civic engagement, and are given six weeks' training in preventative and curative medicine (Davis, Hulme, and Woodhouse 1994). Perceived as a panacea for a weak and underfunded health system, the VHWs receive no payment from the state but rather nominal compensation from members of the community who seek their care (Menon 1991). Occasionally VHWs are hired by MRC projects to serve as reporters, informing researchers of cases occurring in their villages that might be relevant for specific investigative purposes.

In the context of the LCP, the VHWs' role surpassed that of reportage. The protocol described a partnership between VHWs and nurses, the latter providing diagnostic support and pharmaceuticals and the former responsible for treatment. The advantages of enrolling VHWs were similar to those afforded by the local spray men: the VHWs' familiarity with their communities bolstered the empirical capacity of research. However, the VHW clinical skills were found wanting. Few were able to read and write; fewer still had any formal education. Moreover, as opposed to the traditional birth assistants (TBAs) who occupied a social role as healers, the VHWs were a new actor in the village political ecology (Cham et al. 1987). The ambiguous position of the VHW between the government, community, and the MRC meant that often, rather than facilitating community access, the VHW entrenched distrust of research, leading to high dropout rates.

Though it posed clear challenges, the VHW-MRC nurse coalition was an investigative priority. At the start of the rains, LCP staff ran a series of workshops in conjunction with the relevant district health teams to retrain VHWs to treat and recognize the signs of malaria. The LCP team devised a three-part treatment strategy, whereby participant mothers were asked to approach project nurses when their children fell ill. Following diagnosis, the nurse would issue the mother a prescription slip to deliver to the VHW, who would issue drugs given to them by the project at the start of the trial.[29] While seemingly convoluted, the system was unilaterally popular. The MRC nurses claimed that VHWs enabled them to reach more patients; the VHWs believed the support from MRC nurses reinforced their practice; the villager residents, who enjoyed continual access to health care, found their children's health, and that of their community, dramatically improved (Kelly 2011). Embedding the experiment within the local health care infrastructure also had positive implications for the trial. The participants regarded the study positively and, consequently, accommodated the spray men on their lands and brought their children to have their fingers pricked on blood-sampling days.

Through the alignment of local and scientific knowledge, the LCP transformed villages and flood plains into venues of knowledge production and disease management. In the project the boundaries between social and scientific orders were porous — the experimental entanglements between local actors and research institution reformatted the public dimensions of health. Again, like the Gambia Experiment, the LCP impact on the community was registered directly, through extension rather than via policy recommendations. However, despite its impressive operational successes, the LCP did not result in a reduction in malaria infections. The relatively stable transmission rate had less to do with the competence of the spray team — after two years of spraying, the presence of *Anophelese* larvae had dropped by 92 percent — than the rather surprising capacity of mosquitoes to fly great distances from areas not covered by the experiment. In the Gambian floodplains whether or not community-led, manually applied larval control was effective could not be demonstrated experimentally. Here, larval control would only work comprehensively, on a national scale: "in areas with extensive flooding, such as river floodplains and major areas of irrigated rice, significant impact might only be achieved with aerial application because large areas can be treated rapidly at full coverage" (Majambere et al. 2010, 183).

These conclusions — along with the results of Lamin's thesis — were presented during the meeting at the CIAM in July 2007. The LCP's negative results and Steve's recommendation to fund for an area application of Bti provoked little response. What interested the audience, particularly those in the Health and Agricultural Ministry, was the connection Lamin drew between farming techniques and malaria incidence. His presentation sparked a heated debate on the state of the agrarian economy under Yahya A. J. J. Jammeh — the Gambia's president following the 1994 military coup. Those critical of the president's development strategy claimed that rice production had fallen dramatically in the last decade and its increasing reliance on technical assistance from Taiwan had failed to yield any real improvements. Proponents of his policies insisted that Taiwanese-sponsored projects had helped the farmers produce more than 10,000 tons of high quality and high-yielding rice yearly. Further, the secretary of state for agriculture, Kanja Sanneh, revealed that the government of Taiwan was prepared to send the Gambia eight tons of DDT as soon as it received a detailed plan from the government for its domestic application. He suggested that the focus of the meeting shift from discussing completed projects to how the MRC and the National Malaria Control Program (NMCP) might take advantage of this opportunity.

As the LCP disseminated its results back to the participant communities, the NMCP, under the behest of President Jammeh, made preparations to target 80 percent of households in the Gambia as the first step in the newly launched, nationwide campaign—Operation Eradicate Malaria. Lamin, who was made a senior officer at the NMCP, enlisted the LCP research team's support in training a new squadron of spray men in the handling and distribution of DDT. In turn, Margaret, Silas, and Steve secured a grant from the MRC to conduct a randomized controlled study on the effectiveness of the spray campaign and whether it provided any additional protection over the current best practice of long-lasting insecticide-impregnated nets (LLIN). Continuing the work begun by the LCP, the new research project (SANTE) has set aside resources to train the VHWs in the use of rapid diagnostic technologies (RDTs) for detecting malarial parasites. However, though their salaries will be paid for through the research project, this time, the spray men will be government employees.

The trajectory of the LCP reveals the ways in which governmental policy and scientific practice intersect in the Gambia today. Though the research conducted under the auspices of the LCP aimed to generate data of global significance, its experimental practices animated government infrastructure. That this experiment-policy overlap was extended after the LCP was deemed a failure makes the pragmatic potential of the project all that more striking. As contributors to this edited volume show, contemporary public health in Africa is characterized by deterritorialized modalities of governance. Funded by private partners, nongovernmental agencies, and transnational bodies, medical research and therapeutic care no longer exist in a space characterized by the "public"; the nation-state, therefore, seems an inappropriate category for conceptualizing biopolitical life (Ferguson 2006). And yet in the context of the LCP, the state continues to operate as a significant imaginary. Here, research emerges as an awkward form of stewardship. As soon as it ended, the LCP was reformulated to respond to the interlocking commitments of the international scientific community, the economic and political interests of governments, and the health of the population.

In pointing to the ways in which international research can become enrolled in national projects, I do not mean to suggest that scientific and governmental practices are in any way isomorphic. Despite its investigative focus on public health management (and here, perhaps malaria control presents a particular case) the primary aim of the LCP was to publish papers, advance the careers of scientists, and generate further funding for research. Whatever improvements it affected through its implementation, the aim of the experiment was not to transform the lives of Gambians as a population. Launched in 2009, SANTE has accentuated that discrepancy. The experiment initiated the national distribution of bed nets, with the understanding that the government would wait on spraying after initial results were generated. But under the time pressures of Operation Eradicate Malaria, the NMCP spray teams ignored SANTE's randomized design, which requires that particular villages be left unsprayed. As Margaret struggles to reformat the experimental protocol so that it can demonstrate the relative effectiveness of the campaign, Jammeh's malaria eradication plan will be scaled up to include all inhabitable houses, but as she points out, without a clear sense of best practice. Once again, the scale of the experiment does not correspond to the needs of government policy.

The campaign marks a critical shift in the history of research in the Gambia. While the MRC has held the monopoly on malaria research and control, recently health has become a charged domain to exercise and demonstrate state power. The question that faces the research community today is what this repoliticization of the bioscience means for the MRC.

Experiments and Exit

Sir, presidents come and presidents go, but the MRC is for the people of the Gambia.
—Sir Christopher Booth, 1981, in Reynolds and Tansey, *British Contributions to Medical Research and Education in Africa after the Second World War*

Though the team did not know it then, the LCP was one of the last trials to be hosted in the Farafenni MRC Laboratories. In February 2009, the country-based MRC staff and scientists were informed that head offices in London had shifted its vision: rather than focus its investments in the Gambia, the MRC would support regional collaborations across West Africa. In addition to closing Farafenni, the MRC will cut the Gambia's budget in half over the next five years. The rationale is to allow MRC researchers to investigate a greater number of people in diverse circumstances and thus enhance the generalizabilty of their research and the speed at which it is conducted.

In a closing ceremony, the MRC donated the station to the University of the Gambia's School of Medicine and Allied Health Sciences. While heralded by the MRC as a new chapter in a long-standing partnership, this plan has not been well received by Gambians. The former head of Farafenni station, now paid to monitor the empty buildings while the university figures out what to do with them (and how much it will cost), has received hundreds of letters from neighboring villagers protesting the closure. "For the most part," he said, "these people feel abandoned. Some feel betrayed. They had participated with the MRC because they believed it was a lasting commitment."[30]

The MRC's decision to pull out of the Gambia characterizes the contemporary biopolitical regime: extending its reach across state spaces, the MRC laboratories in the Gambia will form just another island in the "archipelago" of international scientific activity (see Geissler, introduction in this volume). If anything, the MRC's long-term commitment to the Gambia is anachronistic. Today, research has less and less to do with specific places than with experimental networks. However, what is particular to the Gambian case is that the MRC's shift in policy is coterminous with Jammeh's increasing interest and involvement in public health issues. More notorious than Operation Eradicate Malaria is the president's claim that he can cure AIDS through a fusion of traditional healing and Koranic-inspired therapies. To administer this "national cure," Jammeh took over a hospital built with foreign donations and enrolled hundreds of HIV patients, who were promptly taken off their ARVs. For criticizing this therapeutic strategy, the president has expelled or detained foreign officials and nationals (Cassidy and Leach 2009). His speech to the Sixty-Fourth United Nations General Assembly in 2009 outlined his position:

> HIV/AIDS, malaria, tuberculosis are killer diseases. While I would like to reiterate my delegation's support for the work of the Global Fund to fighting these diseases, I wish to call for concerted efforts at resource mobilization to support international research on traditional medicine and alternative diseases treatment programs. These traditional systems are in most instances more cost-effective, yet abandoned for the sorts of criticisms that come from multinationals who feel threatened that certain traditional breakthroughs would be detrimental to their corporate existence and interests. These multinationals value their monetary gains more than human life. They should not be allowed to hold humanity for ransom. Their insatiable appetite for massive wealth at any cost has pushed them

to the point of blindness and insensitivity to human suffering and loss of human life in the developing world, especially in Africa.[31]

According to Jammeh, the pursuit of health and wealth short-circuits the well-being of Africans, a biopolitical arrangement that he will aim to undo. Though his methods are reckless and his regime repressive, Jammeh's decision to flex national power through therapeutic practice makes political sense, particularly against the longue durée of biomedical intervention in the country. In their analysis of Jammeh's motivations, Cassidy and Leach (2009, 561) suggest that "they can be read, in part, as a consequence of global scientific governance: as backlashes which contest its power." In other worlds, Jammeh's "cure" is a way of wrestling back sovereign power from the grasp of philanthro-capitalist visions of "grand health challenges."

The MRC's response to Jammeh's assertion has been muted. Their silence can be read as either a pragmatic effort to protect their HIV research activities or as an ideological stance regarding institutional integrity and its distance from political affairs, articulated by Christopher Booth (quoted in Reynolds and Tansey 2001, 38) in the quotation above. Whatever the logic, the MRC is finding a way to disentangle its operations from the political context of the Gambian state, completing a process of separation that began seventy years ago.

Notes

Research and writing of this chapter was supported by Wellcome Trust GR081507.

1 Immediately following the independence of Senegal from France in 1960, the British attempted to develop a formal association—Senegambia—to bolster the Gambia's economy, taking some of the financial pressure off the UK. While Senegal had several reasons to support a fuller integration, including clamping down on smuggling and securing its own political security against the more radical West African governments, for the Gambia, the advantages of being absorbed into another country with a different language, ethnic composition, and higher tariff structures were less clear. The Gambia government rejected the UN's recommendations for a merger and in 1965 the British agreed to grant the Gambia independence regardless of any agreement reached with Senegal. The Senegambia Federation was briefly reinvigorated in 1982, when President Jawara asked for support of the Senegalese army to suppress a coup, but ultimately dissolved six years later after conflicts over the degree of military support

provided by the Gambia to Senegal. Under the current president, Jammeh, relations have soured further, as he is believed to be supporting rebels in the southern Senegalese district of the Casamance (Hughes and Perfect 2006, 254–59).

2 For instance, to prevent direct competition with hospitals for labor, the MRC will only hire clinical staff six months after they have terminated their governmental appointments. Because nurses are only contracted by particular research projects, this policy places nurses in a precarious situation, whereby they might work for the MRC for twenty years or more but only in erratic two- to three-year stints.

3 Sir Ian McGregor comments: "So much research depends, in its interpretation, on accurate knowledge of vital statistics of the communities under study—birth rates, death rates, the effect of season on these particular rates, how individuals grow, what is the nutritional status, what are the standards. In the years following the Second World War such information did not exist for communities in rural areas in West Africa. . . . There was a need to create a facility whereby this information could be supplied accurately. We tried to do this in the Gambia through long-term studies investigating a series of villages" (Reynolds and Tansey 2001, 24).

4 Though the Gambian population is not as genetically homogeneous or isolated as the Icelanders (in the late 1990s, DeCode Genetics, a start-up genetics company, endeavored to combine the genetic identity of the population of Iceland into a single database [e.g., Pálsson and Rabinow 1999]), its significance for the biomedical research enterprise can equally be understood in terms of the completeness and accuracy of its epidemiological history.

5 Though the Gambia only became a colony in 1893, Great Britain administered the territory surrounding Bathurst since the early 1820s, immediately after it had founded the city. For the latter part of the nineteenth century, this cluster of land was administered from Britain's more important possession Sierra Leone. Because the British government would not provide any financial support outside of military costs, Bathurst was built with revenue derived from tax on imports (Gailey 1964, 37, 62–65).

6 By the mid-seventeenth century, indigenous rice seeds had been replaced by Asian varieties (Wright 2010, 81).

7 Over four hundred Gambians served in the British West African Frontier Force, which was stationed in East Africa during the war (Gray 1940, 485).

8 The subsequent tightening of boundaries between the Gambia and Vichy-ruled Senegal during the Second World War added further strain to the groundnut market, as it brought a halt to the seasonal migration of workers from neighboring territories—"strange farmers" (*samalaalu*)—upon whom groundnut production had come to depend (Webb 1992).

9 Following the Second World War, the British were also under considerable pressure from the international community to improve the situation of colonial subjects, a point explicitly raised in connection to the Gambia, which Franklin D.

Roosevelt described to Churchill as "that hell-hole of yours called Bathurst" (Wright 1995, 47–58).

10 Motivated by concerns over Britain's unemployment, the primary aim of the 1929 act was "to aid and develop agriculture and industry in the Colonies, Protectorates and Mandated Territories, and thereby promote commerce with or industry in the United Kingdom" (Colonial Office Memoranda, 1921, quoted in Meredith 1975, 486). The act of 1939 also wrote of over eleven million pounds of debt incurred by colonial governments.

11 The protectorate was, for the most part, left undeveloped and, as it was never entirely certain that the colony would stay in British hands, reluctant to invest in any public works or infrastructural improvements that would ultimately be to a French advantage. In 1925 the total budget for the Gambia was £273, 284, and only £13,996 was budgeted directly for provincial administration (Gailey 1964, 234).

12 The Department of Agriculture, established in 1924, conducted experiments in diversifying agricultural production throughout the 1930s. These attempts had largely been unsuccessful, for despite efforts to encourage farmers to plant other seed varieties or pursue other crops, groundnuts remained the most lucrative—if not always stable—form of income (Gailey 1964, 144).

13 *The Gambia Experiment* (Berry 1998), edited and published by the wife of the team leader, Dr. William Berry, describes the last of three surveys conducted under the direction of Human Nutrition Research Unit and funded by the Medical Research Council.

14 Tested through a series of "wall building trials," described by Berry: "In one such test seventy-five hours were spent building twelve-foot-high walls, over a period of ten days, with a gang of six Africans working on contract. African compared favorably with the European," Report May 1947–1948, in Berry (1998, 44).

15 The extension of the experiment from rice to all crops commonly grown in the Gambia—and, in particular, groundnuts—was the explicit recommendation of the Colonial Office, which felt it necessary to ensure that nutritional investigations addressed economic output (Berry 1998, 23–24; 33–35).

16 W. T. C. Berry and A. H. Bunting, 1946, "Suggestions for a Field Working Party in Gambia Protectorate," in Berry (1998, 25). Bunting had previously worked at the Rothampsted Experimentation Farm in Harpenden, Hertfordshire (1940–43), where R. A. Fischer had recently developed and piloted the experimental design for randomized controlled trials.

17 Kenneth L. Little, April 1, 1948, Report on a visit to the Gambia in connection with the appointment of a Sociologist to the Nutritional Field Working Party: "its significance so far as the sociological process of 'grafting' new methods of life and organization on to the old, may not be conclusive, but its real value will undoubtedly lie in demonstrating what potentially can be achieved in terms of social and nutritional improvement as a result of much increased agricultural productivity. There may still remain, therefore, the fundamental problem, be-

cause the ultimate success of all such developmental work depends upon the community itself shouldering responsibility for the necessary changes, expansion and social improvement" (quoted in Berry 1998, 169).

18 Both of these projects ended in disaster; the losses were a source of considerable embarrassment for the Colonial Office (Cohen 1984, 68–70).

19 Margaret Haswell continued to conduct detailed research on the socioeconomics of Genieri over the following decade.

20 This interpretation that at the basis of problems was the individualist farmer tallies with the commonly held belief on the part of the Colonial Office of the disjuncture between developmental schemes and local practices. As Raymond Firth writes: "Much experiment, demonstration, and extension work has been carried on, and some of the results . . . have been very fruitful. At the same time one is forced to the conclusion that the response of the African farmers has been extremely slow; that the vast majority of them are not convinced that the methods advocated by government are capable of being applied to their own circumstances" (Firth 1947, 78).

21 For a discussion of how the MRC gained a foothold in tropical medicine despite the efforts of the Colonial Office to retain control of the research facilities, see Sir Ian McGregor's comments in Reynolds and Tansey (2001, 20–24).

22 Roger Whitehead, MRC unit director in Kampala, 1959, recalls: "In general, the MRC were more interested in fundamental research, developments of importance to fundamental science. . . . I think the MRC's record in Africa, when viewed internationally in terms of contributions to international science, is preeminent. Perhaps in terms of applying that knowledge, the MRC's record was not so good" (Reynolds and Tansey 2001, 58).

23 According to Foucault (2007, 18), biopolitics is a matter of achieving equilibrium between people and available resources by "organizing circulation, eliminating the dangerous elements, making a division between good and bad circulation, and maximizing the good circulation and diminishing the bad." Science, Foucault suggests, becomes the instrument through which these complex adjustments to the dynamics of exchange, accumulation, propagation, and sanitation are made, rendering the population intelligible for management.

24 The CIAM is one of four training centers built by the Gates Malaria Partnership in Africa intended to strengthen public health services by forging links between international and national researchers, funding bodies, policy makers, and health practitioners. The relationship the CIAM poses between science and government is one of infrastructural stimulation: "with its roots embedded in human resource strengthening," the CIAM hopes to reduce malaria through "equipping individuals and communities with the necessary skills"; see the CIAM website: www.ciam.gm.

25 The scheme has come under scrutiny by the IFAD (2005), whose evaluation of projects funded in the Gambia described the bunds as "in need of refashioning" and "only half-done" because—and here the report echoes the Colonial Office's

comments about rice schemes in the 1950s—"the villagers have no real sense of ownership of the schemes . . . they await the next dose of help and seem unwilling to take any initiative themselves" (IFAD 2005, 21).

26 CIAM research meeting, July 14, 2007.

27 In a Foucauldian sense, Lamin's thesis is an exemplar of the tête-à-tête of truth and the art of government (Foucault 2007). However, whereas Foucault grounded his analysis of governmentality in the context of European nation-states, the interventions Lamin describes are predicated on a political economy shaped by colonialism and forged through the global development regime.

28 The concept of the VHW was made famous by the Chinese barefoot doctor program, which made use of village volunteers as health auxiliaries in the mid-1950s. The dramatic success of this program inspired a number of other countries to follow the Chinese example, particularly those with large underserved areas and where the political agenda centered on eradicating social inequities.

29 As VHWs were, for the most part, illiterate, to ensure the accurate delivery of medicine at appropriate doses, treatment sheets and prescription slips had pictorial representation (e.g., suns for chloroquine and stars for fansidar).

30 Interview with author, May 25, 2009.

31 President Jammeh's Address to the General Assembly of the UN, September 24, 2009. http://www.un.org/en/ga/64/generaldebate/GM.shtml.

References

Beckerleg, Susan, Steve Austin, and Laurence Weaver. 1994. "Gender, Work and Illness: The Influence of a Research Unit on an Agricultural Community in the Gambia." *Health Policy and Planning* 9:419–28.

Berry, Veronica, ed. 1998. *The Gambia Experiment, 1946–1950, and Other Papers*. London: Academy Books.

Bonneuil, Christophe. 1999. "Penetrating the Natives: Peanut Breeding, Peasants and the Colonial State." *Science Technology Society* 4:273.

Bonneuil, Christophe. 2001. "Development as Experiment." *Osiris* 14:258–81.

Burgess, Richard C. 1956. "WHO and Nutrition." *Proceedings of the Nutrition Society* 15:13–21.

Carney, Judith A. 2008. "The Bitter Harvest of Gambian Rice Policies." *Globalizations* 5, no. 2: 129–42.

Carney, Judith A., and Michael Watts. 1991. "Disciplining Women? Rice, Mechanization, and the Evolution of Mandinka Gender Relations in Senegambia." *Signs* 16, no. 4: 651–81.

Cassidy, Rebecca, and Melissa Leach. 2009. "Science, Politics, and the Presidential AIDS 'Cure.'" *African Affairs* 108, no. 433: 559–80.

Cham, Kabbir, Carol MacCormack, Abdoulai Touray, and Susan Baldeh. 1987. "Social Organisation and Political Factionalism: PHC in the Gambia." *Health Policy and Planning* 2, no. 3: 214–26.

Conway, David J. 2007. "Molecular Epidemiology of Malaria." *Clinical Microbiology Reviews* 20:188–204.

Cowen, Mike. 1984. "The Early Years of the Colonial Development Corporation." *African Affairs* 83, no. 330: 63–75.

Davis, Daniel, David Hulme, and Philip Woodhouse. 1994. "Decentralization by Default: Local Governance and the View from the Village in the Gambia." *Public Administration and Development* 14:253–69.

Ferguson, James. 2006. *Global Shadows: Africa in the Neoliberal World Order*. Durham, NC: Duke University Press.

Firth, Raymond. 1947. "Social Problems and Research in British West Africa." *Journal of the International African Institute* 17, no. 2: 77–92.

Foucault, Michel. [1977–1978] 2007. *Security, Territory and Population*. Edited by Michel Senellart. Translated by Graham Burchell. New York: Palgrave Macmillan.

Gailey, Harry A. 1964. *A History of the Gambia*. London: Routledge and Kegan Paul.

Geissler, P. Wenzel, Ann Kelly, Robert Pool, and Babatunde Imokhuede. 2008. "'He Is Now Like a Brother, I Can Even Give Him Some Blood'—Relational Ethics and Material Exchanges in a Malaria Vaccine 'Trial Community' in the Gambia." *Social Science and Medicine* 67:696–707.

Geissler, P. Wenzel, and Sassy Molyneux, eds. 2011. *Evidence, Ethos, and Ethnography: The Anthropology and History of Medical Research in Africa*. Oxford: Berghahn.

Gilson, Lucy, Gill Walt, Kris Heggenhougen, Lucas Owuor-Omondi, Myrtle Perera, David Ross, and Ligia Salazar. 1989. "National Community Health Worker Programs: How Can They Be Strengthened?" *Journal of Public Health Policy* 10, no. 4: 518–32.

Gray, John M. 1940. *A History of the Gambia*. London: Frank Cass and Company.

Greenwood, Brian M., A. K. Bradely, A. M. Greenwood, Peter Byass, K. Jammeh, Kevin Marsh, S. Tulloch, F. S. J. Oldfield, and Richard Hayes. 1987. "Mortality and Morbidity from Malaria among Children in a Rural Area of the Gambia, West Africa." *Transactions of the Royal Society of Tropical Medicine and Hygiene* 81, no. 3: 478–86.

Hansen, Thomas B., and Finn Stepputat. 2001. *States of Imagination: Ethnographic Explorations of the Postcolonial State*. Durham, NC: Duke University Press.

Haswell, Margaret R. 1953. *Economics of Agriculture in a Savannah Village: Report on Three Years' Study in Genieri Village and Its Lands, the Gambia*. Colonial Research Study No. 8. London: HMSO.

Haswell, Margaret R. 1975. *Nature of Poverty*. London: Macmillan.

Havinden, M. A., and D. Meredith. 1993. *Colonialism and Development: Britain and Its Tropical Colonies, 1850–1960*. London: Routledge.

Herbst, Jeffrey. 2000. *States and Power in Africa: Comparative Lessons in Authority and Control*. Princeton, NJ: Princeton University Press.

Hughes, Arnold, and David Perfect. 2006. *A Political History of the Gambia, 1816–1994*. Rochester, NY: University of Rochester Press.

Iliffe, John. 1969. *Tanganyika under German Rule, 1905–1912*. Cambridge: Cambridge University Press.

International Fund of Agricultural Development (IFAD) Report. 2005. *Republic of the Gambia Rural Finance and Community Initiatives Project Interim Evaluation, April*. Loan No 486 GM.

Jarju, Lamin B. S. 2009. "Utilization of 'Swamp' Rice Fields by Members of the Anopheles Gambiae Complex in the Gambia." PhD diss., Durham University.

Jarju, Lamin B. S., Ulrike Fillinger, Clare Green, Vasilis Louca, Silas Majambere, and Steven W. Lindsay. 2009. "Agriculture and the Promotion of Insect Pests: Rice Cultivation in River Floodplains and Malaria Vectors in the Gambia." *Malaria Journal* 8:170. DOI:10.1186/1475–2875–8-170.

Kelly, Ann H. 2011. "The 'Project' of Medical Research: Experimental Publics in the Gambia." In *Differentiating Development: Beyond an Anthropology of Critique*, ed. Thomas Yarrow and Soumhya Venkatasan. Bloomfield, CT: Kumerian Press.

Kelly, Ann H. 2011. "Will He Be There? A Meditation on Immobility and Scientific Labor." *Journal of Cultural Economy* 4, no. 1: 3–10.

Kelly, Ann H., and Uli Beisel. 2011. "Neglected Malarias: The Frontlines and Back Alleys of Global Health." *Biosocieties* 4:71–87.

Lezaun, Javier, and Yuval Millo. 2006. "Regulatory Experiments: Genetically Modified Crops and Financial Derivatives on Trial." *Science and Public Policy* 33, no. 3: 179–90.

Majambere, Silas, Steven W. Lindsay, Clare Green, Balla Kandeh, and Ulrike Fillinger. 2007. "Microbial Larvicides for Malaria Control in the Gambia." *Malaria Journal* 6:76.

Majambere, Silas, Ulrike Fillinger, David R. Sayer, Clare Green, and Steven W. Lindsay. 2008. "Spatial Distribution of Mosquito Larvae and the Potential for Targeted Larval Control in the Gambia." *American Journal of Tropical Medicine and Hygiene* 79, no. 1: 19–27.

Majambere, Silas, Margaret Pinder, Ulrike Fillinger, David Ameh, David J. Conway, Clare Green, David Jeffries, Musa Jawara, Paul J. Milligan, Robert Hutchinson, and Steven W. Lindsay. 2010. "Is Mosquito Larval Source Management Appropriate for Reducing Malaria in Areas of Extensive Flooding in The Gambia? A Cross-over Intervention Trial." *American Journal of Tropical Medicine and Hygiene* 82, no. 2: 176–84.

Malowany, Maureen. 2001. "Introduction." In *British Contributions to Medical Research and Education in Africa after the Second World War*, ed. Lois A. Reynolds and E. M. Tansey. London: Wellcome Trust Centre for the History of Medicine at UCL.

McGregor, Ian A. 1982. "Malaria: Nutritional Implications." *Reviews of Infectious Diseases* 4:798–804.

Menon, A. 1991. "Utilization of Village Health Workers within a Primary Health

Care Programme in the Gambia." *Journal of Tropical Medicine and Hygiene* 94, no. 4: 268–71.

Meredith, David. 1975. "The British Government and Colonial Economic Policy, 1919–39." *Economic History Review* 28:484–99.

Molyneux, Sassy, and P. Wenzel Geissler. 2008. "Ethics and the Ethnography of Medical Research in Africa." *Social Science and Medicine* 67, no. 5: 685–95.

MRC. 2007. *Leading Relevant, Cost-Effective Research: Annual Report of the UK Medical Research Council Laboratories, the Gambia.* London: MRC.

Pálsson, Gisli, and Paul Rabinow. 1999. "Iceland: The Case of a National Human Genome Project." *Anthropology Today* 15, no. 2: 14–18.

Reynolds, Lois A., and E. M. Tansey, eds. *British Contributions to Medical Research and Education in Africa after the Second World War.* London: Wellcome Trust Centre for the History of Medicine at UCL.

Sharma, Aradhana, and Akhil Gupta, eds. 2006. *Anthropology of the State: A Reader.* Oxford: Blackwell.

Snow, Robert W., Kathryn M. Rowan, Steven W. Lindsay, and Brian M. Greenwood. 1988. "A Trial of Bed Nets (Mosquito Nets) as a Malaria Control Strategy in a Rural Area of the Gambia, West Africa." *Transactions of the Royal Society of Tropical Medicine and Hygiene* 82, no. 2: 212–15.

Suffian, Sandra. 2007. *Healing the Land and the Nation: Malaria and the Zionist Project in Palestine, 1920–1947.* Chicago: University of Chicago Press.

Sumberg, James. 1998. "Mixed Farming in Africa: The Search for Order, the Search for Sustainability." *Land Use Policy* 15, no. 4: 293–317.

Tilly, Charles. 1990. *Coercion, Capital, and European States, A.D. 990–1990.* Cambridge, MA: Basil Blackwell.

United Nations Development Programme. 2010. *The Real Wealth of Nations: Pathways to Human Development, Human Development Report.* New York: Palgrave Macmillan.

Webb, James L. A. 1992. "Ecological and Economic Change along the Middle Reaches of the Gambian River, 1945–1985." *African Affairs* 91, no. 365: 543–65.

Welch, Claude E., Jr. 1966. *Dream of Unity: Pan-Africanisms and Political Unification in West Africa.* Ithaca, NY: Cornell University Press.

Wright, Donald R. 1995. "'That Hell-Hole of Yours.'" *American Heritage* 46:47–58.

Wright, Donald R. 2010. *The World and a Very Small Place in Africa: A History of Globalization in Niumi, the Gambia.* 3rd ed. New York: M. E. Sharpe.

CHAPTER 11

Adventures of African Nevirapine:

The Political Biography of a Magic Bullet

Didier Fassin

In 2002 a woman from the township of Alexandra gave birth to a healthy boy in the hospital of Soweto. This ordinary event in a country where almost 2,500 children are born every day would not be noteworthy had not the baby already had, at the very moment he came into the world, a long history, which made his birth a small secular miracle for those who were aware of it. His mother's life had been particularly grim. As a child she was frequently abused by a close relative, as an adolescent she was the victim of her stepfather's sexual violence, and as a young woman she survived in the city by prostituting herself. When she finally found some economic security and affective stability, she became pregnant and gave birth to a girl. At the age of nine months, her daughter fell sick. AIDS was the diagnosis. The mother and her boyfriend had blood tests. Both were HIV positive. Their relationship became difficult and, shortly after the baby's death, they broke up. The woman started to work in a home-based care program for the terminally ill patients of her neighborhood. She also became involved in the Treatment Action Campaign, a national movement fighting for universal access to antiretroviral drugs. At that time the South African government was still reluctant to provide treatment to patients. Well connected among AIDS activists, she was recruited to participate in a clinical trial and her medical condition dramatically improved. When she became pregnant a second time, she was included in a protocol for the prevention of mother-to-child transmission, consisting of a single dose of drug given to the mother during delivery and to the child immediately after birth. A few weeks later, blood tests confirmed that the boy was not infected. Although he was officially given a Christian name, his mother affectionately nicknamed him Nevirapine after the wonder drug that she thought had spared him the infection.

This non-nucleoside reverse transcriptase inhibitor was at the time considered to be a major breakthrough, not so much for its use in the treatment of AIDS patients, because of its troublesome side effects, but more so for its use in the prevention of mother-to-child transmission of HIV, at least in developing countries. During the second half of the 1990s, substantial progress had been made in the reduction of the so-called vertical transmission of the virus after the AIDS Clinical Trials Group (ACTG) trial in the United States and France had demonstrated that two-thirds of infections could be avoided when zidovudine was given to mothers during pregnancy and to children after birth (Connor et al. 1994). However, this preventive procedure remained difficult to implement and too expensive for poor countries, which explains the enthusiastic interest raised by the HIVNET 012 trial conducted in Uganda with a single dose of nevirapine to mothers and children that claimed to reduce by half the proportion of infected babies (Guay et al. 1999). It was estimated that 600,000 mother-to-child transmission cases were occurring each year, 90 percent of them on the African continent (UNAIDS 1998). The rate of vertical transmission in the absence of treatment was between 15 and 30 percent, reaching 30 to 45 percent in the case of prolonged breast-feeding (De Cock et al. 2000). The prospect of reducing by half this proportion with a simple (one dose for the mother, one dose for the baby) and cheap (US$4 per treatment) protocol aroused hope, suggesting that prevention could be generalized to all HIV-positive pregnant women or even to all pregnant women, irrespective of HIV status (Marseille et al. 1999). Actually this new preventive model only concerned the developing world, and more specifically sub-Saharan Africa, where the epidemic was extremely preoccupying, since more effective strategies had been established for Western countries: this explains why the regimen was often termed *suboptimal* (Gibb and Tess 1999). Implying distinct normative foundations for medicine in rich and poor countries, single-dose nevirapine therefore raised ethical issues similar to those previously discussed around other clinical trials designed for the reduction of mother-to-child transmission: although zidovudine had been proved effective in this prevention, all but one experimental regimen in developing countries were still using placebo in order to establish the efficacy of the drug in this specific context (Lurie and Wolfe 1997). However, the case implied difficult ethical questions beyond the trial: on the one hand, one could plead for an ideal universal ethics, since a much more effective combination of drugs existed, but their cost and use made them almost entirely inapplicable in African countries; on the other hand, one could defend a realistic differentiated ethics, considering how simple and cheap the new regimen was. In fact, this discussion was hardly opened, because nevirapine imposed itself—or was imposed—as the only possible, if not the best, solution, in spite of concerns raised from the beginning about probable viral resistance to the drug.

One country soon became the epicenter of a global controversy about nevirapine: South Africa. There were several reasons for this. First, the epidemic there had reached an unprecedented level: with almost five million infected persons, a 20 percent seroprevalence rate in the adult population, and a twenty-year estimated decrease of life expectancy in the next two decades, the situation was more serious than anywhere else in the world (Dorrington et al. 2001). Second, the government had recently been involved in a series of scandals related to the infection, promoting a fake cure named virodene, contesting the viral origin of the disease, and denouncing the toxicity of antiretroviral drugs (Schneider 2002). Third, the biomedical community was forming a solid network of well-equipped public research institutions and hospitals, staffed by highly qualified doctors and scientists, with no equivalent on the rest of the continent, thus allowing the development of clinical trials (Thiers et al. 2007). This unique configuration, inscribed in the immediate post-apartheid era, explains the sense of emergency, the atmosphere of controversy, and the expectations of medicine, respectively, around the epidemic.

It is in this context that the new drug was announced in South Africa during the second half of 1999. It was immediately presented in the specialized circles and the public sphere as a "magic bullet" (Brandt 1987) for developing countries: inexpensive, simple, effective. Hence the incredulity of physicians, researchers, activists, and journalists when they realized that the South African government and its official organization, the Medicines Control Council, did not share their enthusiasm, asked for more evidence, and, after the death of several women involved in a clinical trial with nevirapine, even interrupted the experimentation. This led to the most impassioned disputes in the media, in the streets, and in the courts that the country has experienced since the end of apartheid. In South Africa the Treatment Action Campaign, which was well connected with international nongovernmental organizations such as Médecins sans Frontières and ACT UP, publicly accused the government of criminal behavior. Although officially behind President Thabo Mbeki, the major party of the African National Congress (ANC) was divided. Opposition leaders, who had been more or less involved in the previous regime, saw the opportunity to regain credibility by denouncing their rivals in power. The Congress of South African Trade Unions (COSATU) backed the activists, while the National Association of People Living with HIV and AIDS (NAPWA) supported the government. Most physicians and researchers defended immediate drug access, whereas many public health specialists expressed concerns about the capacity of the health system to implement such a program on a wide scale. Within a few months, nevirapine became the subject of a major controversy in both political and scientific realms. It is this battle that involved tens of thousands of human lives that I want to recount.

The historian of science Lorraine Daston (2000) opens an illuminating perspective on this story with her "biographies of scientific objects," considering such objects as "simultaneously real and historical," thus avoiding the pitfalls of naïve realism as well as extreme constructionism. In a similar vein, I would like to reconstitute elements of the biography of a biomedical object. Nevirapine is a molecule active against reverse transcriptase, the enzyme that is specific to retroviruses. Soon after the publication of the results of the Uganda clinical trial, however, it appeared to be much more than a biochemical element (Phillips 2009). It embodied the hopes of patients and doctors, symbolized for the activists the stubbornness and cruelty of the government, and epitomized for the government the irresponsibility and hostility of the activists. Its scientific life became political, revealing tensions and divisions inherited from the recent past of the country and still profoundly inscribed in the present (Fassin 2007). It is therefore the inseparably scientific and political biography of nevirapine I am interested in. I will first narrate how the drug came to be at the center of a national social drama, revealing the tension between two ethics, which in the end can be understood as two politics. I will then trace its career between medical circles and the public sphere, in a context of uncertainty in science and conspiracy in politics. Finally, I will follow the recent developments of knowledge and recommendations for the prevention of mother-to-child transmission leading to increasingly cautious and restrictive indications of nevirapine, giving the final word to politics.

The rise and fall of the wonder drug is the fate of many treatments in various domains of medicine once believed to be magic bullets but later rejected because of serious side effects. And it is the life of science to continuously challenge its truths of the day and establish new ones, frequently forgetting its previous certainties. The singularity of the South African story of nevirapine resides, however, in the confusion it revealed between government and science, the intensity of the affects it mobilized, the violence of the reactions it aroused, and, in the end, the crisis of the state and of the nation it provoked.

A Social Drama

On April 7, 2001, the auditorium of the Humanities Building at the prestigious University of Witwatersrand in Johannesburg was the scene of a social drama that rarely occurs in academia. This was on the final day of the AIDS in Context Conference, which had brought together social scientists from southern Africa to discuss the historical, political, cultural, and social dimensions of the epidemic, until then generally neglected, the emphasis having previously been exclusively focused on its biomedical aspects. One year prior, the country had suddenly become aware of the gravity of the sanitary situation, with the publication of alarming morbidity and mortality data by the Ministry of Health and the Medical Research Council, but the country had also become conscious of the tensions raised by the interpretation of the disease and its treatment, with the convening of a presidential panel held in parallel to the official International AIDS Conference in Durban and attended by both orthodox and heterodox specialists.

On the last day of the conference, a round table was dedicated to AIDS policies and the politics of AIDS. The first speaker, Zackie Achmat, chair of the Treatment Action Campaign, launched a virulent attack against the government and accused those in charge of the management of the epidemic of being responsible for a "Holocaust against the poor." Citing the case of a recently deceased woman who had left three infected children behind, he denounced these officials as "accomplices in the deaths of all these children." His speech was warmly applauded. Taking the floor immediately after him, Nono Simelela, director of the National AIDS Program, affirmed, her voice broken by sobs, that being a gynecologist and a mother, she felt profoundly hurt by this incrimination. Having recalled the legacy of apartheid in the health system, she asserted that she did not want to repeat the mistakes of the past and had to assume full responsibility for her action, both in terms of efficacy and justice, adding that it was "a question of equity and ethics." At the end of her talk, she left the auditorium without waiting for questions.

This dispute could have been seen as one more episode in the harsh battle between AIDS activists and AIDS officials in South Africa. For at least four years, polemics had arisen on numerous occasions, and the recent shift of the government toward the scientific dissidence emanating from the United States resulted in more aggressiveness and hostility on both sides. However, this unusual scenario in an academic environment and the two orators' surprising notes of sincerity gave me—and many others in the audience that day—the feeling that we had experienced a historical moment. Rather it was a sort of epiphany: the revelation that the battle was not merely truth against error, ethics versus the unethical, as it was usually represented, but that two truths and two ethics were at stake. In terms of scientific truths, was single-dose nevirapine an effective and innocuous intervention or should it be still tested to make sure the side effects, including viral resistance, would not put a strain on the future of the epidemic? In terms of political ethics, was the priority to consider individual saved lives due to the provision of single-dose nevirapine or should one be concerned about the risks of increasing the social and racial divide across the country by an insufficiently prepared program?

The results of the HIVNET 012 trial in Uganda had been announced less than two years earlier. In July 1999 at the Sixth Conference on Retroviruses and Opportunistic Infections in Chicago, a team of researchers led by Dr. Laura Guay from the Johns Hopkins University School of Medicine made a sensation by declaring that a single dose of nevirapine given to HIV-infected mothers and to their newborn babies reduced the risk of vertical transmission by 47 percent. This efficacy was all the more impressive since, first, it was compared with zidovudine, which was then considered the best prevention for the developing world, and second, it was measured for breast-feeding women, a well-known risk factor for late infection of children through maternal milk. Considering that it was not only simple and effective but also cheap ("around US$4.00 wholesale cost") and safe ("well-tolerated"), the conclusion was obvious: "single-dose nevirapine given to the mother and the child is likely to be one of the few deliverable and sustainable strategies for prevention of perinatal HIV transmission in resource-poor settings" (Guay et al. 1999). On July 15, the good news was released in the South African press. The next day, Manto Tshabalala-Msimang, the health minister, announced she would go to Uganda for a direct appraisal of the efficacy of the drug, commenting that it could "represent an unbelievable opportunity for our country to save lives" (SAPA, July 16, 1999). Soon after, the director of the perinatal unit at Soweto's Baragwanath Hospital, Professor James McIntyre, declared that the prospect of the new treatment was "very dramatic," since it "could well be a solution for us" (*IOL*, July 17, 1999). One learned then that the SAINT trial, including nevirapine compared to other therapies, had started a few weeks earlier in several South African hospitals and that the implementation of the new program on a large scale would depend on the results of this clinical experimentation. Things seemed to be on their way.

In March 2000, as activists were pressuring the government to inaugurate a national policy, the specialists involved in the trial called for caution, with Professor Marian Kruger reminding that "we can't say for sure until we've analyzed the results" (*IOL*, March 22, 2000). In April the minister announced the deaths of five women in a distinct trial, STC, conducted with nevirapine, in association with two other drugs, and designed by Triangle Pharmaceuticals, a company described as being from the United States, leading a prominent figure in the Pan-Africanist Congress, Patricia de Lille, to denounce foreign researchers "exploiting" African patients (*SAPA*, April 6, 2000). After the great expectations generated by the wonder drug, suspicion was now growing about the ethical conditions of the trials and the potential risks of nevirapine, whose liver toxicity was well documented. In July, just before the Thirteenth International AIDS Conference, the executive director of UNAIDS, Peter Piot, admitted that "more needs to be known and done before nevirapine can be safely administered on a wide scale in many countries," especially since evidence of resistance to the drug already existed in Uganda (*SAPA*, July 7, 2000); meanwhile, the German pharmaceutical company Boehringer Ingelheim declared that "the amazing drug," in Professor Salim Abdool Karim's words, would be given free for five years in the prevention of mother-to-child transmission (*Daily News*, July 11, 2000). As enthusiasm was rapidly increasing, the results of the SAINT trial presented at the conference seemed to confirm the lessons of HIVNET. The press triumphantly announced that nevirapine could save the lives of 20,000 babies per year, a figure that mushroomed in the media, soon reaching 30,000 (*Star*, November 30, 2000) and then 50,000 (*SAPA*, December 14, 2001) young victims spared.

In this context there seemed to be no good reason for the government to continue delaying the general implementation of the drug. Facing constant attacks from indignant activists and confronted with the increasing convergence of political opposition, the Medicines Control Council agreed in November 2000 to allow the distribution of the drug under the condition that the drug company would monitor the after trial for viral resistance, whereas the Health Department affirmed two months later it would extend its delivery to eighteen hospitals (SAPA, January 26, 2001). In April 2001, however, when the AIDS in Context Conference was held, the final approval of the government was still to be given, as Boehringer Ingelheim did not display any evidence of accepting the condition of the Medicines Control Council, while physicians and scientists appeared to be increasingly confident about its benefits (*Cape Argus*, April 7, 2001). At this point not only were the activists pressuring public authorities but also the health secretaries in several provinces, Gauteng and KwaZulu-Natal in particular, were threatening to distribute nevirapine in their hospitals without waiting any longer for the authorization of the national state, which replied by threatening them with legal actions (*Star*, April 10, 2001). From that point onward tensions were at their peak.

The altercation between Zackie Achmat and Nono Simelela thus took place at this juncture, when positions, although still confused and evolving, were in the process of becoming congealed and radicalized. Two sides were progressively forming, which were increasingly unlikely to converge or even converse. On the one hand, prudent declarations about the new drug were turning into confident affirmation of a decisive discovery. On the other hand, hesitations about its possible side effects evolved into explicit mistrust toward its defenders. The confrontation between the charismatic AIDS activist and the stern AIDS official not only revealed this changing landscape but also crystallized it. The dramaturgy of the public dispute at the University of Witwatersrand echoed a broader social drama occurring in South Africa at that time: the local scene reproduced and illuminated the national scenery. Following Victor Turner (1980, 150), we can interpret this conflict as the "expression of a deeper division of interests and loyalties than appears on the surface," and it therefore unveils "some dominant cleavages in the widest set of relevant social relations to which the parties in conflict belong." The dispute over nevirapine uncovers and reopens a profound breach in the idealized community of the post-apartheid era. Suspicions and accusations that one thought definitively buried reappear with nevirapine serving as a pretext for the manifestation of virulent dissensions. Behind the suspicions that the drug might be dangerous for the population and, symmetrically, the accusations that deferring its use could be assimilated to genocide, there are the wounds of the past.

The Politics of Science

The weekly *Mail and Guardian* is considered to be the most serious reference in South African journalism. Liberal oriented, it has been deeply engaged in the cause of AIDS since the beginning of the epidemic and has constantly challenged the dissident statements and hesitating policies of the government. Yet on April 7, 2000, as the world was learning of the heterodox affinities of the president who announced he would convene a panel with orthodox and heterodox scientists, the journal devoted an entire page to the AIDS situation with three articles written by renowned journalists whose curious association only added to the already extreme confusion over the epidemic and, more specifically, nevirapine.

The first article, under the headline "It's the Trials, Not the Drugs," referred to the decision of the minister of health to interrupt the clinical trials with nevirapine after the deaths of the five women who participated in one of them. "Tshabalala-Msimang spoke in Parliament of a 'problem with the proliferation of clinical trials,'" wrote David Le Page. "Her speech suggested that South Africa has proved to be a fertile source of trial subjects for international drug companies, but that South Africans are unlikely to benefit in the long run from being guinea pigs for the rest of the world." The journalist explained that the scientists in charge of the SAINT trial, in particular Professor Jerry Coovadia, were distancing themselves from the incriminated STC trial, thus appearing to confirm the existence of questionable experimentation being conducted in the country by some of their colleagues. The second article, titled "Furore over Testing on Humans," started with these words: "A leading United States university has been using human guinea pigs to test the rate at which HIV can be transferred from infected to uninfected partners—without appraising the uninfected partners of the risks involved." Evoking the recent editorial of the renowned *New England Journal of Medicine*, Belinda Beresford quoted the editor in chief, Marcia Angell, who, after having criticized the study carried out by researchers from Johns Hopkins University, defended equal ethical standards for research in rich and poor countries: "Any other position could lead to the exploitation of people in developing countries in order to conduct research that could not be performed in sponsoring countries." Such a declaration by an authoritative scientific personality had not passed unnoticed among medical researchers, but it was now put to the fore of the South African public sphere, revealing to large audiences dubious practices in clinical experimentation. The third article, which had for its title "AIDS a Threat to Democracy," presented a report on the situation of the epidemic in the world, underlining in particular the risk of demographic, economic, and political destabilization in developing countries and even more specifically in South Africa. "The CIA has warned that the HIV/AIDS pandemic sweeping sub-Saharan Africa will lay waste to the ruling political and military elite in the region, provoking damaging power struggles over scarce state resources," commented Jaspreet Kindra. That it was the U.S. intelligence agency predicting such catastrophic perspectives was not trivial for most readers in South Africa. It implied an invisible and threatening presence.

The juxtaposition of the three articles therefore suggested a global project and gaze over the African continent emerging in large part from the United States, with the convergent strategies of drug companies, research teams, and secret services that transformed South Africans into experimental subjects and observed populations. Although nevirapine was explicitly mentioned only in the first article, it was in the background of the second, through the theme of the unethical clinical trials, and of the third, because of the links it established between the worlds of medicine and intelligence. The heated debates about the new drug, the doubts permanently raised by health officials about its efficacy and innocuousness, the virulent attacks led by the activists against the government, accused of passivity if not of crime against humanity for not implementing a national program, all contributed to making nevirapine not only a public concern but also a familiar topic. Consequently, suggesting, as the journalists did, that Africans could be exploited as guinea pigs for the rest of the world, possibly as part of a broader plot, immediately made sense for most people in relation to nevirapine.

Besides, in this same period, a story was recounted by a journalist, Edward Hooper (1999), about the origin of the AIDS epidemic, which he attributed, jointly with the famous evolutionary biologist William Hamilton, to the polio immunization campaigns conducted in Africa during the 1950s with an experimental vaccine grown in cells derived from chimpanzee kidneys. As the Thirteenth International AIDS Conference opened in Durban, on July 7, 2000, the weekly *Mail and Guardian* published as a cover story a three-page article under the headline "The True Origin of AIDS," thus appearing to provide an official credence to the idea of a man-made epidemic. If scientists had accidentally provoked the emergence and dissemination of HIV as a result of an experiment on Africans, why would nevirapine not be the latest case of them being used as "guinea pigs" for medical research? Again, this theory, since then abandoned, was given remarkable credibility by a newspaper considered an intellectual and moral authority on AIDS.

This configuration, of which this series of articles offers just an illustration, can be partially inscribed in the recent transformation of clinical trials, which Adriana Petryna (2009, 89) analyzes, with its externalization of the search for "human subjects." But the case of nevirapine under study is different in two ways. First, the clinical trials I am referring to are large international trials almost exclusively funded in the United States by the National Institutes of Health, even when the researchers are Africans or Europeans: therefore, nevirapine is not only globally present but also publicly exposed. Second, the signification of these trials in the South African environment where I discuss them exceeds the scientific and economic realm: as is shown by the development of conspiracy theories, it is also enshrined in profound political and historical networks.

At the time of the disputes over the benefits and risks of nevirapine, a trial was proceeding in Pretoria High Court. The accused was Dr. Wouter Basson, a physician frequently referred to as "Doctor Death" in the South African press. The final hearings of the Truth and Reconciliation Commission in 1998 had revealed the existence of the so-called Project Coast, a secret chemical and biological warfare program created under the apartheid regime with the objective of inventing and testing new weapons to eliminate enemies of the white supremacist regime and also to eradicate the African, that is, black, population of the country (Burger and Gould 2002). Among many other deadly inventions, anthrax was used against political opponents, cholera served to poison wells in refugee camps, and sterilizing oral contraceptives were under study for African women. Each day the accounts of the trial in the press brought to light new revelations about the program and its links with the United States, Britain, and Israel. In the same period, another plot was discovered. It concerned the infamous paramilitary group Vlakplaas, whose leader, Eugene de Cock, envisaged disseminating HIV among African men via infected prostitutes from Johannesburg (Carter 2006). Most of these programs, developed in the 1980s and 1990s, that is, in the dying years of the apartheid regime, remained experiments and/or mere fantasies. However, their coverage, as well as that of several similar narratives, in the media lent a grim background to the nevirapine controversy that blurred the border between the factual and the imaginary and made conspiratorial ideas possible. That drug companies could manipulate South

Africans as guinea pigs to test drugs, and that foreign researchers and agencies could serve as accomplices of the plot was not far-fetched for those who knew, more frequently from rumors than through the press, about much more dreadful plans that had been documented. People I interviewed in the townships as well as scholars I met in academe would often refer to these plans. Conspiracy theories were nourished by revelations of real plots and expressions of enduring doubts. A climate of suspicion enveloped the whole question of AIDS.

In this context, biomedical science had a difficult time making its truth audible, even more so since this truth was not entirely established. If the Bangkok CDC trial with formula feeding (Shaffer et al. 1999) and the Ivory Coast CDC trial with breast-feeding mothers (Wiktor et al. 1999) had proved the efficacy of zidovudine provided during several weeks before birth and, above all, if the Uganda HIVNET 012 trial (Guay et al. 1999) had demonstrated the benefit of single-dose nevirapine, much was yet to be known about the feasibility of scaling up these measures to a regional or national level and about the long-term consequences of these drugs, particularly in terms of viral resistance. The report of a panel convened by the World Health Organization in March 2000 was clear on the subject (UNAIDS 2000): "There is currently insufficient information to recommend wide-scale implementation of nevirapine for mother-to-child transmission prevention." Similarly, all the scientific reviews published during this period were extremely prudent, clearly distinguishing the situation of "developed countries," where antenatal testing could be generalized, multiple drugs could be used during pregnancy, cesarean section could be practiced at birth, and breast-feeding could be replaced by formula feeding, versus "developing countries" where none of these conditions were met and simplified protocols had to be implemented as a substitution without real assurance of the long-term benefits (Mofenson and McIntyre 2000). Even later assessments with new results of clinical experimentations, including the SAINT trial in South Africa (Moodley et al. 2003), remained cautious as the evidence of viral resistance became increasingly problematic (Cunningham et al. 2002; Jourdain et al. 2003). Thus, as late as four years after the initial publications and two years after the court case started by the activists against the South African government, AIDS specialists continued to express circumspection about the best strategy to promote (Scotland et al. 2003). Certainly, since the end of 2000, the World Health Organization had been recommending short courses of antiretroviral drugs in late pregnancy and during labor but always mentioning the possible immediate toxicity, especially for the baby, and long-term potential resistance of the virus induced by single-dose nevirapine, which would have severe consequences for mothers or infected children when they would need to be treated (WHO 2001, 2002). In sum, scientists and officials within the international community of AIDS specialists were both optimistic and careful about the wonder drug.

The contrast was striking with the public discourse of physicians and activists, generally followed by journalists, during the same period. The initial reaction after the announcement of the results of the HIVNET 012 trial in 1999 was of enthusiasm, but it soon turned into indignation when the South African minister of health interrupted nevirapine regimens after the deaths of the five women in the STC trial; this decision being interpreted as one more piece of evidence of the government's dissidence. In July 2000 one of the most prominent scientists in the field, Dr. Glenda Gray, who was involved in the SAINT trial at Baragwanath Hospital, declared in a public event that she had "good news for South Africa and the world," proudly insisting that it came from "studies run in Africa by African scientists" and dramatically calling nevirapine "a vaccine to prevent mother-to-child transmission." Two months later, she confirmed in another press meeting that "data are clear: nevirapine is safe and effective" and that "there is no resistance," even considering this question as "irrelevant" (*Mail and Guardian*, September 8, 2000). Progressively, any question regarding side effects and viral resistance was erased to give way to the representation of the magic bullet. Evoking a religious nurse who was coordinating the program Born to Live at St. Mary's Hospital near Durban to prevent transmission from mother to child, a journalist commented that "unlike government officials who have questioned the toxicity, efficacy and use of nevirapine, Sister Jones has no reservations about the use of the drug. 'Nevirapine is a godsend,' she says" (*Mail and Guardian*, March 1, 2002). Most media thus presented the drug as miraculous. Its efficacy seemed absolute: newspaper articles generally implied that "the trial was a lifesaver" for uninfected babies born to infected mothers, forgetting that the rate of infection at birth without treatment is about one in five (*Star*, July 8, 2002). Similarly, its innocuousness appeared to be established: by contrast, delays in the implementation of the program to explore risks of viral resistance were said to "kill ten babies a day" (*Independent*, March 1, 2002). In the context of the emergency of the epidemic and confronted by the necessity of imposing the new drug against the bad will of the government, researchers and doctors transform their scientific uncertainties into public certainties. Explaining medical facts to general audiences is always a process of translation, which involves the simplification of complex realities and the consolidation of provisional knowledge. In South Africa, this translation had become political.

The Last Word

On the June 24, 2004, the French National AIDS Council published its recommendations on the management of HIV-infected pregnant women in developing countries (Conseil national du sida 2004). This consultative institution, of which I had just become the vice president, was created to advise the government on its policies regarding the AIDS epidemic both at home and internationally. Each report on a given subject followed months of exploring available bibliography, listening to world experts, and defining guidelines. This *Avis suivi de recommandations*, which I had not contributed to and discovered when taking my new position, was considered to be important because of the involvement of French research in several pioneering programs of prevention of mother-to-child transmission, most notably in Thailand and the Ivory Coast.

After having reviewed the side effects of single-dose nevirapine, the document asserted: "if the introduction of simplified regimens of prevention have constituted an important step toward the awareness of the importance of combating AIDS, it does not suffice anymore." It went on to affirm: "it has become unacceptable to expose pregnant women and infected children to the risk of resistances, which compromise the future efficacy of treatment." Actually, besides immediate toxic effects, such as hepatitis and rashes, which could exceptionally cause the death of women, the main problem was resistance of the virus not only to nevirapine but also to the whole class of non-nucleoside transcriptase reverse inhibitors, which include some of the most commonly used antiretroviral drugs in developing countries. Nevirapine was regarded as particularly problematic, since a single mutation of the virus leads to a high level of resistance, as opposed to zidovudine, which needs several mutations to confer resistance. Only two years after the initial publication, the pioneer HIVNET 012 trial in Uganda indicated respectively 20 percent and 46 percent of viral resistance among mothers and children after single-dose nevirapine, although the stability of this resistance over time was not clearly known (Eshleman et al. 2001). Based on these results and others, the French National AIDS Council consequently recommended the development of multidrug regimens, which were more effective and less problematic in the long run.

In fact, the National AIDS Council was for the most part following the new guidelines promoted by the World Health Organization (2004), only making more explicit the questioning of single-dose nevirapine. This signaled the beginning of a progressive shift from monotherapy to multi-therapy, even in developing countries, which were thus considered to fall under the same ethical principles as developed countries, a position that had been previously criticized for failing to take into account the specificities of the Global South in terms of financial and human resources. From then on, what was good for the Global North was good for the Global South. Single-dose nevirapine could only remain as a second or even third best choice, far behind the complex regimens adapted from rich countries.

At the Fifteenth International AIDS Conference in Bangkok, where the latest results of the clinical trials and the new official recommendations were announced in July 2004, South African Health Minister Manto Tshabalala-Msimang exulted: Was the World Health Organization not confirming the risks of single-dose nevirapine, which her department had contested precisely because of potential viral resistance? Certainly her denial of the role of HIV in the disease and her promotion of the African potato as a treatment did not vouch for her scientific rigor (*IOL*, September 1, 2003). But she seized the opportunity to recall that monitoring of viral resistance was the condition the Medicines Control Council had imposed on the drug company to obtain its authorization. As the authority of the government had been challenged not only by international drug companies but also by U.S. funding institutions and medical researchers allied with local scholars and activists, she did not miss the occasion to say that her ministry may have been right in raising doubts about the drug and also to reestablish the sovereignty of the state. Asked about these developments, the spokesperson for the Treatment Action Campaign, Mark Heywood, soberly commented that "there was nothing startling in the report, as it had been known for four or five years that nevirapine by itself was not the most efficient medication for the prevention of mother-to-child transmission," but he added that "monotherapy using nevirapine was better than nothing at all" (*SAPA*, July 12, 2004). Yesterday a godsend, nevirapine had become a stopgap.

Yet this change from a maximalist assertion to a minimalist affirmation was never acknowledged as such by physicians and activists. There was no public recognition that medical truths were not eternal and that the confidence with which nevirapine had been presented as a magic bullet was excessive considering the problems it posed. No one apologized for having accused the South African government of crime, infanticide, and Holocaust because it did not implement a treatment that was in fact much more problematic than what was initially thought. Symmetrically, no one admitted that the president and his health minister had made crucial errors in the management of the epidemic with serious consequences for the South African population. There was no independent assessment of the incapacity of the government to address this major crisis. Nevirapine had been at the epicenter of a political war in the AIDS world: its waning did not signify peace.

The controversy swirling around nevirapine had nevertheless a merit. The emphasis on the issue of viral resistance and future treatment failure for mothers and their possibly infected children unveiled an unspoken fact: the lack of consideration for women, with the initial focus of trials and programs being almost exclusively on newborns. The objective was to reduce new infantile cases, not to treat more patients; the rhetoric was about saving babies, not alleviating the suffering of mothers. This logic has a long history in public health, which has always justified interest in maternal health by the benefits for the offspring. It was revealed by the cynical statement the president's spokesman, Parks Mankahlana, made in an interview with the international journal *Science*: "A country like ours has to deal with that," he was quoted as saying. "That mother is going to die and that HIV negative child will be an orphan. Who is going to bring that child up? It's the state. That's resources, you see" (*Sunday Independent*, July 15, 2000). The reasoning was cruel, but it had some tragic reality in the conception of most trials.

In fact regimens in the late 1990s and early 2000s did not necessarily include antiretroviral treatment of the infected mothers, since the clinical trials were limited to preventing mother-to-child transmission. The emergency concerned the future generation. Significantly the authors of the 2004 recommendations made public by the French National AIDS Council had to reemphasize the obligation to treat women, although it had by that time become part of most trials. But of course, the problem was even more complicated, since the single-dose nevirapine regimen did not only passively neglect mothers: it also actively compromised the efficacy of their future treatment. The implications were all the more tragic since the resistance of the virus was not expressed against only nevirapine but concerned its whole family of antiretroviral drugs, which were precisely the most commonly used in developing countries. This, and the similar problem for infected children, albeit in much smaller proportions because of the low transmission rate, became the crucial issue, which, in the end, condemned nevirapine as a single treatment. Having been considered a magic bullet in reproductive health, it was viewed as a harmful medicine for women. This shift thus revealed that the politics of AIDS had long been more a question of generation than an issue about gender.

The wonder drug died a natural death. Not that nevirapine disappeared. It remained in the antiretroviral pharmacopeia, often in association with others, but the regimen that had been boasted as so simple, effective, and inexpensive progressively became past history. Single-dose nevirapine is now a solution for the poorest who, due to a lack of infrastructures or funds, cannot afford the complex multiple-drug regimens and will have to continue to have it rather than "nothing at all." The most recent clinical trials conducted in Africa with women and children who have been exposed to single-dose nevirapine and have later needed treatment confirm the existence of high proportions of viral resistances and treatment failures leading to complex and expensive multiple-drug therapies. Commenting on these trials, the authors of the editorial "Preventing Mother-to-Child Transmission of HIV" (Lallemant and Jourdain 2010) in the *New England Journal of Medicine* observe that they represent a "paradigm shift away from interventions incorporating single-dose nevirapine to interventions comprising highly active antiretroviral drugs." They still admit that "in resource-limited settings, where many women still present late for antenatal care and too few are screened for CD4+ cell count, single-dose nevirapine will most likely remain an important component of the toolkit for the prevention of mother-to-child transmission." But ten years before, one was rejoicing about this possibility. Now one laments it, pleading for new strategies with long duration treatment associating several substances obviously at a higher cost: exactly the opposite of what had been the dream of nevirapine. The drug remains, but the wonder has gone.

However, I would not like to leave the reader under the impression that, at the end of the day, nevirapine was much ado about nothing. In the early 2000s, when the regimens experimented in Europe and North America for the prevention of mother-to-child transmission were so costly and complex, one can understand the expectations raised by the inexpensive and simple procedure tested in Uganda, especially if one thinks about the millions of infected women and the rate of transmission of at least one in five babies on the African continent. Enthusiastic researchers and activists certainly shut their eyes to the predictable viral resistances and treatment failures (identified quite early in scientific publications), but they contributed, by the continuous pressures they exerted on public authorities and the pharmaceutical industry, to put prevention on the political agenda (even leading to new ethical principles reflected in the multiple-drug regimens now recommended). Symmetrically, the reluctance of the government cannot be attributed only to judicious precaution (which still existed among many I met in the health administration) but must also be considered as a result of its cognitive dissidence (at least among certain members of the cabinet). Just as one could say that during the 1832 cholera epidemic the wrong belief of the hygienists (who adhered to the anticontagionism paradigm) had good effects on public health (through the improvement of the sanitary conditions of cities, since they assumed that lack of hygiene was the source of infection and not human contact), one could assert that the incorrect evaluation of viral resistance problems by researchers and activists had positive consequences both immediately (reducing transmission even if this had a medical cost for mothers and infected children) and in the long term (challenging ethical relativism in developing countries). However, whether medicine and its champions learned prudence and modesty from the refutation of their certainties remains an open question.

———————

The little boy named Nevirapine in my initial story had received single-dose nevirapine at birth: he was thought to be the miraculous child of the announced magic bullet. Yet the fact that he was not infected was more likely the result of chance than of the drug: had he not benefited from any prevention, his probability of not having been infected was four out of five. But having received single-dose nevirapine had reduced by half the risk of him being among the one baby in five developing AIDS: this probability had therefore decreased to one out of ten for him. However, if he had unfortunately been infected, the prospect of treatment failure because of viral resistance induced by single-dose nevirapine at birth would have been multiplied threefold. This calculation with alternatively hopeful (diminished risk of infection) and grim (augmented risk of resistance) outcomes indicates the complexity of the analysis of potential benefits and dangers related to the use of nevirapine. But this difficult question of evaluation of dangers and benefits and even this possible dilemma between a risk associated with abstention and a risk caused by action could still be solved by a combination of mathematical models and ethical principles. Much more complicated, however, were the political issues that it raised or crystallized, reawakening wounds of the past. The disputes were not only about scientific truths: they were also about historical ones.

Attempting to make sense of the story of nevirapine, one should avoid two pitfalls: localism and anachronism. On the one hand, drugs have a global life. My South African depiction of the biography of nevirapine only gives its local dimension. There is a larger picture. The National Institutes of Health, the Centers for Disease Control, and major North American universities, as well as multinational pharmaceutical companies, were crucially involved in the funding of the main clinical trials, while USAID, PEPFAR, the Global Fund, and the Bill and Melinda Gates Foundation promoted most prevention of mother-to-child transmission programs. This international backdrop should be taken into account to grasp not only the design of the trials and programs but also the imaginary of uncertainty and suspicion. On the other hand, the temporal reality of the story is even more complex to grasp. It is about the changes occurring in the realm of knowledge as well as in the problematization of issues. When the single-dose regimen was announced as a magic bullet, prevention of mother-to-child transmission in Africa was a depressive desert in which nevirapine appeared as an oasis of hope. Only a few years later, the experience acquired through the multiplication of trials had made it a medical field full of blossoming expectations and emerging deontologies. The relegation of nevirapine to the status of a suboptimal and problematic drug becomes all the more visible to us now that new regimens are available, which are not only more effective and innocuous but which we also regard as possible treatments in spite of their cost and intricacy. Treatments have changed indeed and so have our attitudes toward them. Realizing how imbricated our objective and subjective assessments are invites us to use the utmost prudence in our moral evaluation.

References

Brandt, Allan. 1985. *No Magic Bullet: A Social History of Venereal Disease in the United States since 1880*. New York: Oxford University Press.
Burger, Marléne, and Chandré Gould. 2002. *Secrets and Lies: Wouter Basson and South Africa's Chemical and Biological Warfare Program*. Cape Town: Zebra Press.
Carter, Chiara. 2006. "Is the TRC Threatening to Become a Cold Case?" In *Truth and*

Reconciliation in South Africa: Ten Years On, ed. Charles Villa-Vicencio and Fanie du Toit, 158–63. Claremont, South Africa: New Africa Books.

Connor, Edward, Rhoda Sperling, Richard Gelber et al. 1994. "Reduction of Maternal-Infant Transmission of Human Immunodeficiency Virus Type 1 with Zidovudine Treatment." *New England Journal of Medicine* 331, no. 18: 1173–80.

Conseil national du sida. 2004. *Promouvoir l'accès aux antirétroviraux des femmes enceintes vivant avec le VIH sida dans les pays du Sud*. Paris: CNS.

Cunningham, Coleen, et al. 2002. "Development of Resistance Mutations in Women Receiving Standard Antiretroviral Therapy Who Received Intrapartum Nevirapine to Prevent Perinatal Human Immunodeficiency Virus Type 1 Transmission." *Journal of Infectious Diseases* 186:181–88.

Daston, Lorraine. 2000. "The Coming into Being of Scientific Objects." In *Biographies of Scientific Objects*, ed. Lorraine Daston, 1–14. Chicago: University of Chicago Press.

De Cock, Kevin M., Mary Fowler, Eric Mercier et al. 2000. "Prevention of Mother-to-Child HIV Transmission in Resource-Poor Countries: Translating Research into Policy and Practice." *Journal of the American Medical Association* 283, no. 9: 1175–82.

Dorrington, Rob, Dawn Bourne, Debbie Bradshaw et al. 2001. *The Impact of HIV/ AIDS on Adult Mortality in South Africa*. Cape Town: Medical Research Council.

Eshleman, Susan, Martin Mracna, Laura Guay et al. 2001. "Selection and Fading of Resistance Mutations in Women and Infants Receiving Nevirapine to Prevent HIV-1 Vertical Transmission (HIVNET 012)." *AIDS* 15, no. 15: 1951–57.

Fassin, Didier. 2007. *When Bodies Remember. The Experiences and Politics of AIDS in South Africa*. Berkeley: University of California Press.

Gibb, Diana, and Beatriz Tess. 1999. "Interventions to Reduce Mother-to-Child Transmission of HIV Infection: New Developments and Current Controversies." *AIDS* 13 (suppl. A): S93–S102.

Guay, Laura, Philippa Musoke, Thomas Fleming et al. 1999. "Intrapartum and Neonatal Single-Dose Nevirapine Compared with Zidovudine for Prevention of Mother-to-Child Transmission of HIV-1 in Kampala, Uganda: HIVNET 012 Randomised Trial." *Lancet* 354:795–802.

Hooper, Edward. 1999. *The River: A Journey to the Source of HIV and AIDS*. Boston: Little, Brown.

Jourdain, Gonzague, et al. 2004. "Intrapartum Exposure to Nevirapine and Subsequent Maternal Responses to Nevirapine-Based Antiretroviral Therapy." *New England Journal of Medicine* 351, no. 3: 229–40.

Lallemant, Marc, and Gonzague Jourdain. 2010. "Preventing Mother-to-Child Transmission of HIV: Protecting This Generation and the Next." *New England Journal of Medicine* 363, no. 16: 1570–72.

Lurie, Peter, and Sidney Wolfe. 1997. "Unethical Trials of Interventions to Reduce Perinatal Transmission of the Human Immunodeficiency Virus in Developing Countries." *New England Journal of Medicine* 337, no. 12: 853–56.

Marseille, Elliot, James Kahn, Francis Mmiro et al. 1999. "Cost Effectiveness of Single-Dose Nevirapine Regimen for Mothers and Babies to Decrease Vertical HIV-1 Transmission in Sub-Saharan Africa." *Lancet* 354:803–9.

Mofenson, Lynne, and James McIntyre. 2000. "Advances and Research Directions in the Prevention of Mother-to-Child HIV1 Transmission." *Lancet* 355:2237–44.

Moodley, D., et al. 2003. "A Multicenter Randomized Controlled Trail of Nevirapine Versus a Combination of Zidovudine and Lamivudine to Reduce Intrapartum and Early Postpartum Mother-to-Child Transmission of Human Immunodeficiency Virus Type 1." *Journal of Infectious Diseases* 187:725–35.

Petryna, Adriana. 2009. *When Experiments Travel: Clinical Trials and the Global Search for Human Subjects.* Princeton, NJ: Princeton University Press.

Phillips, Alton. 2009. "The Life Course of Nevirapine and the Culture of Response to the Global HIV and AIDS Pandemic: Travelling in an Emergency." In *The Fourth Wave: Violence, Gender, Culture and HIV in the 21st Century*, ed. Vinh-Kim Nguyen and Jennifer Klot, 189–216. Paris: UNESCO.

Schneider, Helen, and Didier Fassin. 2002. "Denial and Defiance: A Socio-Political Analysis of Aids in South Africa." In "A Year in Review," special issue, *AIDS* 16 (suppl. 4): S45–S51.

Scotland, Graham, et al. 2003. "A Review of Studies Assessing the Costs and Consequences of Interventions to Reduce Mother-to-Child HIV Transmission in Sub-Saharan Africa." *AIDS* 17:1045–52.

Shaffer, Nathan, et al. 1999. "Short-Course Zidovudine for Perinatal HIV1 Transmission in Bangkok, Thailand." *Lancet* 353:773–80.

Thiers, Fabio, Anthony Sinskey, and Ernst Berndt. 2008. "Trends in the Globalization of Clinical Trials." *Nature Reviews Drug Discovery* 7:13–14.

Turner, Victor. 1980. "Social Dramas and Stories about Them." *Critical Inquiry* 7, no. 1: 141–68.

UNAIDS. 1998. *Mother-to-Child Transmission of HIV: Technical Update.* Geneva: UNAIDS.

Wiktor, Stefan, et al. 1999. "Short-Course Oral Zidovudine for Prevention of Mother-to-Child Transmission of HIV1 in Abidjan, Côte d'Ivoire." *Lancet* 353:781–85.

World Health Organization. 2001. *Prevention of Mother-to-Child Transmission of HIV: Report of a Technical Consultation.* Geneva: WHO.

World Health Organization. 2002. *Strategic Approaches to the Prevention of HIV Infection in Infants: Report of a WHO Meeting.* Geneva: WHO.

ULI BEISEL is assistant professor of culture and technology in Africa at Bayreuth University, Germany. Her work is interested in the conditions of coexistence between humans, mosquitoes, and parasites, the ways in which biological resistance reconfigures disease control technologies and practices, and uneven geographies of access to health in sub-Saharan Africa.

DIDIER FASSIN is James Wolfensohn Professor of Social Science at the Institute for Advanced Study and director of studies at the École des Hautes Études en Sciences Sociales. Anthropologist, sociologist, and physician, he was the founding director of the Interdisciplinary Research Institute for Social Sciences and vice president of Médecins Sans Frontières. He is currently president of the French Medical Committee for Exiles. His field of research is political and moral anthropology and he is interested more specifically in various forms of inequalities.

P. WENZEL GEISSLER is professor of social anthropology at the Department of Social Anthropology, University of Oslo, and also works part time as director of research at the Department of Archaeology and Anthropology at Cambridge. He has studied for several years transnational scientific collaboration in medical research in various locations around the continent. His ongoing research focuses on the remains, and memories, of medical science and, in particular, of scientific research stations.

RENE GERRETS is Assistant Professor of Anthropology at the University of Amsterdam. His current research interests include the relation between science and governance and memories generated by biomedical interventions in Tanzania.

ANN H. KELLY is lecturer in anthropology in the Department of Sociology, Philosophy, and Anthropology at the University of Exeter. Her work centers on the practices of public health research, with special attention to the built environment, material artifacts, and affective labors of entomological inquiry in sub-Saharan Africa. She has recently written on the epistemology of makeshift experiments, the disentanglement in human and nonhuman encounters, and the memories of colonial and postcolonial medical research in the tropics.

GUILLAUME LACHENAL is lecturer in history of science at the University Paris Diderot and a fellow of the Institut Universitaire de France. His research is on the history and anthropology of biomedicine in Africa, especially Cameroon. He combines the approaches of science studies, anthropology of health, and colonial and postcolonial studies to examine biopolitics and biosciences in Africa.

JOHN MANTON has conducted fieldwork in Nigeria and Cameroon. His doctoral work in history at Oxford investigated leprosy control in southeastern Nigeria, in its public health, medical research, and missionary manifestations, an investigation that was broadened in postdoctoral work funded by the Wellcome Trust. Subsequent investigations into the relations between agronomy, plant breeding, and nutrition in Nigeria and recollections and remnants of medical research in Cameroon reflect an overarching concern in his work with the interactions between medical research, clinical practice, and welfare and development in Africa from historical and anthropological perspectives.

LOTTE MEINERT is professor of anthropology at the Department of Culture and Society, Aarhus University, Denmark. She is currently visiting scholar at the Anthropology Department at Johns Hopkins University. Meinert leads a research project on recovery after war in northern Uganda, as well as a Center for Cultural Epidemics (EPICENTER). She has carried out long-term fieldwork in Uganda since 1993.

VINH-KIM NGUYEN is a medical anthropologist and an HIV physician. He practices at the Clinique Médicale l'Actuel and in the Emergency Department at the Jewish General Hospital in Montreal. He is a researcher at the Centre de recherches du Centre hospitalier de l'Université de Montréal and is associate professor in the Department of Social and Preventative Medicine at the University of Montreal, where he heads the PhD program in Health Promotion.

BRANWYN POLEYKETT is research associate at the University of Cambridge. Her current research focuses on the historical and anthropological study of scientific capacity building and on the visual representation of plague in Africa.

SUSAN REYNOLDS WHYTE, professor in the Department of Anthropology, University of Copenhagen, carries out anthropological research in East Africa on social efforts to secure well-being under adverse circumstances. Her publications deal with misfortune and uncertainty, the social lives of medicines, disability, and changing kinship practices.

biopolitics, 2–3, 8, 35, 328n23; in Africa, 6–8, 10, 106; colonial, 25; in transnational medical research, 17–18, 29, 315

biosecurity, 105, 106, 118–19, 127, 132

biosociality, 71

Biya, Chantal, 122, 123

blood: compliance to testing of, 250, 252; health care in exchange for, 61–62, 63–65, 121; importance/value of, 113, 120, 134n21

Blood, Hillary, 305

blueprints, architectural, 160–63, 172–73n17

Boehringer, Ingelheim, 339, 340

Bonneuil, Christophe, 83, 300n9, 314

Booth, Christopher, 323, 325

Browne, Stanley G., 93, 94, 97n12

Bti, sprayed to control malaria, 318

building materials, atemporality of, 172n12

Bunting, A. H., 327n16

Burke, Donald, 113

bushmeat, 133n4; testing of blood of, 117; theories on viral hazards of, 105, 118–19, 124–25; criticism of, 126–27; racism in, 120, 135n31

Cameron, Edwin, 213

Cameroon: medical research in, 103–5, 107, 109–19, 132; criticism of, 120–23; and neoliberalization policies, 108–9, 127; public health policies in, 105, 114; avian flu crisis responses, 128–31; to fight HIV epidemic, 123–28

capacity building, 36n3

care: conceptions of, 29–30. *See also* health care

Carson, Rachel, 287, 294

Cassidy, Rebecca, 325

CDC (Center for Disease Control, United States), malaria research cooperation in Tanzania, 185

celebrations, anniversary, 145, 149–53, 158–59, 165

Centre Pasteur du Cameroun (CPC), 110, 113, 114, 115–16, 117, 122, 128

Chang, Y. T., 92

Chantler, Tracey, 173n20

Cheah, Pheng, 253

China, barefoot doctor program in, 329n28

chloroquine, continued use of, 189–90

circumcision, male, to prevent HIV infections, 51–52, 56–57

citizens/citizenship, 3, 18; therapeutic, 275, 277n5

civil servants, 207, 209–12, 220–22, 229–30nn3–4, 330n6, 330n10; and ART, 215–19, 222–29

Clarke, Sabine, 88

class, notions of, 216–17, 230n9

clients of medical research projects, 265–67, 269, 271–72, 276; health care access for, 274–75; noncompliance by, 267–68; patron-client relationships, 269–70, 273

clinical trials: in Africa, 20–21, 37n10, 38n13, 62, 63–64, 66–67; ethical issues, 334–35, 341; patient records, 78–81, 91; social consequences of, 64–65, 67, 71–72

—of HIV drugs/treatments: antiretroviral drugs, 52, 54, 55, 66–71, 333–35, 338–39, 343, 344; criticism of, 341–42, 348–49; TasP, 56, 68–71

—of leprosy drugs, 78, 82–83, 86–88, 90–92, 93–95; of malaria drugs, 185–86, 187–98, 200–201nn3–4; methodology/regulatory protocol of, 37n6, 57, 64, 73n2; multisite/transnational, 22–23, 27, 29–30, 38n13, 70, 146, 171n6; and population trials, 70; of vaccines, 51, 63–64

clofazimine, 78, 88, 92–94, 95

cluster randomized trials, 68, 69–70

Cochrane, Robert, 90, 91, 93, 97n6
Cohen, Myron, 57–58
collaboration in transnational research, 13, 88, 103–5, 113, 115, 146–48, 149–60, 161, 162–69, 171n5, 171n8, 172n13, 172nn15–16, 173n18, 173n20, 184, 186, 321; inequalities in, 20–21, 23–24, 144, 148, 149–50, 166, 172n11
Colonial Development Corporation (Great Britain), projects in Gambia, 313–14, 328n18
colonialism, 304; British, 83–84, 299n1, 307–9, 326n5, 327nn9–11; French, 241; health care/public health in, 83–84, 107–8, 237, 242; legacy of, 240, 241–42, 252–53, 304; medical science in, 14–15, 83, 88, 126
Comaroff, Jean and John, 133, 217
commemoration. *See* memorialization
communities, trial, 63–64, 67
community engagement, and science, 166–69, 173n20, 321
consent procedures, for participation in research programs, 243, 266–67
conspiracy theories, development of, 343–44
CONTACT (transnational malaria research partnership), 181, 185–88, 199, 200; adaptations in, 188, 191; organizational aspects of, 192–98
continuities, and discontinuities, 35
Coovadia, Jerry, 341
Corbin, Alain, 240–41
corporate social responsibility (CSR) activities: malaria control program as part of, 281, 284–91, 299n1, 300n11; in para-statal cooperation projects, 283–84; public engagement with, 289–91, 297–98, 300n7
counseling, in HIV research projects, 265, 266, 267–69, 271
CSR. *See* corporate social responsibility

Dakar, architecture in, 241
dances, epidemics linked to, 130
dapsone, 78, 87, 89
Daston, Lorraine, 336
data: global processing of, 37n7, 146, 171n6; protests against experiments as part of, 293
DDT: sprayed to control malaria, 287, 299–300n6, 322; sprayed to control sleeping sickness, 299n6
De Cock, Eugene, 343
De Lille, Patricia, 339
Delaporte, Eric, 112
democracy, 1; in corporate public health programs, 32, 295
demographic surveillance systems (DSS), 201n5, 201n8
deterritorialization, of medical science, 17, 22, 32, 33, 322
development, 166–67; as experiment, 300n9; and malaria control, 317; and research, 312–13
— plans/projects, 264; funding of, 211–12; shortcomings of, 186–87, 314, 328n20
developmental(ist) states, 2–3, 81, 83. *See also* postcolonial states
disclosure, of HIV+ status, 225–27
discontinuities, and continuities, 35
Durkheim, Émil, 73n5

Eastern Europe: AIDS epidemic in, 48; transnational medical research in, 19–20
Eboko, Fred, 115
economic value: of blood/serum samples, 113, 134n21; of virus discoveries, 111–12
economic zones, 17
economy, global: in blood and body parts, 62, 63–64, 65; of survival, 5
education/training: of African scientists, 36n3; of malaria control sprayers,

education/training (*continued*)
284–85, 318, 319, 322; of volunteer
health workers, 320
emergency situations, 17, 37n8, 85–86
employment, 215; of HIV/AIDS infected
persons, 212–15, 260–61; in HIV/AIDS
treatment/research programs, 219–20,
258, 264–65, 273, 276; in malaria control programs, 284–85, 318–19; in
para-statal research institutes, 326n2;
in Uganda, 27, 208, 209–12, 216–17,
220–21, 229–30n1, 230nn3–4, 230n6,
230n10
enclosures, 15, 16–17, 30
epidemics, dances linked to, 130. *See also*
HIV/AIDS
ethical issues, in medical research, 91,
120–21, 334–35, 341–42, 348–49
ethnography: of HIV medical research,
29–31, 61–71, 144, 237–40, 243–52,
257–58, 263–77; of living with HIV/
AIDS, 214–20, 221–29; of malaria
control programs, 284–87, 289–91,
299n2; malaria medical research,
188–98
Europe, post-welfare societies in, 7. *See
also* Eastern Europe
exception, states of, 17
expatriate staff, 172n14; in transnational
medical research, 147, 157–58, 159,
171n8, 172n16
experimental societies, 47, 71, 72–73,
292, 300n9, 311
experimentality, 71–72, 148, 253–54,
300n9
experimentation: Africa as site for, 7–8,
36n1, 47, 148, 170n2, 300n9; enclosures necessary for, 16–17; and laboratory metaphor, 69; in malaria control
programs, 283, 284, 285–87, 292–96;
pharmaceutical (*see* clinical trials);
population-based, 47, 68–69; as social
good, 250

exploitation, transnational medical research accused of, 120–21

Fairhead, James, 61–63
families: polygynous, 259–60; relation-
ships in, 258; and HIV, 261–62, 263,
265–66, 269, 272–73, 276
Faraja (Gambia), MRC complex in, 62
Farmer, Paul, 107
Fassin, Didier, 10, 33–34, 107
Ferguson, James, 283, 298
field sciences, 293
field trials, 292
Fingon Tralala, 130–31
First World War, 308, 326n7
Firth, Raymond, 303, 304, 328n20
Fisher, R. A., 327n16
Folks, Thomas, 112
food insecurity, research. *See* nutrition
research
Foucault, Michel, 71, 106, 328n23,
329n27
France: colonial rule by, 241; National
AIDS Council in, 346–47; state regula-
tion of prostitution in, 240–41
Freeman, Denis, 90–91
funding: of African medical research,
36n4, 143–44, 211–12, 343; of malaria
research, 184, 317; of public-private
partnerships, 180; of response to HIV/
AIDS-epidemic, 213–14
future, past as reservoir for, 144, 170

Gallo, Robert, 122, 123
Gambia, 303; agricultural production in, 308, 312–15, 321, 327n12,
327n17; colonial rule of, 307–9, 326n5,
326nn9–11; health care system in,
319–21, 324–25; limited size of, 304–5;
national identity of, 305, 325n1
—medical research in: 32–33, 62–65,
303–4, 305–6, 315–16, 323–24,
326nn3–4, 328n21; community en-

gagement with, 321; government interference with, 319, 322–23, 325; malaria research, 306–7, 316–23, 328n24–25; nutrition research (Gambia Experiment), 306, 307, 309–16, 327nn14–17, 328n19

gambling, self-employment as, 217–19

Garret, Laurie, 106

Gates Malaria Partnership in Africa, 316, 328n24

Geigy, 92–93

Geissler, Paul Wenzel, 26, 27, 63–64

Gerrets, Rene, 27, 28–29

Ghana, malaria control programs in: corporate controlled, 281–83, 284–87, 289–91, 299n1, 300n7, 300n11; public-private partnerships, 296–99; as real-world experiment, 292–96

Gilbert, Hannah, 239

global economy: in blood and body parts, 62, 63–64, 65; of survival, 5

Global Fund, grants, 281, 282, 296, 298

global health governance, and nation-states, 28–29, 180

Global Program on AIDS (WHO), 110

Global Viral Forecast Initiative, 103, 105

globalization, 5; of clinical trials, 70

Good Clinical Practice (GCP) protocol, 37n6

governance, and experimentality, 253–54, 300n9

governmentality, 25, 35, 71, 329n27

governments: employees of (civil servants), 207, 209–12, 220–22, 229–30nn3–4, 230n6, 230n10; and ART, 215–19, 222–29; and science, 3–4, 35, 162, 173n17

—interventions by: dramatizing of, 133; in medical research, 319, 322–23, 325, 335–37, 345, 347. *See also* states

Gray, Glenda, 345

Great Britain: colonial rule by, 83–84, 299n1, 307–9, 326–27n5, 327nn9–11;

MRC's research in Africa, 62, 63–65, 303, 305, 309, 315–24, 325, 328nn21–22

Greater Involvement of People with AIDS (GIPA), 219

Greene, Graham, 107

Greenhough, Beth, 250

Grillo, R. D., 222, 230n9

"Grippe Aviaire" (song), 130, 131

Guay, Laura, 338

Guggenheim, Michael, 69

Gurtler, Lütz, 109

Hahn, Beatrice, 118–19, 134n25

Hamilton, William, 342

Haswell, Margaret, 311–12, 313, 323, 328n19

Hayden, Cory, 38n12

health care: colonial, 83–84, 107–8; in exchange for blood and bodily substances, 61–62, 63–65, 121; Gambian system of, 319–21, 324–25; Tanzanian system of, 182–83, 189–91, 192, 193, 194–95, 200n2, 201nn6–7; and transnational medical research, 16, 27, 62–63, 67, 147, 166–69, 171n7, 173n19, 267–68, 273–75

health workers, volunteer, 219–20, 228, 319–20, 329nn28–29

Herbst, Jeffrey, 304–5

herd immunity, 51, 58

Heywood, Mark, 347

Hibou, Béatrice, 115

historical analyses, 34–35

HIV/AIDS: conferences, 47–48, 73n1, 109, 213, 337–38, 339, 340, 342, 347; counseling, 265, 266, 267–69, 271; epidemic, 48, 118; in Africa, 50, 260–62, 324, 335, 337–38, 342; bio security concerns, 118–19; medicalization of, 59–61; nihilistic responses to, 107; public health interventions, 123–28; social consequences of, 58–59, 212–15,

Kelly, Ann H., 32, 35, 299n3
Kikwete, Jakaya, 197
Kindra, Jaspreet, 342
kinship idiom, used in medical research, 63–64
kinship networks, and medical research networks, 269–72
Klein, Naomi, 72
knowledge production, 8, 300n9, 321, 351. *See also* scientific knowledge
Krohn, W., 292, 300n9
Kruger, Marian, 339
Kufuor, John, 284
Kyaddondo, David, 216

laboratory: Africa as, 7, 300n9; Gambia as, 32, 303–4, 305, 309, 310; notion/metaphor, 69; "without walls"/population, 70–71, 292. *See also* experimental societies
Lachenal, Guillaume, 26–27
Lane, T. D. J., 97n4
Leach, Melissa, 61–63, 325
Leibowitch, Jacques, 126
leprosy research, 86–88; in Africa, 26, 65–66, 78–88, 89–92, 93–96; and treatment, 91, 93
Lewis, D. J., 130, 131
life, government of, 6–7
Lindsay, Steve, 318–19
Little, Kenneth L., 327n17
local communities, and science, 166–69, 173n20, 321
local health care, and transnational medical research, 16, 27, 62–63, 67, 147, 166–69, 171n7, 173n19, 267–68, 273–75
localization, of celebrations, 150–51

Mail and Guardian (newspaper), 341–42, 345
Majambere, Silas, 316, 318
makeability, of public-private partnerships, 181

malaria control, 317, 321; corporate control of, 31–32, 38n14, 281–83, 284–87, 289–91, 299n1, 300n7, 300n11; insecticide spraying, 287–89, 294–95, 318–19, 322; public-private partnerships in, 28–29, 281–82, 296–99; as real-world experiment, 292–96
malaria research: clinical trials, 63–64, 185–86, 187–98, 192–98, 200–201nn3–4; funding of, 184, 317; in Gambia, 306–7, 316–23, 328nn24–25; in Ghana, 285–87, 299n4; in Tanzania, 28, 181, 182, 188, 191
malaria treatments, 189–91; distribution of, 192–98, 201n10
male circumcision, to prevent HIV infections, 51–52, 56–57
malnutrition. *See* nutrition research
Mankhalana, Parks, 348
Manton, John, 25–26, 35
Marchoux, Emil, 65
Mauclere, Philippe, 115
Mbeki, Thabo, 58–59, 335
Mbembe, Achille, 108
Mboup, Souleymane, 238
McGregor, Ian, 306, 326n3
McIntyre, James, 338–39
media coverage, of medical research, 108–9, 122, 339, 341–44, 345
medical care. *See* health care
medical knowledge. *See* scientific knowledge
medical nihilism, 26, 107–8, 122–23, 124, 126, 132
Medical Research Council (MRC, Great Britain), 62, 63–65, 328n22; research program in the Gambia, 303, 305, 306, 309, 315–24, 325, 328n21
Medical Research Council of Ireland (MRCI), 87–89, 92, 95
medical science, 2; and anthropology, 24; deterritorialization of, 17, 22, 32, 33, 322; media coverage of, 108–9,

medical science (*continued*)
122, 339, 341–44, 345; temporality of,
22, 30, 150–51
—in Africa, 2–6, 8, 20, 81, 96, 155,
172n10; colonial, 14–15, 83, 88; and
neoliberalization, 28–29, 38n11,
106, 132; postcolonial, 155, 161, 162,
173n17, 316; social studies of, 61–73.
See also para-statal scientific institutes
—transnational research in, 14, 17,
20–21, 37n7, 143, 324; biopolitics in,
17–18, 29, 315; clinical trials, 22–23,
27, 29–30, 38n13; collaboration,
13, 20–21, 88, 103–5, 113, 115, 144,
146–48, 149–60, 161, 162–69, 171n5,
171n8, 172n11, 172n13, 172nn15–16,
173n18, 173n20, 184, 186, 321; criticism of, 120–23, 144, 148, 339, 341–44,
345; ethical issues, 91, 120–21, 334–35,
341–42, 348–49; ethnographies of,
29–31, 61–71, 144, 188–98, 237–40,
243–52, 257–58, 263–77; funding of,
36n4, 143–44, 211–12, 343; government interference with, 10, 33–34,
319, 322–23, 325, 335–37, 345, 347;
and local health care, 16, 27, 62–63,
67, 147, 166–69, 171n7, 173n19, 267–
68, 273–75; public-private partnerships, 19–24, 28, 38nn11–12, 109–19,
179–81, 184–85, 187, 198–99
medicalization, 59–61, 73n4
Meinert, Lotte, 29, 30–31, 228
memorial celebrations. *See* anniversary
celebrations
memorialization, 145, 165
memories, 10, 31, 145, 160, 169, 170; of
medical research, 61, 152, 154–55, 158,
161, 165
metacodes, 187, 188
microbicides, 51
missionaries/missionary resources, in
African medical research, 87, 88, 96

mobility of people, and medical research
requirements, 30, 266, 268, 273
modernization, 142, 163
Montagnier, Luc, 122–23, 135n39
Moser, Ingunn, 250
mosquito collecting, 285–86, 299n3
Mosse, David, 181, 186
mother-child HIV transmission prevention, 54, 333–35, 344–45, 350–51
Mpudi-Ngolle, Eitel, 112
MRC. *See* Medical Research Council
multinational corporations, 31
Museveni, Yoweri, 211

naming, politics of, 146
nation-building, in Africa, 3
nation-states. *See* states
nationalism, in public health/science
policies, 33–34, 155, 162, 173n17
natural history research, of HIV, 238
Ndoye, Ibra, 242
Ndumbe, Peter, 112, 134n20
neoliberal societies/states, enclosures/
enclaves in, 15–16
neoliberalization, 5, 26, 72, 142; and science, 142–43; and transnational medical science, 28–29, 106, 132, 143–44
—in Africa, 108–9, 161; civil service,
211; public health, 106, 114–15, 128,
132
networks, 276; of medical research
projects, 266, 268–72, 276–77, 324; of
transnational research, 14, 96
nevirapine, 33; clinical trials of, 333–35,
338–39, 343, 344; controversies over,
335–36, 339–51; risks of, 346–47, 348–
49, 350–51
NGOs, employment by, 212, 260–61,
264
Nguyen, Vinh-Kim, 24, 25, 35, 36n1,
209, 275
Nigeria: civil war in (1967/68), 80–81;

leprosy research in, 26, 78–88, 89–92, 93–96; malaria control programs in, 294; meningitis research in, 37n10; nihilism, 106, 127; medical, 26, 107–8, 122–23, 124, 126, 132

nonintervention, 26–27, 106–7, 124, 126, 132, 135n49

nostalgia. *See* memories

novelty claims, 35

nutrition research, in Gambia (Gambia Experiment), 306, 307, 309–16, 327nn14–17, 328n19

Nyerere, Julius, 182

Obama, Barack, 156

objects, scientific, 292, 293, 300n10, 336

Obote, Milton, 210

Omari, Dr., 193, 194, 195, 196, 197–98, 199

otherness, 151

outsourcing, of medical research, 23, 38n13, 172n10

Page, David le, 341

para prefixes, 1, 6, 9–10, 11, 224

para-statal partnerships. *See* public-private partnerships

para-statal scientific institutes, 14, 36n2; capacity building by, 36n3; and local health care, 16, 27, 62–63, 67, 147, 166–69, 171n7, 173n19, 267–68, 273–75

—in Africa, 10–12, 14–16; descriptions of, 143, 145–47, 170–71nn4–5, 305; funding of, 143–44, 211–12; and neo-liberalization, 106, 113, 143–44

—transnational collaboration in, 12–13, 37n5, 115, 146–48, 149–60, 161, 162–65, 171n5, 171n8, 172n13, 172nn15–16, 173n18, 173n20, 184, 186, 321; inqualities in, 20–21, 23–24, 144, 148, 149–50, 166, 172n11

para-states, 1–2, 4, 9–10, 26, 36, 207, 211, 228; and experimental societies, 47, 72–73

para-work, 211

Parkin, David, 215, 216, 217, 221

participants in medical research programs: communities of, 63–64, 67; inclusion criteria, 265–66, 267–68, 272–73; patron-client relationships, 269–70, 273; surveillance issues, 30, 72, 73n6, 146, 266, 268, 273

partnerships, 183, 200n1. *See also* public-private partnerships

past: and present, 145, 169–70; as reservoir for the future, 144, 170

Pasteur Institutes, 110, 113

Pasteurian strategies, 69

patents, on viral proteins, 111–12

patient records, of clinical trials, 78–81, 91

patron-client relationships, in medical research projects, 269–70, 273

Paulson, Tom, 303

peanut production, in Gambia, 307–8, 313, 314, 326n8

Peeters, Martine, 112

Perfect, David, 305

Peterson, Kris, 65, 72

Petryna, Adriana, 70, 172n10, 343

Pfizer Trovan trial (Nigeria, 1996), 37n10

pharmaceutical trials. *See* clinical trials

pharmaceuticalization, 60

Pinder, Margaret, 318

Piot, Pierre, 339

plantation economy, 312

Platt, Benjamin Stanley, 309, 310, 313, 315

Poleykett, Branwyn, 29–30

politics: African, 304; of HIV drugs, 336; of naming, 146. *See also* biopolitics

Pols, Jeannette, 250

polygynous families, 259–60

population trials, 61, 68–71, 73n2; control/surveillance issues in, 72, 73n6

post prefixes, 5

post welfare societies, 7

postcolonial states, 108, 210; medical research in, 155, 161, 162, 173n17, 316. *See also* colonialism, legacy of; developmental(ist) states

power relations, transnational, 283, 298, 325

PreP (pre-exposure prophylaxis), to prevent HIV infections, 52, 54–55

private science, 21–24, 38n12. *See also* public-private partnerships

privatization, of the state, 115. *See also* neoliberalization

prostitution. *See* sex workers

protests against experiments, as research data, 293

public, notions of, 18, 19, 21, 38n12

public health: colonial, 107–8; deficient, 26–27

—interventions, 31–32; in avian flu crisis, 128–30; experimental, 283; in HIV epidemic control, 123–27; in malaria control programs, 38n14, 281, 293–94, 295, 297; noninterventions, 26–27, 106–7, 124, 126, 132, 135n49; and transnational virus research, 105–6

—policies: antiscientific, 33–34; nationalism in, 33–34, 155, 162, 173n17; and neoliberalization, 106, 114–15, 128, 132

—research/science, 18–19, 21, 24, 37n7, 156; in Africa, 20, 23–24, 85, 322–23; public-private divide in, 21–24, 38n12; simulation exercises, 128–29

public science, 19, 21, 291–92, 294, 297, 298–99

public-private partnerships, 283–84; in malaria control programs, 28–29, 281–

82, 296–99; in transnational medical research, 19–24, 28, 38nn11–12, 109–19, 179–81, 184–85, 187, 198–99

Rabinow, Paul, 71

racism, 120, 135n31

randomization methods, 68

real-world experiments, 292, 293. *See also* experimental societies

Redfield, Peter, 106, 172n14

Renaud, Michelle Lewis, 243–44

research: and development, 312–13; funding of, 36n4, 143–44, 211–12, 343; global processing of data of, 37n7, 146, 171n6; object and subject in, 292, 293, 300n10; sites of, 12–13; transnational (*see* transnational medical research)

resistances of viruses: against drugs, 346, 348–49; against insecticides, 287, 288, 294, 295

retrovirus research, 103–5, 109–19; criticism of, 120–22

rice production, in Gambia, 308, 310, 313, 321

risk assessments, 350–51

The River (Hooper), 116–17

Roosevelt, Franklin D., 326n9

Rose, Nikolas, 6

Rottenburg, Richard, 81, 96, 170n2, 181, 187

rural areas: colonial neglect of, 304; development of, 306, 307, 309–16, 327nn14–17, 328n19

Russell, Steven, 216

Sahelian style architecture, 241

Sanneh, Kanja, 321–22

Sanofi (pharmaceutical company), 113, 115, 187, 192–93, 196, 197, 198

Schoofs, Mark, 134n27

science: advancement/modernization,

142; African, 142, 143, 162, 170; and biopolitics, 328n23; community engagement with, 166–69, 173n20, 321; government/and government, 3–4, 35, 162, 173n17, 336–37; and local culture, 151; and neoliberalization, 142–43; public/public engagement with, 19, 21, 291–92, 294, 297, 298–99, 300n8. *See also* medical science

scientific knowledge, 3, 8; traffic in, 85

scientists: African, 36n3, 110, 147, 155, 171n8; transnational, 14, 23, 38n13

security, bio, 105, 106, 118–19, 127, 132

Seeley, Janet, 216

self-employment, as gambling, 217–19

Semali, Dr., 197–98

Senegal: HIV research among sex workers in, 29–30, 237–40, 242–43, 249–52, 253; state regulation of prostitution in, 237, 240–42, 243–49, 252–53

Senegambia, 305, 325n1

serums, importance of access to, 113, 134n21

sex workers: HIV research on, 29–30, 237–40, 242–43, 249–52, 253; state regulation and registration of, 237, 240–42, 243–49, 252–53

sexual transmission of HIV, and antiretroviral therapy, 55–56

Shaw, Thomas, 241

The Shock Doctrine (Klein), 72

Silent Spring (Carson), 287, 294

Silla, Eric, 66

Simelela, Nono, 337, 340

simian immunodeficiency virus (SIV), 105, 117–19

simulation exercises, 128–29

SIV. *See* simian immunodeficiency virus

sleeping sickness, DDT spraying against spread of, 299n6

the social, 59–60, 61

social good, experimentation as, 250

social studies: of HIV epidemic, 337, 342; and laboratory metaphor, 69; of medical research in Africa, 61–73

sociality, research driven, 71

societies, 6–7, 60; experimental, 47, 71, 72–73, 292, 300n9, 311

sociology, 73n5

somatic individuality, 7

South Africa: apartheid era scandals in, 343; HIV/AIDS epidemic in, 337–38; treatment availability, 10, 333, 339–40; HIV/AIDS research in, 68, 335, 339; government interference with, 10, 33–34, 335–37, 341, 345, 347; public controversies over, 339–51

Southeast Asia, transnational medical research in, 19–20

SP (sulphadoxine-pyrimethamine), 189, 190, 191, 195–96, 200n3, 201n10

states, 3, 6–7, 25; African, 3, 8–9, 25–26, 229n5, 304 (continued relevance of, 4, 13, 27–29, 31, 34, 35, 115, 180–81, 200, 207–8, 209, 229, 252, 283, 298, 322); postcolonial, 108, 210; weakening of, 37nn6–8, 106, 132–33, 273–74; developmental, 2–3, 81, 83; and global health governance, 28–29, 180; para, 1–2, 4, 9–10, 26, 36, 207, 211, 228; and experimental societies, 47, 72–73. *See also* governments

states of exception, 16, 17

Stengers, I., 300n10

Strathern, Marilyn, 253, 257

structural adjustment policies. *See* neoliberalization

subjects, scientific, 292, 293, 300n10

surveillance systems/techniques: demographic, 201n5, 201n8; in medical research, 14, 15, 22, 68, 72, 73n6, 123–24, 146, 294, 319–20; and mobility of participants, 30, 266, 268, 273

Synergies Africaines, 122
Szerszynski, B., 292, 293

Tagne Condom, 130–31
Tanzania: health care system in, 182–83,
    189–91, 192, 193, 194–95, 200n2,
    201nn6–7; malaria research in, 28, 181,
    182, 188, 191, 192–98; role of state in,
    199–200; stability in, 29
TasP (treatment as prevention) for HIV,
    47, 52–53; clinical trials of, 56, 68–71;
    criticism of, 58–59; effectiveness of,
    57–58, 68–69, 73n3; origins of, 48, 49,
    53–56; social consequences of, 72
temporality, 6; of medical research, 22,
    30, 150–51; multiple, 144
tenofavir, 52, 55
therapeutic citizenship, 275, 277n5
Tilley, Helen, 83, 84
Titmuss, Richard, 8, 19
traditional medicines, used in HIV/AIDS
    treatments, 324–25
transformation narratives, 142
transnational medical research, 14, 17,
    20–21, 37n7, 143, 324; biopolitics in,
    17–18, 29, 315; clinical trials, 22–23,
    27, 29–30, 38n13; criticism of, 120–23,
    144, 148, 339, 341–44, 345; ethnogra-
    phies of, 29–31, 61–71, 144, 188–98,
    237–40, 243–52, 257–58, 263–77;
    funding of, 36n4, 143–44, 211–12,
    343; government interference with,
    10, 33–34, 319, 322–23, 325, 335–37,
    345, 347; and local health care, 16, 27,
    62–63, 67, 147, 166–69, 171n7, 173n19,
    267–68, 273–75; public-private
    partnerships in, 19–24, 28, 38nn11–12,
    109–19, 179–81, 184–85, 187, 198–99
—collaboration in, 13, 88, 103–5, 113,
    115, 146–48, 149–60, 161, 162–69,
    171n5, 171n8, 172n13, 172nn15–16,
    173n18, 173n20, 184, 186, 321; in-

equalities in, 20–21, 23–24, 144, 148,
    149–50, 166, 172n11
Treatment Action Campaign (South
    Africa), 333, 335
trial communities, 63–64, 67
Triangle Pharmaceuticals, 339
Tshbalala-Msimang, Manto, 338, 341,
    347
tuberculosis research, in Ireland, 88–89,
    97n3
Turner, Victor, 340

Uganda: employment in, 27, 208,
    209–12, 215–17, 220–21, 229–30n1,
    230nn3–4, 230n6, 230n10; neoliberali-
    zation in, 211; state/government in,
    28, 207–8, 210, 211, 229, 229n5
—HIV/AIDS in, 212–14; research, 334,
    338; treatment availability, 208–9, 213,
    223, 230n11
United Kingdom. See Great Britain
United States, transnational medical re-
    search funding by, 343

vaccine research, 50–51, 63–64
vampire rumors, and Western medical
    research in Africa, 62
video clips, of African songs mocking
    avian flu crisis, 130–31
viral forecasting projects, 124, 127
virus research: in Africa, 26, 103–5,
    109–19, 132; criticism of, 120–23;
    economic value of virus discoveries,
    111–12
Vlakplaas paramilitary group (South
    Africa), 343
volunteer health work, 219–20, 228,
    319–20, 329nn28–29

Weyer, J., 292, 300n9
White, Luise, 62
Whitehead, Roger, 328n22

WHO: Global Program on AIDS, 110; on HIV/AIDS treatments, 344–45, 347; malaria eradication programs of, 287

Whyte, Ikoli Harcourt, 79

Whyte, Susan Reynolds, 27–28

Wolfe, Nathan, 103–4, 105, 108, 112–13, 119, 121, 128, 132

women, HIV research's neglect of, 348

wonder drugs, 336, 339, 345, 349, 350

World Health Organization. *See* WHO

Wynne, B., 291

Zekeng, Leopold, 109, 112, 135n31, 135n49

zidovudine, 334, 338, 344, 346

zoonosis, AIDS as, 118, 124, 126